When AiDS Began

When AIDS Began

San Francisco and the Making of an Epidemic

Michelle Cochrane

ROUTLEDGE
NEW YORK AND LONDON

Published in 2004 by
Routledge
29 West 35th Street
New York, New York 10001
www.routledge-ny.com

Published in Great Britain by
Routledge
11 New Fetter Lane
London EC4P 4EE
www.routledge.co.uk

Routledge is an imprint of the Taylor & Francis Group.
Printed in the United States of America on acid-free paper.

10 9 8 7 6 5 4 3 2 1

Library of Congress Cataloging-in-Publication Data

Cochrane, Michelle.
  When AIDS began : San Francisco and the making of an epidemic /
Michelle Cochrane.
      p. ; cm.
Includes bibliographical references and index.
  ISBN 0-415-92429-4 (hardcover : alk. paper) — ISBN 0-415-92430-8
(pbk. : alk. paper)
1. AIDS (Disease)—California—San Francisco—History. 2. AIDS
(Disease)—California—San Francisco—Case studies.
  [DNLM: 1. Acquired Immunodeficiency Syndrome—epidemiology—San
Francisco—Case Report. 2. Acquired Immunodeficiency
Syndrome—etiology—San Francisco—Case Report. 3. Acquired
Immunodeficiency Syndrome—history—San Francisco—Case Report. 4.
Homosexuality, Male—San Francisco—Case Report. 5. Sentinel
Surveillance—San Francisco—Case Report. 6. Sociology—San
Francisco—Case Report. WC 503.4 AC2 C661w 2003] I. Title.
  RA643.84.C2C636 2003
  616.97'92'00979461—dc21
                                                2003010928

To Joe M. (1948–1992)

I observe the physician with the same diligence as he the disease.

—John Donne, "Devotions Upon
Emergent Occasions" (1624, n.6)

Contents

Illustrations

Tables

Preface

John Doe was admitted to the emergency room at San Francisco General Hospital at 10:40 P.M. on July 17, 1994. His "pupils were 7mm dilated, fixed," he had "poor peripheral pulses," blood pressure was falling and near zero.

Upon entry to the operating room 21 minutes later, John Doe was pronounced "DOA" (dead on arrival). He was 38 years old. The Coroner's Property receipt for him listed "no propirty [sic]" other than a wristwatch.

John Doe was the 261,000th American to die from acquired immune deficiency syndrome (AIDS) since surveillance for the epidemic began in 1981.[1]

I was sitting in a San Francisco bar perusing the gay weekly newspapers when I first learned of this man's death one evening in July 1994. I could not have been more shocked to see John Doe in the little gray box bordered in black, as I knew him as a charismatic San Francisco writer and AIDS treatment activist who had lived with a diagnosis of AIDS for almost half his life. He was renown in San Francisco's AIDS community for surviving that life/death sentence. Diagnosed with "gay pneumonia" (*Pneumocystis carinii* pneumonia; also known as PCP) in the early 1980s and given six months to live, Doe had survived to write a weekly alternative treatment column for a gay newspaper and held frequent community forums on the immune-restorative properties of DNCB, a photochemical applied topically to the skin that is purported to jump-start the immune system of persons with AIDS (PWAs).[2]

I often perused John Doe's weekly treatment column and had last seen him speak at a DNCB forum held at a San Francisco church in the Tenderloin district one summer afternoon in 1993. He was a dynamic and aggressive speaker; the tenor of the treatment forum brought to mind a Southern Baptist revival in Missouri. Doe indicted the establishment of AIDS researchers and clinicians as "doctors of death" who had fashioned professional careers and lucrative salaries from an investment in "our deaths." At the conclusion of his speech, following his scathing attack on the science of AIDS medicine and its orthodox treatments, I half expected more debilitated members of the audience to throw away their crutches and leap dancing into the aisles.

But did John Doe die of AIDS? It all depends on your "social location" in the debates surrounding AIDS pathogenesis and treatment; it depends on who you are, whom you ask, and which questions you pose. For the doctor on duty in the emergency room at SFGH, this "middle-aged man was brought in by paramedics" after apparently falling (30–40 feet) down some stairs. Cause of death: "probable secondary to head/chest injuries. Anatomical findings: severe head trauma, cyanosis with bloody tracheal aspirate."[3]

Translation: John Doe died of a broken neck after tripping and falling 35 feet down a staircase.

For the Department of Public Health's AIDS Office Seroepidemiology and Surveillance Branch (ASSB), which has responsibility for capturing and reporting all AIDS diagnoses in the city/county and collating deaths from the disease, John Doe was just another unfortunate mortality statistic, the most recent of more than 12,762 residents who had died of AIDS in San Francisco as of July 1994.[4]

As I had been conducting research in the AIDS dissident community for a number of years and knew several of Doe's friends, I learned that his death was an ironic tragedy and macabre joke for his peers and compatriots in the alternative treatment community. Here was a vigorous and articulate advocate for alternative treatments, a veritable living testament for twelve years to the possibility of surviving and thriving with AIDS, a man who seemingly overcame the disease and partially restored the function of his immune system only to die suddenly and ignominiously by tripping and falling down the stairs of his boarding house. Although they made no secret of his battles with addiction to intravenous drugs and recent bouts of depression, these were perceived only as additional struggles that John would overcome with the help of his friends.

Some of Doe's closest confidantes were less optimistic and admit the possibility of suicide that Thursday night. John had recently fulfilled his life's goal by writing and researching his "magnum opus" on alternative AIDS theory and treatment practice; thereafter, he lost any further purpose for living. Doe had previously struggled with thoughts of suicide and had recently, once again, fallen off the wagon in his struggle with drugs; his second trip to the detox center had proven no more of a permanent solution to his addictions than had the first. Perhaps he tripped and fell 35 feet by mistake . . . perhaps he had been careless . . . perhaps the vodka and Valium had clouded his vision or judgment.

To enemies within the AIDS community who resented his evangelical zeal in proselytizing about DNCB and had suffered from Doe's scathing ad hominem attacks about their co-optation by "AIDS Incorporated" and global pharmaceutical companies, his death confirmed the common fate that awaited all HIV-positives; both those that assented to the power of HIV and those who denied it. They read Doe's death as a confession of both cowardice and hypocrisy. They claimed that his blood counts had been falling despite his treatments with DNCB, and concluded that John Doe had cowardly returned to "using" after berating members of the gay community for being co-opted by the pharmaceutical companies and acquiescing to the "death culture" of AIDS. In the end, he took his own life rather than admit he was dying of HIV/AIDS.

Did John Doe die of AIDS? His life history, his diagnosis, his alternative treatment activism, and even his death map the terrain where battles are waged between orthodox AIDS researchers and public health officials on the one hand and those referred to as AIDS dissidents on the other. Whether John Doe was sick and, if so, why he was sick and why he died are questions that bring into stark relief the role of social location in the production of knowledge on HIV/AIDS, suggesting that one's answers are contingent not only on where you are, but on where you want to go.

Acknowledgments

I would like first to thank my parents for their emotional and financial support, which has buoyed me through nearly a decade of research, fieldwork, and writing. I could never have completed this manuscript without their love and support. Friends who have also stood by me as I pursued my dream of writing include Barbara, Christine, Joe, Karla, Parto, and Richard.

Research and travel funds for the dissertation upon which this manuscript is based were provided in part by the following donors: a University of California at Berkeley Provost Award (1993); a Rocca Scholarship for Advanced Study on Africa (1992); a University of California Humanities Travel Grant (1993); the Society for Women Geographers (1994); and a grant from the National Science Foundation "Ethics and Values Studies Program" (1994). Fieldwork at the San Francisco Department of Public Health (SFDPH) was partially funded by a work-study award from the University of California at Berkeley and supplemented by an AIDS Task Force stipend for the summer of 1994. I would also like to personally thank Dean Joseph Cerny for his support in obtaining a University of California at Berkeley Chancellor's Dissertation Award (1995–1996) that was critical for completing my fieldwork at the AIDS Office Seroepidemiology and Surveillance Branch (ASSB) and writing up my initial findings. Without the institutional support listed above, my research would never have begun, let alone been completed within a reasonable time frame.

In the Bay Area, Mr. Kevin McKinney, formerly AIDS Surveillance field unit coordinator at the ASSB, and presently at San Francisco General Hospital, proofread this text in order to rectify any inaccuracies, and I subsequently met with him at the SFDPH to clarify difficult passages. It should be noted that the original text of several of the conversations related verbatim in this book were awkwardly written and disjointed in parts because they reflected the difficulty of taking field notes in a hectic AIDS surveillance office with staff who were simultaneously speaking with me while responding to telephone calls and the demands of their jobs. I was fortunate to have been supervised by Mr. McKinney, for despite our different aims (he a civil servant and myself a social scientist) and contentious arguments over the cause, treatment, and bureaucracy of surveillance for HIV/AIDS, he was always helpful, gracious, and generous with his time and expertise. Paul O'Malley and Tim Piland of the San Francisco AIDS Office also generously agreed to be interviewed and provided material documentation to help in reconstructing data on sexually transmitted diseases, Hepatitis B, and HIV/AIDS during the late 1970s and early 1980s. I am also grateful to ASSB staff such as epidemiologists and disease surveillance investigators (DCIs) who tutored me in the mechanics of seroepidemiology and surveillance practices and policies in San Francisco and willingly endured my endless questions; special gratitude goes to DCI Craig Clevenger, who was an exceedingly collegial tutor in surveillance practices during my internship at San Francisco General Hospital and the AIDS Office.

I would also like to express my personal gratitude to Drs. Michael Watts, Michael Johns, Allan Pred, and Paul Rabinow, and Warren Winkelstein at the University of California at Berkeley (UCB) for help in obtaining the necessary institutional affiliations and money needed to conduct this research. Michael Watts was especially instrumental in delivering all of the grants received and noted above. He is also a vibrant example of the very best teaching that a renown university has to offer, and I have never known another academic mentor who has given so freely of his professional and personal life and asked so little in return for his efforts. Michael Johns helped to focus this project before I began fieldwork, and thereafter helped to structure its narrative. He provided needed critiques of the text's style and thematic continuity, and was always available to turn to for provocative discussions about my research and innovative solutions for writing slumps. In turn, Drs. Pred and Rabinow provided copious theoretical critique and advice throughout my research. I owe a special thanks to Dr. Warren Winkelstein, professor emeritus in the Department of Public Health (epidemiology) at UCB, who secured for me the internship at the ASSB, and then directed me to additional valuable resources on the AIDS epidemic in the Bay Area.

I would also like to acknowledge and publicly thank the staff at the Department of Geography at the University of California at Berkeley; Natalia Vonnegut for expediting all manner of graduate work and scholarship; and Don Bain, a Macintosh virtuoso, for his help with computer-video transfers and Adobe Photoshop color scanning. My gratitude also goes to Dallas Dishman, and Drs. Michael Dear and Jennifer Wolch at the Department of Geography at the University of Southern California for their editorial suggestions, fellowship support for postdoctoral research on AIDS in Southern California, and for ensuring that I found a suitable publisher for this research. In that regard, I would like to thank my editor Ms. Ilene Kalish for providing me with the opportunity to publish with Routledge—and for her forbearance as I missed deadline after deadline. Finally, a handful of anonymous reviewers have labored over drafts of this manuscript at various stages of publication; I am deeply indebted to these reviewers for their frank critiques of the text, their advice on strengths and weaknesses in the manuscript, and most of all, for their implicit encouragement to bring the book to publication. I am also grateful to Tom Norris for his help in configuring graphics at the last minute and creating an electronic file of illustrations used in this text.

While many friends, fellow graduate students, informants, institutions, and activist organizations helped me to obtain source material and provided editorial advice, several individuals have truly changed the way I think about AIDS. Thank you to Richard Berkowitz, a freelance author in New York City, for years of weekly correspondence that has kept me abreast of AIDS activism, politics, and art. I would also like to express my gratitude to New York City's Dr. Joseph Sonnabend, formerly medical director of the Community Research Initiative on AIDS (CRIA) and now an AIDS clinician at St. Luke's Hospital, for access to personal files and unpublished papers, valuable research leads on AIDS treatment and surveillance sources, and for his generosity in interviews and vis-à-vis the occasional dinner cheque.

Billi Goldberg of the DNCB Study Group in San Francisco has posted daily email correspondence regarding the rapid developments in AIDS treatments, immunology, and virology, and was often available for lengthy dinners in the Castro to tutor me on the finer points of P24 antigen or the mechanisms of action of the new protease inhibitors. I cannot think of a single HIV/AIDS treatment or research forum or conference that I attended in the mid-1990s without finding Billi Goldberg in the audience; if there is such a thing as an AIDS maven, Billi is it. My views on HIV and the AIDS epidemic have also been fundamentally influenced by the contribution of time, archives, and critical dialogue of Drs. Steven Epstein (UCB sociologist), Peter Duesberg (UCB microbiologist), and the recent research and publications of the Bancroft Library's Regional Oral History Office at the University of California at Berkeley. Those readers familiar with Steven Epstein's work on the sociology of knowledge on this epidemic (*Impure Science,* Berkeley: UC Press, 1996) will recognize his considerable influence on my own research. He was an especially generous colleague to me in the summer of 1993, providing contacts and an initial draft of his unpublished dissertation in sociology before I began preliminary fieldwork on AIDS dissident organizations in the United Kingdom. While in London, I bummed cigarettes from the entire team of Meditel Productions Inc. (Joan Shenton, Hector, Pascal, and Michael), who also lent me the use of their offices, FAX machines, and access to a plethora of video, audio, and print archives on HIV/AIDS dissidents in the United States and England.

In conclusion, I want to emphasize that none of the organizations or individuals cited above bears any responsibility whatsoever for the contents or conclusions of this text, and perhaps few would agree with its arguments.

Introduction

Do we really need another book on this disease? Arguably AIDS is the most studied epidemic in history; bookshelves abound with numerous histories of the disease,[1] sociological and cultural treatises and anthologies, specialized epidemiological and biomedical texts,[2] and studies of the global HIV and AIDS pandemics.[3] The ideologies of prevention and education discourse and the impact of the disease on American culture have been critically dissected in works by social theorists such as Cindy Patton, Paula Treichler, Simon Watney, Sander Gilman, Leo Bersani, Jeffrey Weeks, and others.[4]

But notwithstanding Steven Epstein's *Impure Science* and its cogent analysis of struggles vis-à-vis the credibility and legitimacy of AIDS science, research, and treatment paradigms and practice, social scientists have largely avoided critical interrogation of the "politics of knowledge" and social construction of the epidemiological reality and empirical facts comprising official scientific discourse and public health data on the AIDS epidemic.[5]

Within my own discipline, medical geographers have given scant attention to the epidemic during the past 20 years. The epidemiology and diffusion of HIV/AIDS is the focus of just two medical geography books and a handful of articles in major geographical journals.[6] While these texts exemplify the traditional strengths of the subdiscipline—spatial analysis, disease mapping, and studies of epidemic diffusion over space and time—medical geographers studying the AIDS epidemic have thus far failed to advance critical theory or participate in the reformulation of a geography of health that incorporates ethnographic and interpretive methods informed by progressive social theories emphasizing studies of identity, gender, deviance, and the politics of knowledge embedded in scientific discourse and research.[7] As Robin Kearns and Wilbert Gesler advocate in *Putting Health into Place*, medical geographers need to "infuse" the field "with broader theoretical concerns" already evidenced in other geographic subdisciplines and in the social sciences at large, thereby advancing our collective understanding of how disease, epidemics, and "health policies are socially produced, constructed, and transmitted."[8] In this vein, *When AIDS Began* comprises a critical interrogation of scientific knowledge of AIDS and an empirical case study of the social construction of epidemiological and surveillance knowledge, data, and discourse on the disease in San Francisco, California, an historical epicenter for producing knowledge on HIV and the AIDS epidemic.

During the past decade, numerous empirical studies by historians of science have critically problematized the rational and linear progression of scientific theory via the progressive and painstaking accumulation of empirical data and the self-evident and objective character of "normal" scientific practice. Consonant with this tradition, I view nature and knowledge as social constructions, and power critically constitutive of both the subjects and objects of knowledge, biomedical knowledge not exempted. While this case study of AIDS in San Francisco is about the social construction of facts, theories, and "situated knowledge(s),"[9] it is also necessarily about consensus, conflict, and voice—in other words, about who has sufficient authority to speak as an expert on the epidemic and who speaks credibly. My thesis is that power and the social relations of science, politics, and culture have constructed an official consensus of knowledge and facts about the cause and course of the AIDS epidemic, legitimating some voices, one historical narrative of the epidemic, and a particular representation of the epidemiological reality of this disease while censoring other claims.

Overview of Research Study, Field Site, and Methods

> If we relinquish the compulsion to separate true representations of AIDS from false ones and concentrate instead on the process and consequences of representation and discursive production, we can begin to sort out how particular versions of truth are produced and sustained, and what cultural work they do in given contexts. Such an approach . . . raises questions not so much about truth as about power and representation.[10]

Following the report of an outbreak of a clinical syndrome of rare disease symptoms occurring among young male homosexuals in New York, San Francisco, and Los Angeles in the summer of 1981, there were several competing theories about the cause(s).[11] While some epidemiologists favored an explanation rooted in the lifestyle of urban homosexual men (e.g., the widespread use of inhalant drugs known as "poppers"), others believed that the cause for the clusters of cancer and pneumonia was some combination of behaviors and rare but previously characterized viruses (such as cytomegalovirus) already known to be immunosuppressive (the multifactorial thesis). A third hypothesis was that a new and virulent disease agent had recently emerged among U.S. populations and was the cause of the epidemic.

For orthodox AIDS science and historiogaphy, the matter was definitively laid to rest when Margaret Heckler, then U.S. secretary of Health and Human Services, stood before a podium at a press conference on April 23, 1984, and announced that HTLV-III (later known as the human immunodeficiency virus or HIV), discovered by Robert Gallo, was "the probable cause" of the acquired immune deficiency syndrome.[12] Thereafter, the majority of AIDS researchers formed a consensus around the hypothesis that the retrovirus HIV, and only HIV, was the cause of AIDS. This theory was further codified in 1985 with the development of a test to detect HIV antibodies that was used to screen blood and to identify persons at risk for developing AIDS.

The single-virus theory has never achieved consensus among all scientists nor among some elements of the public, however. Challenges to the theory that HIV is the single primary cause of the AIDS epidemic have arisen from "heretics" within the biosciences and from independent researchers, individuals, and organizations outside of institutionalized science. In 1992, a coordinated assault to the theory that HIV causes AIDS was mounted by participants at the Alternative AIDS Conference in Amsterdam[13] and representatives from the Group for the Scientific Re-appraisal of the HIV-AIDS Hypothesis.[14] These events were followed by a flurry of organizational activity by AIDS dissidents, increased attention paid to dissidents' views in the popular and scientific media, and the emergence of several new sites of opposition to "expert" AIDS science.[15]

The continuing production of knowledge around alternative theories of AIDS pathogenesis and the longevity of this dissent from the "HIV causes AIDS" theory drew me to examine the social construction of knowledge on AIDS in epidemiological research, in the medical charts of AIDS patients in the early years of the epidemic, and in AIDS surveillance activities in San Francisco. Almost certainly, the failure of Western researchers to adequately describe the way in which HIV causes AIDS or to develop an AIDS vaccine has contributed to the persistence of alternative theories of treatment and pathogenesis. But acknowledging the reality of imperfect knowledge about AIDS and the impact of other developments, such as the discovery of HIV-negative cases of AIDS at the Ninth International Conference on AIDS (1992), does not provide a sufficient explanation for continuing challenges to the hypothesis that HIV, and HIV alone, causes AIDS. Instead, one must return to the early years of the epidemic to reexamine the empirical evidence that undergirded the lifestyle and multifactorial theories of AIDS and how those theories were eclipsed by the emergence of the theory that HIV causes AIDS.

The same issues of credibility and power that legitimated the voices affiliated with institutions most aggressively pushing the "one sexually transmitted virus–one fatal disease" hypothesis continue to play an explanatory role today in reproducing and maintaining a consensus about the cause and pathogenesis of the disease. And AIDS surveillance data and epidemiology from San Francisco have been critically constitutive of the global consensus on orthodox AIDS historiography and science. Thus, local and global orthodox representations regarding the evolution of AIDS, the epidemiology of risk factors for acquiring the disease, and the central role played by the infectious retrovirus HIV display a remarkable coherence and internal theoretical consistency that is collectively marshaled to censure or refute alternative theories of the AIDS epidemic.

Apropos Paula Treichler's quote above, *When AIDS Began* is a case study of the very real politics of the disease and the politics of culture embedded in official AIDS discourse, science, and representations of the epidemic that have contributed to advance a politics of sexuality that has increasingly medicalized gay male sexuality since the 1970s. As far as it succeeds in advancing a credible thesis, this book comprises an historical study of the ways and means by which the social relations of science, power, and the political economy of public health in San Francisco have shaped the fundamental character and content of what we believe we know about HIV and AIDS.

Two decades after the epidemic began, the cumulative toll of AIDS in the United States is 793,026 cases and 457,667 deaths.[16] Because of the city's historical preeminence as one of the epicenters of the epidemic, knowledge on HIV/AIDS derived from epidemiological cohort studies and surveillance data in San Francisco is central to the construction of AIDS historiography, research on the natural history of the disease, and is used as a harbinger of national trends in the epidemic.[17] With a cumulative total of 27,982 cases and 18,957 official deaths from the disease at present, and the nation's highest per capita incidence of the disease until 1994,[18] the city/county of San Francisco constitutes a premier field site for a case study of AIDS surveillance practices and politics and the production of qualitative and quantitative knowledge on the emergence, evolution, and epidemiology of HIV/AIDS in one urban region heavily impacted by the epidemic.

Given the wealth of AIDS clinical, historical, and epidemiological resources in the Bay Area, I was able to interview public health officials, attend research and treatment forums, and readily access early epidemiological studies and transcripts of oral histories given by physicians, researchers, and those public health leaders who first discovered the disease in 1981 and established surveillance policies to monitor and contain the epidemic. Securing a nine-month internship at San Francisco's AIDS Office Seroepidemiology and Surveillance Branch (ASSB) for research and study in the summer of 1994 and the spring of 1995 enabled me to conduct an ethnography of HIV/AIDS surveillance practices at the ASSB.

The ASSB is the repository for San Francisco's AIDS case registry database (i.e., HARS), and the central official public health agency responsible for producing and disseminating public and internal reports on surveillance practices and policies, HIV seroprevalence, AIDS incidence, data on cumulative caseloads and mortality, retrospective analyses and future projections of epidemiological trends in the city.[19] Working as a disease control investigator in training, I reviewed patients' medical records and laboratory reports, captured and documented new AIDS patients, abstracted information to update prior AIDS case files, and observed the social construction of facts and the production of knowledge on the AIDS epidemic in situ and the dissemination and reification of this local knowledge in national and global forums. My sources included medical charts for the first AIDS patients reported in San Francisco in 1981 and 1982; internal documentation on these cases at the Department of Public Health; interviews with disease surveillance Investigators and AIDS prevention officers; and recently published transcripts from the AIDS Oral History Project at the Bancroft Library at the University of California at Berkeley. Triaging these primary resources enabled me to critically analyze, cross-reference, and juxtapose empirical data and historical documents against public representations and official historiography on the epidemic.

The Book's Organization

When AIDS Began is an interdisciplinary synthesis of disparate scholarship from the fields of geography, social epidemiology, cultural studies, and the sociology of scientific knowledge. This empirical and ethnographic case study of the social construction of scientific knowledge on AIDS and the politics and practice of AIDS surveillance activities in San Francisco extends the recent theoretical turn in the social sciences that challenges notions and narratives of neutral and objective science, the rational progress of scientific theories via a progressive accumulation of empirical evidence, and the apolitical character and content of scientific research, discourse, and data.

Arguing that nature and knowledge are social constructions and that power and social relations influence the constitution of both the subjects and objects of (biomedical) knowledge, *When AIDS Began* reveals the social construction of clinical, epidemiological, and surveillance knowledge on HIV/AIDS during two paradigmatically critical, yet contradictory, phases in the epidemic. The first half of the book excavates materials from 1981 through 1983, when the earliest official reports of AIDS diagnoses were registered in the city's Public Health Department, a bureaucracy of surveillance emerged to report cases and monitor the impact of the disease on the city's residents, and epidemiological studies were initiated among gay men. The latter half of the book describes my ethnography of the mechanics of AIDS surveillance practice and the production of official statistics and public representations of the epidemic by the ASSB in 1994 and 1995—well after the epidemic's peak, as it began to sharply decline. Juxtaposing research from these different phases of the epidemic demonstrates the ideological and theoretical continuities of orthodox discourse and representation of the AIDS epidemic and reveals how power and politics sustain particular representations of the disease even in the face of empirical contradictions or inconclusive or anomalous epidemiological and surveillance data and research.

When AIDS Began begins with a brief theoretical review of the sociology of scientific knowledge and an argument for the methodological utility of constructivism for advancing our understanding of the "facts" of AIDS epidemiology and public health surveillance practices, policies, and data. Chapter 2 comprises a brief summary of how a theoretical consensus on the cause and risk factors for AIDS was socially constructed, concretized, and disseminated in scientific, public, and government discourse on the disease between 1981 and 1983; traces the emergence of a city's bureaucracy of surveillance for monitoring and characterizing populations perceived to be at risk for acquiring the disease; and demonstrates how local cohort studies among gay men in San Francisco contributed to rapidly codifying epidemiological risk factors for the disease and circumscribing the demographics of risk for the disease, both regionally and nationally. This chapter also includes a review of the increasing medicalization of gay men in the national hepatitis B vaccine trials of the late 1970s and early 1980s before the emergence of a syndrome of opportunistic infections and cancers in gay men in 1981. Together, these chapters demonstrate that the medicalization of gay desire and contentious debates over the spaces of gay eroticism and lifestyle preceded the emergence of the AIDS epidemic.

Chapters 3 and 4 deconstruct medical documentation and/or AIDS case reports for all 24 AIDS cases that the San Francisco Department of Public Health reported in 1981. These chapters largely complement one another by methodically documenting and critically interrogating the social construction of individual diagnoses for some of the nation's earliest recorded AIDS patients in the first year of the epidemic. While this exhumation of medical records for gay patients belies any declarative claim, in toto these chapters advance my thesis that surveillance practices and policies jointly produced and continue to produce representations of the AIDS epidemic that overtly simplify the demography of risk for acquiring the disease.

The roots of contemporary dissent about the cause and risk factors for acquiring the disease and prevention strategies also lie in the contentious debates from these early years of the epidemic. In contradistinction to texts that chronicle the theoretical plurality of the initial years of the epidemic between 1981 and 1983, *When AIDS Began* demonstrates that the construction of the central tenets of clinical, epidemiological, and surveillance knowledge that established the unambiguous infectious nature and risk for the sexual transmission of AIDS began immediately and in earnest in the first months of the official discovery of the epidemic. These years therefore constitute a critical historical juncture when some epidemiological data, and some voices articulating alternative theories for the emergence of the epidemic and correlates for acquiring and transmitting the disease were marginalized or silenced in a process of scientific gatekeeping as a hegemonic discourse and representation of the epidemic was codified. *When AIDS Began* argues that local knowledge produced in this one city was both constitutive of, and reciprocally reinforced by, a national and a global consensus on the epidemiology and historiography of this disease.

The second half of the book includes more contemporaneous material derived from an ethnography of HIV/AIDS surveillance practices at the ASSB in San Francisco between 1994 and 1995. Chapter 5 comprises an ethnography of embodied biomedical practices and the ambiguities attendant upon ascribing the most likely mode of transmission for HIV/AIDS cases at San Francisco General Hospital and the ASSB. By cross-referencing patients' medical charts with AIDS case report files and juxtaposing primary data to official HIV/AIDS surveillance statistical reports and projections of epidemic trends, this chapter shows how surveillance officers necessarily employ subjective and often competing criteria to interpret and attribute a given patient's risk factors for acquiring the disease.

I demonstrate that the sexual transmission of this disease is more often assumed than empirically documented and that HIV/AIDS surveillance practices have shown remarkable continuity through time, demonstrating both immediate and persistent tendencies toward systematically overestimating the risk for contracting AIDS solely through sexual activity, while simultaneously underestimating the proportion of the HIV/AIDS caseload in San Francisco (and the nation) that is attributable to intravenous drug use and/or socioeconomic factors that condition access to health-care services, treatment, and care. The political economy of the bureaucracy of public health and AIDS surveillance also leads to gatekeeping and skewed trend analyses of the evolution and trajectory of the epidemic. Chapter 6 demonstrates how the public's perception of an exponential explosion in AIDS cases has been augmented considerably by the multiple and extensive changes in methods by which the Centers for Disease Control (CDC), and thus local health departments, have captured and recorded patients during the past two decades. The frequent elaboration of the clinical criteria for diagnosing AIDS patients complicates historical analyses of the epidemiology and diffusion of AIDS and is largely responsible for the general impression that the epidemic's growth is unabated and that the demography of risk for the disease has shifted.

In conclusion, chapter 7 acknowledges that although challenging the material foundations of several key tenets of AIDS historiography and epidemiology is risky business, examining the social construction of AIDS surveillance knowledge and data also introduces the possibility that there might be alternative explanations for why AIDS emerged when it did and superior explanations of why, even into the new millennium, the HIV/AIDS epidemic remains firmly ensconced in the same "high-risk" populations of intravenous drug users and gay men comprising the initial groups at risk for "acquired immune deficiency" in 1981.

To foreshadow my concluding remarks, this empirical study of the social construction of scientific knowledge on AIDS challenges orthodox discourse and representations of the history and epidemiology of this disease by directing our attention to the "more immediate practical and explicitly political considerations of the scientific practices by which the facts of science are actually produced."[20] Moreover, *When AIDS Began* argues that orthodox science and official public health surveillance practices often elide or wholly neglect analysis of the social factors that gave rise to and abet this epidemic, the socioeconomic correlates of the disease, and the epidemiological evidence of patients' multiple and synergistic risk factors for immune deficiency. The dangerous reductionism of orthodox AIDS science, epidemiology, and surveillance practices structurally produced and sustains an artifactual simplicity in HIV/AIDS surveillance data and public health discourse, promotes diffuse public health interventions that fail to target prevention and education resources effectively, and narrowly circumscribes the range and scope of interventions that could more effectively lead to the end of this scourge. Conversely, a richer and more critical theory of health and disease posits more complex models of social agency and structure that incorporate multiple and varied correlates of individual risk for acquiring and transmitting AIDS, generates better predictions of the historical and temporal trends in the epidemic, and can point the direction to more comprehensive, effective, and targeted prevention programs.

I repeat: *Did John Doe die of AIDS?* It all depends on your social location—who you are, whom you ask, and which questions you pose.

A Note on Methods and Patient Confidentiality

This ethnography could never have taken place without the training, advice, cooperation, and graciousness of the staff at San Francisco Department of Public Health's AIDS Seroepidemiology and Surveillance Branch. The research itself adhered to university standards for protecting the rights of human subjects and was supervised and reviewed in process and amended prior to publication by staff at the ASSB. While working as an intern, I respected the ASSB's stringent confidentiality policies, which include neither revealing nor disclosing any patient's identification or health status, and never using a computer for any confidential data or analysis. I also assigned unique and arbitrary codes to my notes pertaining to individual case reports to avoid any possibility that they could be cross-referenced to official ASSB case files. I submitted both a research progress report and a copy of the original manuscript to Kevin McKinney, AIDS surveillance field unit coordinator at San Francisco's ASSB, for his editorial review and corrected or deleted any inaccuracies in quotes or empirical data from the text at that time; altered portions of the manuscript were then resubmitted to McKinney for a second editorial review. All quotes used in the text were either transcribed verbatim from tapes when available, or from the author's extensive notes when recording was prohibited or impractical. As a final note, I have inserted brackets [ ] at various points in the text to clarify medical terminology, translate specialized jargon into vernacular language, and to indicate where the author has added parenthetical comments to correct grammar and lend greater context and clarity to an informant's comments or to excerpts from published research or media accounts.

I
The Sociology of Knowledge on HIV and AIDS

The Sociology of Scientific Knowledge

In the most general sense, the critique of empiricism and "ethically neutral"[1] scientific practices is a theoretical argument about the way in which the structure of science at a macro level of analysis influences the choice of the object(s) of study and conditions and constrains the nature and interpretation of the product(s) of that research. Moreover, it is a critique of the ideologies and the politics embedded in scientific research that are structurally reproduced through the professional training of scientists and are materially reproduced when institutions determine which research is to be funded and how research findings will be disseminated.

In *The Social Construction of Reality: A Treatise in the Sociology of Knowledge,* Berger and Luckmann provide a brief historical chronology of this critical theoretical tradition by locating the immediate progenitors of a sociology of knowledge (Marx, Nietzsche, and Dilthey) and identifying their contributions of a trilogy of constructs: "superstructure/substructure," "anti-idealism," and "historicism."[2] A formal discipline of the sociology of scientific knowledge was born in the 1920s when first Scheler, then Mannheim, extended Marx's material analysis of "ideology (ideas serving as weapons for social interests)" and developed a philosophy of inquiry to study the history of ideas, exempting the natural sciences and mathematics.[3]

Much of the sociology of biomedical knowledge and the sociology of knowledge on AIDS has continued in the tradition of Mannheim, largely adhering to the study of ideology and its attendant functions of legitimating class relations and economic exploitation, maintaining the status quo of privilege and authority in society, and normalizing "deviant" social behavior. A plethora of case studies have been published that elaborate the function of ideology and social control in constructing medical knowledge and in contextualizing and even defining illness,[4] and unveil the implicit ideological arguments[5] contained within models of the pathogenesis of disease.

In one text exemplifying this theoretical tradition, Howard Waitzkin analyzed the role of medical ideology in normalizing social and sexual behavior and reifying symbolic discourse and medical technology.[6] Using the Frankfurt

School's critical theory to elaborate upon Marx's initial conception of ideology as a system of beliefs that "sustain and reproduce the social relations of production, especially patterns of domination," Waitzkin advances his argument about the individualizing techniques of medical language and the way in which medical behavior achieves its politically neutral guise. These techniques enable "scientific medicine" and its practitioners to obfuscate their class interests and to elide their role in legitimating the social status quo. In particular, Waitzkin marshals the arguments of Habermas in support of this latter point, as the Frankfurt School's critical theoretical approach produced the most sophisticated analysis of the way in which "[science] and cultural symbols in the mass media, educational system, and technical organization of the workplace [legitimate] current patterns of domination [in society] and depoliticize [social problems]."[7]

> To study ideology is to study the ways in which meaning serves to establish and sustain relations of domination. Ideological phenomena are meaningful symbolic phenomena *in so far as* they serve, in particular social-historical circumstances, to establish and sustain relations of domination. (This is a question which can only be answered) by examining the ways in which symbolic forms are employed, circulated and understood by individuals situated in structured social contexts.[8]

This broader definition of ideology, as articulated by John B. Thompson in *Ideology and Modern Culture,* informs our understanding of how the Public Health Service, the Centers for Disease Control, and local public health disease investigators who initially identified the emergence of the AIDS epidemic in metropolitan areas throughout the United States, constructed a system of surveillance for the disease and imputed various meanings to the clinical symptoms manifest among gay men suffering from immunological deficiencies at the beginning of the 1980s.

But for Waitzkin, the premier theorist in analyzing how social control is operationalized in medicine is not Habermas but Michel Foucault, who produced a number of exhaustive historical case studies of the exercise of social power and domination in constructing definitions of deviance and normality and establishing their parameters. According to Foucault, power is predominantly exercised in modern times via the operation of "discourse through which professionals communicate their special knowledge [which] enhances their ability to intervene in and control others' behavior." The absence of "intentionality" in the way in which medical discourse reproduces and achieves social control means that in large part, this discourse takes place with little self-reflection on the part of medical practitioners or patients as to the way in which diagnosis, treatment, and theories of etiology of disease sustain relations of social domination.[9]

Social control is thereby operationalized within medicine via the explicit directives that a patient is given to relieve their symptoms, and warnings given regarding adverse consequences of a patient's present course of behavior. Of equal import for Waitzkin, however, is the manner by which social control is achieved implicitly by excluding certain lines of inquiry or privileging some interpretations over alternative constructions of reality. This point is central to my analysis of the character and form of epidemiological research on AIDS from the initial moment that the "disease syndrome" was "recognized." And medicine's specific symbolic and ideological functions in AIDS research and discourse will be a theoretical touchstone for my analysis of cultural studies that follow.

There is currently a large body of literature on the sociology of AIDS and analyses of the role of the media in representing and disseminating information about the disease, which has developed a critique of the social and political consequences produced by ideological and metaphorical representations of the AIDS epidemic.[10] While explicit about their grounding in the study of ideology and social control in science, many literary and cultural theorists writing on AIDS are more heavily indebted to Foucault's study of power and an "archaeology of medical perception,"[11] and they frequently employ the methods of textual deconstruction and linguistic analysis pioneered by poststructuralists.

In *Inventing AIDS*, for example, Cindy Patton uncovers and directly indicts the entrenched racist biases that lie behind the facade of altruistic biomedical research in Africa. "Western science today is slowly consolidating around a particular construction of 'African AIDS,' which elaborates on the colonialist mystifications of the past century . . . carried by Western ethicists and researchers who speak of an 'African culture' based largely in their fantasies. . . . (These) Western representations of the national and sexual cultures of postcolonial Africa direct the international AIDS research and policy agenda."[12]

Patton recounts the ubiquitous themes implicit in most representations of African AIDS: the high-risk cultural homogeneity of the continent and its peoples; the continent's aversion to or incompetence in recognizing and reporting AIDS; the futility of educational interventions to reduce African's risks; and narratives constructing the origin of AIDS in Africa as a product of nature as much as culture—"conjured out of the primordial [jungle] or caught from animals imagined to live side by side with Africans." Though she does not deny the stark political-economic realities of illness in many African countries, Patton's larger point is that AIDS is represented iconographically as emblematic of Africa's underdevelopment, "as if a lack of Western-style industrialization, rather than a virus, were the cause of AIDS in Africa."[13]

The material consequence of these pervasive images fuels Western initiatives to conduct vaccine trials on the continent at the expense of cheap African lives. . . . "African research subjects are thus constructed simultaneously as noble savages helping science improve the lot of humanity, and as a sort of postmodern Agar plate, a halfway house between humans and the animals conventionally used in drug testing." As Patton argues, "an HIV/AIDS vaccine [can] only leave Africans where they were before the epidemic, (whereas) by contrast, an investment in education, clinics and health awareness programs [could conceivably] create baseline knowledge and interest that other health-related programming could build on."[14] Nonetheless, an exclusive emphasis on the unlikely development of an effective and affordable vaccine against AIDS is consistently advocated over alternative research on treatments for the opportunistic infections that actually kill people with AIDS in Africa. As she deconstructs the present course of AIDS research on the continent, Patton claims that:

> [Implementing vaccine] trials in Africa rests on two assumptions which reveal the complicity of science in actually making AIDS in Africa worse: 1) vaccine trials are based on the assumption that Africans will continue to be exposed to HIV in large numbers, [e.g. that education] "for risk-reduction is destined to fail;" and 2) "the high risk involved [in vaccine trials] is obscured [by the] widely promoted image that Africans are already lost to the HIV epidemic. This is combined with the controversial new ethical concept of catastrophic rights, according to which trials which don't quite pass ethical muster should be allowed as "compassionate," [thereby releasing] Western researchers from liability.[15]

Patton argues that this convoluted logic of "ethical experimentation" can be rationalized—or as Waitzkin would say, "ideologically legitimated"—by the construction of a catalog of African difference. Unlike populations in the West, Africans cannot be successfully educated to reduce their risk of exposure to HIV; and fundamentally contrary to the Western form of the disease, African AIDS is almost exclusively a heterosexually transmitted disease and as such is potentially a larger and more threatening epidemic than that in the West. Moreover, a central argument about AIDS in Africa is that the disease is in some way explicable by cultural differences in African sexual behavior (a predilection for anal intercourse and "dry sex") or African genital health (a preponderance of ulcers and epidemic STDs).[16] This "hyper-heterosexualization of African AIDS" does violence to the reality of modes of transmission of HIV that may be of greater consequence for the health of Africans (e.g., blood transfusions, male homosexual behavior, injections, and IV drug use) and sets up a tragically comedic mythology based on the assumption that prostitutes are the vectors of HIV/AIDS in Africa—a notion "that flies in the face of epidemiological [data]" and common sense, as it cannot be empirically supported by the observed AIDS case ratio for males and females on the continent.[17]

Patton provides a powerful analysis of the persistence of mythologies in texts on African AIDS, fantastic narratives that gain their longevity from the strength of their articulation with, and appropriation of, entrenched tropes, metaphors, and themes that pervade other "knowledge" and bodies of discourse on Africa, disease, race, and the nature of plague.[18] But when she speaks as an activist engaged in the work of AIDS prevention, Patton's political commitment to subverting metatheoretical discourses (patriarchy, for instance) leads her to promulgate entirely new epidemiologies of risk grounded in the very same form of identity politics that she previously undermined. In her most recent work, *Last Served? Gendering the AIDS Epidemic,* Patton's thesis rests on the "invisibility" of women with AIDS and the "heterosexualization [or] banish[ment]" of lesbians:

> A major reason for the failure to situate women in their various contexts is the heavy reliance of HIV policy and education on the ideas of risk groups and target groups. Given the focus on these related but not identical statistical concepts, women fade from view in HIV epidemiology for two reasons: first, considered by source of infection, women continuously appear to be statistically small in number, especially when broken down into gender subcategories of risk behaviour groupings. Second, when "targeted" by potential to become infected, the group "partners of," despite containing a small number of men thought to have been infected by women, is so vague that it seems only to mean "not men": male partners of men get their own category—"homosexual" or "bisexual." "Lesbians" are either heterosexualized or banished as "other."[19]

In other words, Patton is simultaneously arguing that men have more categories of risk differentiation, thereby validating the fluidity of their sexual desire, while the magnitude of female AIDS cases is erased by their gender subcategories. Her solution? Create additional subcategories, such as lesbian, that are based on the very same reification of permanent categories of difference and desire that she previously deconstructed. Implicitly, Patton concludes that official AIDS surveillance data underestimates the size of the epidemic, and by its conservatism fails to capture the real and significant risk for the disease to "nontraditional" populations.

Other social scientists, while authoring brilliant analyses of the iconography of AIDS and deconstructing the latent texts within AIDS discourse and media representations, have been similarly reluctant to commit themselves completely to a deconstruction of biomedical texts and representations of the reality of the disease. In other words, although there are a number of sophisticated critiques of the ideologies that direct research interests, inform the direction and character of government AIDS prevention policies, and imbue media discourse on AIDS with symbolic meaning(s), much of the literature on the sociology of knowledge of AIDS exempts the practices, discourse, and product of (at least some) of epidemiology and AIDS surveillance activities from critical inquiry.

For example, with his writings on "moral panics," Jeffrey Weeks argued that this disease "became the bearer of a number of political, social and moral anxieties, whose origins lay elsewhere, but which were condensed into a crisis over

AIDS."[20] He referred to Erving Gusfield's formulation of the legitimating functionalism and instrumental control of particular symbolic moral crusades (for instance, the temperance movement) in maintaining society's status quo power relations in order to explain the way in which the moral panic over AIDS produced a "symbolic resolution" of profound anxieties in the United States over race, sexuality, and social order.[21] However, despite Weeks's admission that, far from being ideologically neutral, "medicine is deeply involved in the relations of power—and hence the morals—of the culture in which it is embedded,"[22] he exempts from critique the biomedical knowledge produced through these social relations of power. Calling for a "more developed and rational response" to the AIDS epidemic, "based on a realistic assessment of risk [and] a balanced understanding of the nature of AIDS and HIV infection" to be implemented, Weeks presumably believes there are those who are able to separate the wheat (the symbolic and ideological meanings of HIV/AIDS) from the chaff (the "objective reality" of the disease).

In contrast, although Simon Watney rejects the model of moral panics, he argues that the regulation and "policing" of desire have provided the raw material out of which AIDS mythologies are constructed.

> We are witnessing the latest variation in the spectacle of the defensive ideological rearguard action which has been mounted on behalf of "the family" for more than a century. . . . Whether they emanate from neo-conservatism, Christian fundamentalism, sociobiology or feminism, all these positions share a common aim to ground a narrow, normative theory of human nature in biology. . . . In this respect we can identify the whole of medical education as it trains doctors and nurses and affects their career prospects, as one major vector of homophobic science, together with all the other academic disciplines—criminology, social psychology, politics, and so on—which possess the power to institutionalize and disseminate evaluative sexual definitions and discourses.[23]

All the same, Watney unabashedly cites epidemiological research on AIDS— for instance, "the statistical likelihood of contracting the HIV virus from a new [gay male] sexual partner in New York is now put at fifty-fifty"[24]—to buttress his central thesis that "safe sex" needs to be eroticized in public health discourse since monogamy is a moot point when half of your sexual partners are likely to be infected. Similarly, he uncritically accepts the epidemiological premise that everyone is at risk for AIDS, "gay or straight," in order to jettison the relevance of identity or sexual orientation for the construction of risk groups: "We need to abandon the insane notion that AIDS is only a threat to 'risk' communities, without neglecting the very specific rights and needs of gay men, who have been most devastated by this catastrophe."[25]

As is evident from this brief review, much of this literature on the "social construction" of AIDS displays extraordinary virtuosity in tracing the archaeology of medical views of homosexuality and of plague, and in utilizing literary theory and cultural or media studies to deconstruct the ideological content and social and political repercussions of AIDS discourse. However, in order to deconstruct the empirical content and data constitutive of the biomedical "reality" of AIDS, we need to reference a more radical theoretical tradition within the history of the sociology of scientific knowledge that foregrounds analyses of the embodied and "situated material practices"[26] of scientists (and physicians) at the micro level of the laboratory (and the hospital bedside).

The Social Construction of Reality

As conceived by Berger and Luckmann, in contrast to the more conservative Mertonian realist tradition, a "radical" school of the sociology of knowledge treats all bodies of knowledge, including laboratory and natural science, as socially constructed and thus amenable to sociological inquiry. And they are less concerned with the epistemological problems of "how do we know that what we know is true" than with case studies of the social construction of reality in scientific practice. In the following text, Berger and Luckmann subtly cleave apart philosophical (epistemological) and metaphysical (ontological) questions from empirical practice within the field:

> To include epistemological questions concerning the validity of sociological knowledge in the sociology of knowledge is somewhat like trying to push a bus in which one is riding. To be sure, the sociology of knowledge, like all empirical disciplines that accumulate evidence concerning the relativity and determination of human thought, leads toward epistemological questions concerning sociology itself as well as any other scientific body of knowledge . . .
>
> The logical structure of this trouble is basically the same in all cases: How can I be sure, say, of my sociological analysis of American middle-class mores in view of the fact that the categories I use for this analysis are conditioned by historically relative forms of thought, that I myself and everything I think is determined by my genes and by my ingrown hostility to my fellowmen, and that, to cap it all off, I am myself a member of the American middle class?
>
> Far be it from us to brush aside such questions. All we would contend here is that these questions are not themselves part of the empirical discipline of sociology. They properly belong to the methodology of the social sciences, an enterprise that belongs to philosophy and is by definition other than sociology, which is indeed an object of its inquiries. The sociology of knowledge . . . will "feed" problems to this methodological inquiry. It cannot solve these problems within its own proper frame of reference.[27]

This focus on "scientific practice . . . and not just with its institutional 'context,'"[28] has revolutionized studies of the history of science and the sociology of knowledge of science during the past 20 years. Although not acknowledged by Berger and Luckmann, Thomas Kuhn's *The Structure of Scientific Revolutions* was contemporaneous with their own work. Referencing the emergence of "a historiographic revolution in the study of science," Kuhn proffered both a philosophical argument and a variety of historical case studies that helped to destabilize wholly positivist and historically progressive accounts of scientific knowledge. He argued instead that the rise to prominence of one particular scientific theory over another (a paradigmatic revolution) could not be attributed to the truth or falsity of that theory, or to a "failure of method" within the paradigm overthrown. Rather, a paradigm shift depended on some "apparently arbitrary element, compounded of personal and historical accident, [which] is always a formative ingredient of the beliefs espoused by a given scientific community at a given time."[29] Thus, not only did Kuhn extend his analysis to include the practices and content of scientific knowledge, but he also advanced the concept of historically contingent "paradigms" that circumscribe the "disciplinary practices" of normal scientific research, characterized as "puzzle-solving."[30]

As Kuhn provided the initial impetus for the rediscovery and translation of *Genesis and Development of a Scientific Fact*[31] he was a central force in introducing historians and philosophers of science to the work of the obscure Polish physician-immunologist Ludwick Fleck. Fleck's musings on the constitutive role of "thought-collectives" in guiding theories about syphilis and directing research on a blood test to detect the disease catalyzed Kuhn to develop the construct of cognitive models which he referred to as "paradigms": "the actual scientific practice[s] . . . from which spring coherent traditions of scientific research."[32]

By his own admission, Kuhn had little to say about the role of social and intellectual contingencies in constituting these paradigms (the traditional province of the moderate school in the sociology of knowledge), yet his research provided a seminal text used in codifying a radical or "strong programme" in the sociology of knowledge that came to be associated with the Edinburgh School in the mid-1970s.[33]

It was the anthropological ethnographies of Donna Haraway and, especially, Latour and Woolgar that provided models to emulate when studying the construction of scientific facts.[34] And case studies of scientific controversies, such as the controversy regarding the role of HIV in the etiology and pathogenesis of AIDS, can be one entry point for examining "science in the making."

> The impossible task of opening the black box [of a scientific fact] is made feasible (if not easy) by moving in time and space until one finds the controversial topic on which scientists and engineers are busy at work. This is the first decision we have to make: our entry into science and technology will be through the back door of science in the making, not through the more grandiose entrance of ready made science. . . .
>
> We start with a textbook sentence which is devoid of any trace of fabrication, construction or ownership; we then put it in quotation marks, surround it with a bubble, place it in the mouth of someone who speaks; then we add to this speaking character another character to *whom* it is speaking; then we place all of them in a specific situation, somewhere in time and space, surrounded by equipment, machines, colleagues; then when the controversy heats up a bit we look at *where* the disputing people go and *what* sort of new elements they fetch, recruit

or seduce in order to convince their colleagues; then, we see how the people being convinced stop discussing with one another; situations, localisations, even people start being slowly erased; on the last picture we see a new sentence, without any quotation marks, written in a textbook similar to the one we started with in the first picture. This is the general movement of what we will study over and over again in the course of this book, penetrating science from the outside, following controversies and accompanying scientists up to the end, being slowly led out of science in the making.[35]

The microtextual analysis of past controversies offers two additional advantages for a sociology of scientific knowledge for historians Steven Shapin and Simon Schaffer. "One is that they often involve disagreements over the reality of entities or propriety of practices whose existence or value are subsequently taken to be unproblematic or settled." The second: "In the course of controversy [historical actors] attempt to deconstruct the taken-for-granted quality of their antagonists' preferred beliefs and practices, and they do this by trying to display the artifactual and conventional status of those beliefs and practices."[36] The "cultural construction" of HIV and the artifactual and contested belief that HIV is the sole cause of AIDS is the object of study for several authors in the following section.

The Construction of HIV and "Facts Settled by Dispute"

In her review of medical sociology, Ilana Lowy lamented the fact that much of the promise inherent in Ludwick Fleck's case study of the social construction of medical knowledge on syphilis had not been realized.

> Fleck, a convinced holist, claimed that the formation of medical knowledge was a time-dependent, dynamic process including many complex interactions and involving not only the limited circle of medical experts but society as a whole. Only the combination of historical, sociological and philosophical approaches into a multi-disciplinary approach, called by him "comparative epistemology," could allow for a proper study of such a complex phenomenon.[37]

Lowy argued that few medical sociologists had built upon the tradition by applying the sociology of knowledge to concrete case analyses of the facts constitutive of contemporary medical practice and theory. As of 1988, she concluded that despite the elaboration of a philosophy of the social construction of scientific knowledge "the developments of the last years cannot . . . justify the idea that the sociology of biomedical research already exists."[38]

With the notable exception of books such as Wright and Treacher's *The Problem of Medical Knowledge*, and Paula Treichler's work on the sociology of knowledge on HIV and AIDS discussed below, Lowy's point is well taken for much of medical sociology and studies in the history of science.[39]

In a succession of texts, Treichler deconstructs orthodox AIDS knowledge while providing numerous examples of "how knowledge is produced and sustained within specific contexts, discourses, and cultural communities."[40] In

"AIDS, HIV, and the Cultural Construction of Reality," Treichler analyses the "correspondence" between various representations of HIV and its reality as espoused by conflicting theories that describe in contradictory ways how HIV causes the clinical symptoms collectively referred to as the acquired immune deficiency syndrome. Building on the critical theory of those such as Gramsci who spoke of the way in which the reification of objects and/or ideas obfuscates power relationships, Treichler examines the "reification of HIV" in various material forms; for example, how the virus is stylistically and theoretically rendered in models and in scientific texts. She then documents how the stability of orthodox representations of HIV and its material reality as an "observable entity" (albeit contested by some persons living with AIDS and by some AIDS dissidents) is sustained by a succession of "gatekeeping operations."

> Scientific inquiry and the study of science always take place within a given context, a context that includes the community of one's peers. . . . [A] scientific laboratory does not simply enter its product—its publications—into open competition in the scientific marketplace; rather the publication is shaped from the beginning by the gatekeeping operations of scientific peer review. Gatekeeping thus influences the entire research process, including what research project is selected and how it is pursued. . . .
>
> Our knowledge of the "life history" [of HIV] has been produced by an intense national research effort focused both on HIV and on drugs designed to disrupt its life history at various points; as the major subject of scientific investigation and pharmaceutical research efforts and major recipient of AIDS research funding, HIV is, therefore, also, as Joseph Sonnabend puts it, "metaphorically representative of other interests."[41]

According to Treichler, this tedious and methodical process of laboratory practice which transforms provisional evidence into facts and artifacts necessarily elides any consideration of the interests that initially directed research and "thus reified, HIV exhibits a number of predictable characteristics. It is referred to by a universally agreed upon signifier; conventional representations for it have been developed in journals, etc. . . . and scientific discourse [emerges] as a form of shorthand in which facts, once admitted, need no longer retain the history of their fabrication."[42]

The specifics of the messy and historically contingent circumstances surrounding the discovery of HIV, and the story of how HIV became known as the singular necessary and sufficient cause of AIDS is provided by Jamie Feldman, a former student of Treichler's in "Gallo, Montagnier, and the Debate over HIV: A Narrative Analysis."[43] À la Latour, Feldman argues that several aspects of the discovery and taxonomy of the human immunodeficiency virus remain contested issues to this very day even though HIV was "black-boxed" as the cause of AIDS more than a decade ago.

> The main difference between literary or social science accounts and scientific narrative is the latter's evolution from one story among many to acceptance by

its community of readers as the singular representation of reality. . . . As we shall see in the dispute over the initial isolation of HIV, the virus involved in AIDS, this transformation is achieved through the work of narrative, competing in a type of marketplace replete with its own set of investments and credits. Once a fact is created, it then becomes divorced from its constructive origins, becoming that which has always been true. As Stanley Fish succinctly puts it, "Disagreements are not settled by the facts, but are the means by which the facts are settled." The Gallo-Montagnier dispute is an excellent example of this process, and also is virtually unique in that the "facts" have not been settled in over seven highly volatile years.[44]

Feldman carefully documents the way in which the material reality of a virus (variously inscribed as LAV or HTLV-III or HIV) was constructed in 1983/ 1984 by specific social actors (Luc Montagnier and Robert Gallo) and biomedical research institutions in France (the Pasteur Institute) and in the United States (the National Institutes of Health). Analyzing popular and scientific publications for "themes, audience, and actors," Feldman notes the rhetorical strategies employed by prominent authors arguing for the primacy of their theoretical interpretations vis-à-vis the specific virus that causes AIDS. Beginning her story with the discovery of *several* retroviruses, Gallo's human T-cell leukemia virus-I (HTLV-I) and Montagnier's lymphadenopathy associated virus (LAV) in the sera of AIDS patients, Feldman traces the subsequent transformation of this "provisional journal knowledge" into the claim that one of these retroviruses (Montagnier's LAV; appropriated and renamed HTLV-III by Gallo) is "the probable cause of AIDS."[45]

To summarize Feldman, in short order the popular and scientific press inscribed HTLV-III as the "AIDS virus," and Robert Gallo as the man who discovered it. Luc Montagnier, the French pretender to the throne of retroviral hall of fame, subsequently challenged the Gallo/U.S. "fiction" in legal venues and before multiple commissions on scientific integrity in the United States. Although it took some time to achieve unanimous consent within the scientific world, the issue of what to call the virus was eventually settled shortly after the International Committee on the Taxonomy of Viruses officially dubbed the novel retrovirus the human immunodeficiency virus (HIV) in 1986. In contrast, credit for the discovery of the virus and patent royalties accruing from the development of an antibody test to detect its presence in blood remained contentious issues for a number of years.[46]

A court battle was avoided in 1987 when the heads of state in the United States (Reagan) and France (Chirac) reached a legal settlement whereby the proceeds from the patent of the antibody test were equally divided between the two countries. But more important, the settlement stipulated that no party to the agreement could discuss the origin of the controversy surrounding the discovery of LAV/HTLV-III//HIV nor independently author an alternative history other than that "sanctioned as the authoritative narrative by the out-of-court patent settlement."[47] This messy and historically contingent account of the discovery of HIV (as published in a special issue of *Scientific American* in 1988) subsequently became the official history of the chronology of AIDS research in the early years of the epidemic, "closing the book on the issue . . . accepted as fact, it need never be referred to again."[48]

Feldman concludes that the dispute between Gallo and Montagnier was especially unsettling to the scientific community at large, first because it "revealed certain excesses of character for which scientists are often criticized," and second because it required the political imposition of an "authoritative narrative" from "outside" science to resolve an internal controversy that should have been adjudicated by reference to truth and objective evidence. Nevertheless, for AIDS researchers and their professional peers the controversy was an exceptional and aberrant episode; one that primarily exemplified a "political dispute" that had little to do with "good science."[49] Furthermore, the personal and professional differences between Gallo and Montagnier were considered irrelevant to the immediate scientific problem of continuing to unravel the mysteries of HIV and explain how it causes AIDS.

This scientific controversy at the very center of AIDS research is anything but exceptional for many AIDS dissidents, however, or for scholars such as Patton, Treichler, and Feldman who challenge authoritative narratives of the emergence, cause, and epidemiology of AIDS.[50] Rather, this contemporaneous and very public debate only makes it relatively easier to recognize how power and prestige influence the content of scientific knowledge and how disagreements settle the facts; thereby creating coherent historical narratives that enable scientists to get on with the normal practice of puzzle-solving within a given paradigm.

> If we relinquish the compulsion to separate true representations of AIDS from false ones and concentrate instead on the process and consequences of representation and discursive production, we can begin to sort out how particular versions of truth are produced and sustained, and what cultural work they do in given contexts. Such an approach . . . raises questions not so much about truth as about power and representation.[51]

Locating the discord in theories of AIDS etiology and pathogenesis in a larger context of studies of dissent in science, Feldman's and Treichler's work brilliantly deconstructs the rhetorical struggles to lay claim to the discovery of HIV, to write the history of the epidemic, and to represent AIDS. Nevertheless, I will extend their work by arguing that not all knowledge claims vis-à-vis AIDS are constructed to the same degree or are equally true, by which I mean that not all theories are internally consistent and not every representation of the epidemic or of AIDS patients is materially grounded. In fact, I examine the material foundations for several key tenets of AIDS epidemiological research and orthodox historical accounts of the epidemic in large measure precisely for the purpose of suggesting that some representations of AIDS and AIDS patients are made *only* for the cultural work they do, as there is little empirical evidence to support them. By doing so, I focus on the very real politics of the disease—the politics of culture that inheres in particular metaphorical representations of HIV/AIDS, and a politics of sexuality that increasingly medicalizes and pathologizes gay men. These twin foci lead us finally to Stephen Murray and Kenneth Payne's anthropological archaeology of AIDS epidemiology in the early 1980s and a study of the way in which power and discourse fundamentally shaped the construction of populations at risk for contracting AIDS in the first years of the epidemic.

The Politics of AIDS: Social Control and the Medicalization of Homosexual Desire

> Historically, the European construction of sexuality coincides with the epoch of imperialism and the two inter-connect.[52]
>
> —Kobena Mercer

In many ways parallel to Patton's work on the African AIDS epidemic, Murray and Payne focus a critical lens on the latent texts, tropes, and colonizing discourses about homosexuality which informed epidemiological research of AIDS in the United States during the early years of the epidemic.[53] Their analysis ventures beyond much of the medical sociology of the disease because it empirically refutes the premise that orthodox epidemiological knowledge of AIDS derives fundamentally from a neutral observation of data, isolated from the social, sexual, and political "zeitgeist" that characterized the early 1980s.[54]

Using Conrad and Schneider's writings on deviance to set up the introduction for their article on the social classifications of AIDS epidemiology in the early 1980s, Murray and Payne correlate the 1981 "remedicalization" of homosexuality on the basis of physical pathology (AIDS) to the hotly contested "demedicalization" of homosexuality on the basis of psychological pathology in 1974. Thus, the male homosexual remains "diseased," but now by virtue of a different biological mechanism; the symptoms of homosexual desire are both more visible (clinical lesions), and subject to greater empirical quantification (CD4 counts).

> Repeating the history of the psychiatric colonial expeditions into male homosexuality, the new medical model of why male homosexuality is unhealthy [also] does not include any cure.
>
> We shall show how the original identification of a syndrome of opportunistic infections in gay men living in the most institutionally-elaborated gay communities made it a "gay plague" and therefore sexually-transmitted, and how such identification constrained conceptualization and research subsequent to the initial "explanation" of "gay promiscuity."[55]

To document the social construction of "the gay disease (dis-ease) syndrome" between 1980 and 1982, Murray and Payne revisit the original case studies of AIDS patients published in the CDC's *Morbidity and Mortality Report* (MMWR) and medical journals of the period. These texts demonstrate that although 20 percent of early AIDS cases were among heterosexuals, and a considerable number of the earliest homosexual AIDS cases were IV drug users, this epidemiological information was rewritten or erased by the risk categories constructed by the Centers for Disease Control.

In point of fact, between 1980 and 1985, the mode of HIV transmission for an AIDS patient who was both a homosexual male and an intravenous drug user was attributed exclusively to his (homo-)sexual orientation, thereby "de-emphasizing and under-representing every patient characteristic except homosexuality"; in other words, "that which is most 'sinful' was presumed to be most dangerous."[56] And as AIDS epidemiological data was written and read, the wages of the sin of anal sex was death. The authors drive this point home through an extensive analysis of the Haitian AIDS risk category, an appellation eventually dropped when political pressure was applied to eliminate this single risk group that was indicted for "who they were rather than what they did."[57]

Continuing their chronological reconstruction of AIDS epidemiological research, the authors reference the development of the HIV test in 1985 as a catalyst for the further medicalization of asymptomatic homosexuals and members of other high-risk groups. After 1985, it was no longer necessary to be clinically ill to be considered at risk for developing AIDS; rather two additional categories of patients were created; asymptomatic persons testing positive for antibodies to the virus became HIV-positive patients, while those with minor symptoms and a positive antibody test were diagnosed with "AIDS-related complex (ARC)." For Murray and Payne (and many AIDS dissidents who came after them), tying a positive HIV-antibody test to a diagnosis of AIDS/ARC/or asymptomatic pre-AIDS fashions a tautological diagnosis that artificially reifies the pathogenic role of the virus; it means that HIV-positive gay males with *no symptoms* are diseased, while HIV-negative persons with clinical symptoms suggestive for AIDS are diagnostically excluded from surveillance data. This tautology not only skews AIDS surveillance statistics and projections of the magnitude of populations at risk for the disease, but also exemplifies an historical exception in the definition and staging of diseases:

> This boundary HIV/ARC/AIDS construction is recapitulated in doctor-patient interactions as the doctor chooses a diagnosis which is heard as a death sentence (AIDS) or as the potentially survivable (ARC)—[therefore] the contention that AIDS is "invariably fatal" is an artifact of the drawing of conceptual boundaries within the "biological facts," and unique in medical practice in that diseases are rarely divided linguistically by their perceived outcome.[58]

Sadly, however, the development of the HIV antibody test neither assuaged patients' suffering nor offered a treatment or a change in prognosis; to the contrary, it only furthered the medicalization of many additional persons, asymptomatic yet HIV-positive, who were now seen as having begun the long descent into sickness and death.[59] If, as AIDS researchers admit, HIV can be carried without effect for eight to twenty years within a host, what is gained by pathologizing and stigmatizing an otherwise healthy, asymptomatic person?

The authors conclude that the gains were solely political: "under the guise of public health, homosexual behavior *en toto* has been remedicalized, making enforcement of and compliance with 'safe sex' guidelines a political issue."[60] As scientific discourse exercises unique powers for social control, and unrivaled credibility for constructing reality in Western life and society, the identification of a "gay plague" in 1981 was initially sufficient to arrest gay demands for greater political liberties and the decriminalization of sexual practices.[61] After a decade subverting social and medical-psychoanalytical constructions of homosexuality as deviant and diseased, gay men were obliged to circumscribe their sexuality in the 1980s in the name of public health, in the name of hygiene, in the name of forestalling the spread of their contamination of other groups in society, and finally for their own survival. If, for Foucault, sexuality is regulated in the modern world through discourse and ubiquitous and constant confession, for Bentham, omnipotent and pervasive surveillance is the manner by which social control is operationalized, as "surveillance confiscates the gaze for its own profit, appropriates it, and submits the inmate to it."[62] In the 1980s, these twin mechanisms of scientific discourse and surveillance for HIV/AIDS were enlisted to sustain the status quo by convincing the male homosexual in the name of public health and the body politic to police himself and remake himself in the image of heterosexual norms.

> All dominant classes have a vested interest in preserving their privilege . . . [T]he bourgeoisie was the first in modern times to invoke the metaphor of health in order to invest its position with legitimacy. What is at once so fascinating and efficient in the use of this metaphor is the combination of reform, discipline, and progress, such that the measures of social control directed toward subordinate and recalcitrant groups in society are also justified as being implemented on their behalf. . . . People would obey public health measures in the event of a plague because both the social institutions and collective mentalities exist that would accord such measures legitimacy.[63]

The conflation of the desire for technical omnipotence over the disease by biomedical practitioners, interests of policy makers for social stability and control, and interests of AIDS patients for miracle treatments and a cure for the disease reproduced and sustained virtually unanimous support for more sophisticated technical initiatives to treat and diagnose AIDS and further medicalized the lives of male homosexuals.[64]

Latent Texts

> Like any complex text, the signs of illness are read within the conventions of an interpretive community that comprehends them in the light of earlier, powerful readings of what are understood to be similar or parallel texts. The medical profession, as well as society in general incorporates such sets of symbolic readings of these signs of pathology in its understanding of the disease. These communal interpretations of the disease, the signs and symptoms, construct the image of illness and the patient suffering from that illness.[65]

The "similar or parallel texts" informing symbolic readings on AIDS are previous scientific tracts that pathologize homosexual desire and expression.[66] Though biomedical discourse is superficially cleansed of these prior medical and moral arguments claiming that homosexual behavior is deviant, physically degenerate, and gravely threatening to the body politic or the moral order, they transmogrify and are subsumed within biomedical texts that seek to objectively explain and/or metaphorically represent the cause and course of the AIDS epidemic and the pathogenesis of HIV.

For instance, the depiction of HIV's latency, and its alleged virulence (all the more insidious because it is hidden and undetected) is linguistically parallel to texts that locate the moral threat of homosexuals in their inversion and their invisibility. And just as the awakening of HIV out of quiescence is the proximate biological cause of AIDS, so the political emergence of gays out of the closet is the proximate political cause of AIDS. San Francisco's Public Health director, Dr. Selma Dritz, explicitly made this argument by citing the decriminalization of sodomy in 1974 in California as the catalyst for unleashing public health emergencies such as the AIDS epidemic.

> In San Francisco the epidemiology of sexually transmitted enteric diseases seems to be related to both political and social changes in the city. In 1974 a change in political atmosphere in the city made it apparent that legal pressures on the homosexual community would be eased. This was accompanied by an increase in the populations of homosexuals in two particular areas of the city. Within six months we noticed the beginning of a rapid rise in reported cases of amebiasis, shigellosis and viral hepatitis.[67]

In a logic parallel to that of Alan Whiteside, who argued that "political isolation and apartheid" may have contained the spread of HIV/AIDS in South Africa,[68] Dritz seems to imply that curtailing gay civil liberties prior to 1974 contributed to a greater measure of public health in the Bay Area during that period. Meanwhile, other authors have located the proximate cause of the AIDS epidemic in the changing sex roles of gay men in the 1970s, arguing if only gay men had remained either exclusively "tops" or "bottoms," then AIDS could never have become an epidemic within the gay community.[69]

In many biomedical texts, symbolic and metaphorical constructions of the latency and pathology of homosexuality permeate scientific discourse on HIV

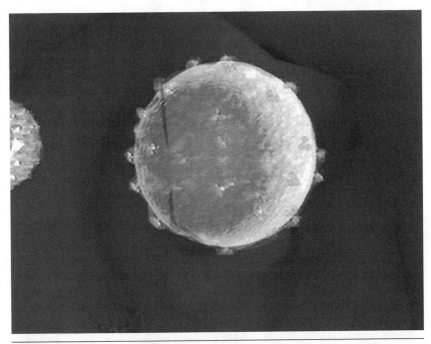

FIGURE 1 "[I]t enters the body in blood or seminal and vaginal fluids and seeks out a key cell in the immune system, a white blood cell called the T-helper lymphocyte 150 times its size."
—narration from "AIDS Research: The Story So Far," KTEH-TV, April 24, 1994,
Copyright © 1994 WGBH/Boston.

and AIDS. Often, lavender colors vividly identify the RNA strands of the virus (the genetic components of HIV) or the enzyme *reverse* transcriptase, and penetration and invagination commonly represent the way in which the virus enters the CD4 T-cell, alluding to the sexual transmission of HIV.[70]

Before my argument is dismissed out of hand as just one alternative reading among many, consider the following computer simulation of HIV infection broadcast on educational TV in the Bay Area. "AIDS Research: The Story So Far," sponsored by the Aaron Diamond Foundation, graphically illustrates the process of HIV infection and reproduction by computer simulation and in Technicolor.[71] The first frame sequence introduces the human immunodeficiency virus stylized as a green, perfectly spherical hand grenade floating languidly through sexualized body vesicles, à la Georgia O'Keefe (Figure 1).

After encountering a human T-cell with a CD4 receptor, HIV then "docks" to the surface of the cell membrane with a neon purple flourish, thereby gaining entry to the inner sanctum of the cell (Figure 2). Now fused with the CD4 T-cell, HIV slips inside the lymphocyte disguised innocuously as something other than what it is. Within minutes, HIV sheds its external coat in a viral striptease revealing its true morphology: a purple triangle (Figure 3).

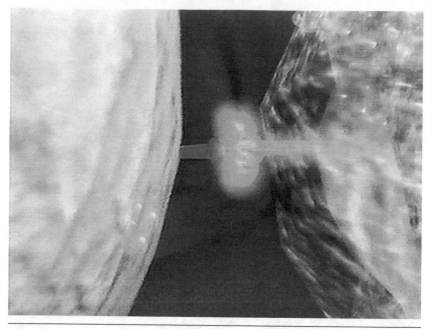

FIGURE 2 "They have on their surface a specific doorway, a specific structure through which this virus can attach and enter."
—narration from "AIDS Research: The Story So Far," KTEH-TV, April 24, 1994, Copyright © 1994 WGBH/Boston.

The narration continues with an explanation of the transcription of viral RNA into DNA, which leads to a colonization of the cell's machinery in the service of producing new HIV progeny. Once this process is complete, the human immunodeficiency virus, stylized once again as a purple triangle, "migrates to the surface of the cell and buds out from the cell membrane." It is now a "free new viral particle which can go infect an uninfected cell and start this whole life cycle over. Before it is destroyed, one infected cell can produce thousands of HIV particles which go on to infect other lymphocytes." This biomedical representation of HIV infection and the manner by which the virus spreads at the micro level of the host mirrors similar epidemiological explanations for HIV's dissemination at the macro level of populations, as "free, new" HIV-positive gay men spread infections to thousands of sexual partners before being destroyed by AIDS. In the words of Professor Opendra Narayan at Johns Hopkins Medical School: "These people have sex twenty to thirty times a night. . . . A man comes along and goes from anus to anus and in a single night will act as a mosquito transferring infected cells on his penis. When this is practiced for a year, with a man having three thousand sexual intercourses, one can readily understand this massive epidemic that is currently upon us."[72] These are just a few examples from among many of the ways in which cultural

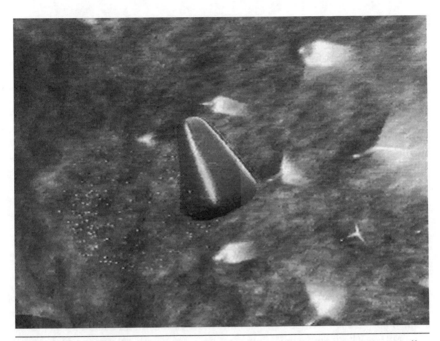

FIGURE 3 "Like many unwanted guests, once it comes in your door it decides to take its coat off and make itself at home. And that's what it does. So it enters the cell at the surface, it sheds its coat, and then it sheds its inner core, revealing its genetic material."
—narration from "AIDS Research: The Story So Far," KTEH-TV, April 24, 1994,
Copyright © 1994 WGBH/Boston.

politics and the politics of sexuality are embedded in scientific discourse on the disease and in the very content of AIDS clinical and biomedical research.

The following chapters examine the geography and epidemiology of AIDS in San Francisco and the city's local role in constituting global claims about the historiography of HIV/AIDS. Juxtaposing primary sources, such as AIDS case reports, internal public health memoranda, and early epidemiological research against public representations of the disease, with an ethnography of AIDS surveillances practices and policies in San Francisco reveals the social construction of knowledge of AIDS in situ and exemplifies Nancy Krieger's thesis that public health data inherently embody political and ideological decisions.

With the following case study of AIDS surveillance in San Francisco I return to the project begun by Ludwick Fleck, and the example he established for an historical description of the reciprocal articulation between medical and social conceptions of disease and his conclusion that professional training and specialization contributes to the acquired ability of some medical specialists to "see" what they were trained to look for, and in so doing, "establish many applicable facts,"[73] albeit while "rendering the recognition of other forms and other facts impossible."[74]

Although there were several hypotheses in 1981 and 1982 about the cause(s) of AIDS that were equally consistent with the empirical evidence (both clinical and epidemiological) on the disease, the specific historicity of AIDS, the state of development of biotechnology, the institutionally mediated authority of some actors and not others, the political economy and ideological structure of public health surveillance and the federal institutions of biomedical research, and complex interactions between society and medical experts combined to produce a near unanimity of consensus around the theory that a retrovirus (HIV), predominantly spread through sexual intercourse, was the single precipitating, proximate, and overwhelming cause of the epidemic of acquired immune deficiency syndrome.

Anticipating Derek Gregory's assertion that "History is never innocent; it is always 'history-for,' "[75] Janet Abu-Lughod argues that:

> All accounts are not only constructed, but, what is worse, are constructed *backwards* . . . That is, it is only "after the fact" that narratives are built, especially narratives that seek to explain. . . . In history also, it is only after events have run their course that we build the narrative that appears to make them inevitable . . . . It is far better to stop along the way, assessing relative conditions at successive points in time and then trying to analyze how these various states could have come about. . . . This is all the more important because interests determine *where* any narrator will begin his/her account.[76]

II

The Medicalization of Gay Desire in San Francisco (1978–1983)

> *Too much is being transmitted (among gay men in San Francisco), we've got all these diseases going unchecked. There are so many opportunities for transmission that, if something new gets loose here, we're going to have hell to pay.*
>
> —Dr. Selma Dritz, 1980

Prefiguring AIDS—Gay Men's Health and Demographics in SF (1974–1980)

In the years immediately preceding the discovery of the first AIDS cases in the United States in June 1981, the Public Health Services issued ominous warnings of sex-related health problems: in 1976, of an epidemic of genital herpes among America's sexually active youth and, two years later, of various STDs, which the agency targeted as the gravest threat facing American health. This position was reiterated in 1980 with the publication of the U.S. Public Health Services "Health Objectives for the Nation," which identified "11 goals relating to the control of sexually transmitted diseases (STD's)"—paradigmatically, in the words of Murray and Payne, a "trendy classification in the *zeitgeist* of 'sexual counter-revolution' " that presaged the way in which AIDS would be interpreted.[1]

National and local public health authorities in San Francisco began to pay increasing attention to gay male sexual practices, targeting surveillance and research of gay men and escalating political efforts to restrict gay sexual license in the name of public health. As assistant director at the Bureau of Communicable Disease Control of the San Francisco Department of Public Health, Dr. Selma Dritz was responsible for monitoring infectious disease outbreaks in the city. As medical epidemiologist for the city, Dritz wrote about the alarming increase of sexually transmitted diseases among gay men there. In her opinion, epidemics had been unleashed by "political and social changes in the city" after 1974, which precipitated rapid increases in enteric diseases (amebiasis, shigellosis) as well as other bacterial and viral infections (hepatitis A and B, and typhoid). Dr. Dritz argued:

> With the relaxation of traditional moral restraints and the emergence of more permissive modes of social and sexual interplay in the past 10 years, some major cities have acquired large, highly visible homosexual communities. This concentration has produced more opportunities for frequent sexual contacts between

21

homosexual men. In a recent profile of one sample of homosexual patients with sexually transmitted diseases, investigators reported that these men visited public bathhouses and had an average of two to three sexual contacts per visit, largely with anonymous partners. . . . The frequent practice of oral and anal intercourse has been accompanied by reports of a rapidly increasing incidence of "classic" venereal diseases (herpes genitalis, herpes proctitis, and gonorrheal proctitis in both men and women), venereal herpes, and enteric disease.[2]

In mid-1974 the gay community began to expand rapidly from an estimated population of 30,000 or 40,000 . . . [until presently in 1979] San Francisco has a total population of 660,000 persons [with] 100,000 predominantly homosexual men. With the expansion of the homosexual community in San Francisco, the number of cases of sexually transmitted enteric disease reported by cooperating physicians and laboratories increased by orders of magnitude: by 1979, amebiasis had risen [by 25 times], giardiasis had risen from one or two per year to 85, shigellosis and hepatitis A had doubled, and hepatitis B had trebled. Similar increases have been reported from other parts of the country. The problem is greater than these numbers suggest, because they represent only cases that were reported as laboratory confirmed . . . the true incidence may be 100 per cent higher. . . . Infections in the homosexual community that are not transmitted sexually may also on occasion present a potential problem for the wider population of a city.[3]

Physicians . . . may be unaware of the role of homosexuality in medical problem[s]. We need effective education for both physicians and the public about the "new" sexually transmitted diseases.[4]

At the Medical Staff Conference in San Francisco in 1979, Dr. Wibbelsman, outgoing chief of the Division of Venereal Disease Control at the city's Department of Public Health (SFDPH), made the following epidemiological and demographic observations:

Dr. Dritz presented an overview of enteric disease trends in San Francisco and conflicting estimates of the gay population which range between 100,000 and 200,000. . . . There are 72,000 patient visits a year to the SFDPH's City [VD] Clinic . . . my impression is that 60 to 80 percent of these patients are gay men. San Francisco leads the US in reported cases of primary and secondary syphilis in cities of 200,000 . . . [and was] fourth in gonorrhea incidence in 1977.[5]

In these various articles, Dr. Dritz personally correlates the temporal rise of sexually transmitted infections among gay men not only to the "emergence of more permissive" sexual mores, but specifically to the coming in 1974 of a more relaxed "political atmosphere" in the city. She is obliquely referring, of course, to the May 1975 decision by the state of California to repeal its 103-year-old sodomy laws. In other words, Dritz is explicitly tying the specter of infectious disease epidemics and declining public health in San Francisco to increased civil rights for male homosexuals.

This is odd for several reasons. Dritz had already noted that the increase of STDs in San Francisco in the 1970s was true for both men and women and oc-

curred nationally as well as in California. But in addition, as a medical specialist in communicable diseases she was well aware that New York City's epidemic
of "gay bowel disease" in homosexual men (which preceded San Francisco's
epidemic) had occurred in the absence of any similar legislation decriminaliz-
ing sodomy. Dritz's logic therefore is inversely analogous to that of Alan
Whiteside when he suggested that "political isolation" and apartheid helped
slow the spread of AIDS in South Africa.

Randy Shilts, a gay reporter for the *San Francisco Chronicle* between 1982
and 1987, is the most widely known and most often cited resource for the sexual and social milieu in San Francisco. Working closely with Selma Dritz, the
CDC, and prominent AIDS researchers in constructing his historical narrative
And the Band Played On (1987), Shilts echoes the SFDPH estimates of epidemic proportions of sexually transmitted diseases among gay men: an 8,000
percent increase in gay bowel disease between 1973 and 1980, a 700 percent increase in shigellosis cases among single men in their thirties, and a fourfold increase in the incidence of hepatitis B between 1976 and 1980.

But in their accounts of the demography and morbidity of gay males in San
Francisco and the United States, neither Shilts nor Dritz acknowledges the already heightened attention on the part of the U.S. Public Health Services to the
prevalence of sexually transmitted diseases in the country in general, especially
among urban homosexual men, nor to biotechnological developments during
the same period (e.g., the hepatitis B antigen test) which increased the number
of cases diagnosed and reported.[6]

This is a glaring omission, as between 1978 and 1981, the Centers for Disease Control of the U.S. Department of Health Services were heavily invested
in researching the incidence of one particular sexually transmitted virus and
were conducting epidemiological studies of hepatitis B in San Francisco, New
York City, Amsterdam, Chicago, and Los Angeles. While the hepatitis B studies
are historically significant for their role in advancing theories of retroviral infections and constructing much of the early hypotheses about the emergence
and sexual transmission of AIDS, they also demonstrate that the U.S. government was heavily invested in a national program for the surveillance of gay
men's health with a specific interest in characterizing the epidemiology of
STDs in these populations in the years immediately preceding the discovery of
AIDS. Both Dritz and Wibbelsman acknowledged these aggressive surveillance
policies when noting that "some of (the SFDPH) morbidity data are statisti-
cally skewed due to an intense epidemiological effort by interested physicians
whose practices include numerous patients who have adopted . . . alternative
life-styles,' "[7] and that the Public Health Department monitored gay bathhouses and used mobile vans to check for STDs in the Tenderloin's "red-light"
district. And well over a year before the first AIDS case was reported in the city,
Dritz and other medical professionals were publicly speculating about the potential threat that homosexuals might pose for public health in San Francisco

in the absence of measures to curtail sexually transmitted infectious disease in the gay community.

In the midst of Reagan's national budget cuts affecting the U.S. Public Health Service, including the elimination of a merchant marine hospital in San Francisco that primarily served indigents and threats to downsize the Centers for Disease Control, and on the heels of a recent CDC survey that concluded "that homosexual men [with] multiple sex exposures are at "high risk for major disease,"[8] the CDC's initial report heralding the discovery of an immunodeficiency syndrome in gay men was published on June 5, 1981 (Figure 4).

"A Pneumonia That Strikes Gay Males"

Given the context described above, the conclusions expressed by the editor of the *Morbidity and Mortality Weekly Report* (*MMWR*) are hardly unanticipated: "The fact that these patients were all homosexuals suggests an association between some aspect of a homosexual lifestyle or disease acquired through sexual contact and [the] pneumonia."

By virtue of concurrent research on hepatitis B and the focus on sexually transmitted epidemics among gay men, government health officials were theoretically predisposed, at the very moment the Los Angeles cases of pneumonia were discovered, to infer that male homosexuality per se was epidemiologically and epistemologically salient for understanding the cause of this syndrome of cellular immune deficiency. This paradigmatic predisposition foreshadowed their official determination only fifteen months thereafter that the "probable mode of transmission" of this new disease was sexual contact.

What does seem incongruous both then and now, however, is that these five homosexual men with pneumonia were characterized as "previously healthy" or "generally healthy young men" in the same breath. Given the state of knowledge and medical scholarship on gay men in the late 1970s and the alleged hyperendemic levels of STDs, meningitis, hepatitis B, cytomegalovirus (CMV), gay bowel disease, and so on within their communities—how is it that these men with pneumonia were, and continue to be, represented as "previously healthy"? Perhaps one could argue that the comment regarding hyperendemic morbidity among gay men was made about aggregate populations and did not accurately describe these specific individuals. Turning to the original *MMWR* report of June 5, 1981, however, reveals that all five patients were characterized as "previously healthy" despite their disparate clinical histories: one patient was an intravenous drug abuser, one had been treated with radiation for Hodgkin's disease, four had evidence of past hepatitis B infection, and all five "reported using inhalant drugs."

The one thing that is not clear from their clinical histories is their promiscuity, as all of the patients differed with respect to past infections with STDs, and only two of the five were reported in the *MMWR* as having had "frequent homosexual contacts with various partners." Yet from these ambiguous observations, the only salient commonality that is adduced in orthodox narratives

CENTERS FOR DISEASE CONTROL   June 5, 1981 / Vol. 30 / No. 21
MORBIDITY AND MORTALITY WEEKLY REPORT

Epidemiologic Notes and Reports
249 Dengue Type 4 Infections in U.S. Travelers to the Caribbean
250 *Pneumocystis* Pneumonia—Los Angeles

Current Trends
252 Measles—United States, First 20 Weeks
253 Risk-Factor-Prevalence Surveillance—Utah
259 Surveillance of Childhood Lead Poisoning—United States

International Notes
261 Quarantine Measures

Epidemiologic Notes and Reports

Pneumocystis Pneumonia—Los Angeles

In the period October 1980–May 1981, 5 young men, all active homosexuals, were treated for biopsy-confirmed *Pneumocystis carinii* pneumonia at 3 different hospitals in Los Angeles, California. Two of the patients died. All 5 patients had laboratory con-firmed previous or current cytomegalovirus (CMV) infection and candidal mucosal infection. Case reports of these patients follow.

Patient 1: A previously healthy 33-year-old man developed P. *carinii* pneumonia and oral mucosal candidiasis in March 1981 after a 2-month history of fever associated with elevated liver enzymes, leukopenia, and CMV viruria. The serum complement-fixation CMV titer in October 1980 was 256; in May 1981 it was 32. The patient's condition de-teriorated despite courses of treatment with trimethoprim-sulfamethoxazole (TMP/SMX), pentamidine, and acyclovir. He died May 3, and postmortem examination showed . . .

Editorial note: . . . The occurrence of pneumocystosis in these 5 previously healthy in-dividuals without a clinically apparent underlying immunodeficiency is unusual. The fact that these patients were all homosexuals suggests an association between some as-pect of a homosexual lifestyle or disease acquired through sexual contact . . .

. . . All the above observations suggest the possibility of a cellular-immune dysfunction related to a common exposure that predisposes individuals to opportunistic infections such as pneumocystosis and candidiasis. Although the role of CMV infection in the pathogenesis of pneumocystosis remains unknown, the possibility of P. *carinii* infec-tion must be carefully considered in a differential diagnosis for *previously healthy ho-mosexual* males with dyspnea and pneumonia.

FIGURE 4   *Morbidity and Mortality Weekly Report*

on AIDS is the homosexual identity of these men; their common medical (CMV infection) and behavioral (inhalant drug use) histories were irrelevant for understanding their illnesses. Male homosexuality itself evidenced the high risk for disease in these men. As further proof of this etiological bias, it was five years into the epidemic before the CDC disaggregated the "homosex-ual/bisexual" risk group for AIDS and created a separate category for gay in-travenous drug users. Therefore, during this period, the way in which the CDC classified and quantified populations at risk for developing AIDS "de-emphasized and under-represented every patient characteristic except homosexuality." And consequently, the nation's surveillance statistics between 1981 and 1985 *overrepresent* the number of AIDS cases attributable to "homosexuality and bisexuality" while simultaneously *underrepresenting* cases attributable to intravenous drug use (or to a history of transfusions or hemophilia) as "the CDC's methodology would not include anyone who could be labeled 'homosexual' in any other risk category."[9]

The Emergence of a Bureaucracy for AIDS Surveillance in San Francisco (1981)

Surveillance is a type of observational study that involves the continuous monitoring of disease occurrence within a population. Routine surveillance data are typically obtained through provider-initiated reports (passive surveillance) or health department–solicited reports (active surveillance). Whatever the method of collection, surveillance data are necessary to portray the ongoing pattern of disease occurrence, which will allow detection of unusual disease patterns and subsequently trigger disease-control and prevention efforts. In addition, these data can be used for resource allocation in public health planning and to evaluate control and prevention measures. Moreover, unusual events detected from surveillance data are often a stimulus for health-related research. Finally, these data provide an important archive of disease activity.[10]

As succinctly summarized by Thacker et al. above, the general mandate of disease surveillance is to monitor the health of a given population by quantifying morbidity (illnesses) and mortality and documenting disease trends over time. And it was as a consequence of this sentinel function of the CDC in Atlanta, Georgia, that "gay-related immune deficiency" (later known as acquired immune deficiency syndrome) first came to the attention of the public on June 5, 1981, in the pages of the *MMWR*.

It is curious that the CDC's report in June 1981 was the first indication that the San Francisco Department of Public Health received alerting them of the discovery of a new disease in the city's gay community. Although Dr. Selma Dritz declined to be interviewed for this book, she confirmed that she first learned of AIDS from "Michael Gottlieb in *The Morbidity and Mortality Weekly Report* . . . that was the first we heard of it."[11] In other words, although she was the assistant director of San Francisco's Bureau of Communicable Disease Control and actively monitored infectious disease in the gay community, Dritz had not received any alarming reports of patients with Kaposi's sarcoma or atypical pneumonia from Bay Area clinicians. Instead, the AIDS epidemic arrived from the top down as the CDC's report of a Los Angeles "cluster" of five gay men with cellular immune deficiency was disseminated nationally via the *MMWR* and catalyzed intense surveillance in San Francisco in the summer of 1981.

Throughout the remaining six months of 1981, Dr. Dritz did painstakingly gather a number of reports from private physicians in San Francisco and staff at the CDC describing gay and bisexual men with Kaposi's sarcoma (KS) and Pneumocystis carinii pneumonia (PCP) who had been treated at clinics and hospitals in the San Francisco metropolitan area the previous year. Randy Shilt's describes the first case of AIDS in the city:

> [Dr. Paul] Volberding was starting his dream job as chief of oncology at San Francisco General Hospital . . . when a veteran cancer specialist slapped him on the back on his first day at work, July 1 [1981], and pointed toward an examining room. "There's the next great disease waiting for you," he said. "A patient with KS." Volberding had never heard the term KS before. [He] walked into the room and, for the first time, saw one of the people who would merge his interests in retroviruses and the terminally ill into a career that would consume much of his life. . . . A friendly down-home accent identified the twenty-two-year-old patient as from the South. He was an attendant in a San Francisco bathhouse and had been admitted to the hospital a few days ago with diarrhea and weight loss; the Kaposi's sarcoma diagnosis had been confirmed just the day before. . . . The youth didn't have many friends in San Francisco and lived in a lonely apartment in the seedy Tenderloin neighborhood. He was estranged from his family, and he didn't understand why he had lost so much weight or where the purple spots had come from.[12]

More than a decade later, Dr. Volberding began a lecture at the Fairmont Hotel in San Francisco in 1994 with a slide show of this very same patient. Informing the audience that he had previously spent two years as a postgraduate in Jay Levy's virology lab at the University of California at San Francisco, Volberding related the following story:

> Really what I wanted to do mostly was take care of patients with cancer. So I took a position taking care of cancer patients at San Francisco General Hospital, and the first day that I was there, this man came to my attention [referring to a slide of a man with purple lesions spread over his trunk, his eyes masked by tape]. And I blocked his eyes . . . for his own privacy, although he's been dead for well over ten years now. But his eyes were really perhaps the most striking feature— haunting eyes, showing . . . with the very first case—you didn't need 1,000 or 10,000 or now 250,000 cases of AIDS in the country to know that this was an important new problem. He was twenty-two years old [groan from the audience] and dying from a disease that was supposed to happen only in very old men . . . we were mystified.
>
> Now, there was working with me a brand-new oncology fellow at the time. . . . And he said, "Gee, I think in the hospital that I was in, in New York, there were some other patients like this." And this was before there was any publication at all, before any, before anything had been written about this disease, and we called New York and compared notes and found out that they were seeing patients, but no one knew what was going on with this disease. And obviously this was the first case that I saw of AIDS, and at the time . . . having time on my

hands just starting at the hospital, it seemed like an interesting thing to become involved in.[13]

In accounts such as these, a mythology of the archetypal AIDS patient is constructed: young, mysteriously ill, and foreboding. Furthermore, the two stories are extraordinarily similar—they corroborate one another; not unexpectedly, as Volberding was most surely Shilts's informant regarding this early AIDS case. But a review of this patient's medical records, and case files in San Francisco's AIDS Seroepidemiology and Surveillance Branch, unravels the coherence of this narrative. First, the historical record contradicts Volberding's claim that nothing had been written about the disease at the time he first met this patient. As previously noted, the initial *MMWR* publication of cellular deficiency among gay men had been released to the press on June 5, 1981, a month prior to this encounter at San Francisco General Hospital and was of sufficient medical importance to catalyze an extensive surveillance effort in San Francisco. Further confirming the power of this news in constructing the syndrome of immune deficiency in gay men was a copy of the *MMWR* that I found pasted in a medical chart to guide in the diagnosis of a gay man who presented to SFGH with a "fever of unknown origin" that very month.[14]

Second, there is the representation of the patient himself. What is and is not said about this man contributes to the mystery and mythology of AIDS. What Shilts and Volberding emphasize is the man's youth (22 years old),[15] his "down-home" accent and demeanor, his connection to the gay bathhouse culture, and the mystery of his debilitated condition. What is omitted from this picture is that this patient was homeless, had only sporadic employment as a dishwasher or janitor (the latter only briefly at a bathhouse where he traded work for a place to sleep), was "sickly from birth," suffered from Marfan's syndrome (a debilitating disease of the connective tissues), and had a history of MDA ("ecstasy") and intravenous amphetamine use which the patient himself correlated with the emergence of his "purple spots."[16] Contrary to Dr. Volberding's story about a prescient colleague who exclaimed "there's the next great disease waiting for you," according to notes in his medical chart this young man was seen as a rather unremarkable and indigent patient with "numerous social problems," probably suffering from lymphoma, gallstones, and septic emboli until June of 1981 when the new syndrome of cellular immune deficiency was lit upon to guide his differential diagnosis. Nor was this man the first AIDS patient diagnosed in San Francisco; the first and second AIDS cases in the city were pediatric siblings diagnosed in 1978 and 1979, information freely available to Volberding and Shilts—the children had been cited in a proposal submitted to the National Institutes of Health in 1983 by a prominent Bay Area epidemiologist studying AIDS in San Francisco.[17] Moreover, the patient was not even the first gay man reported with the disease or the first case of the disease seen for care at San Francisco General Hospital.

Within three months of this case (October 1981) epidemiologists from the CDC arrived in San Francisco to interview AIDS patients regarding risk factors for the disease. For the purpose of surveillance, the new syndrome of immune deficiency was operationally defined as the occurrence of Kaposi's sarcoma, atypical pneumonia, or a handful of other opportunistic infections "moderately predictive of a defect in cell-mediated immunity, in a person with no known cause for diminished resistance to that disease."[18] As of December 31, 1981, the San Francisco Department of Public Health had reported 24 AIDS cases in the city, all of them eventually identified as male homosexuals or bisexuals. The CDC's patient interviews were subsequently incorporated into a national case-control study whose results were published in August 1983. This report concluded that "certain lifestyle factors were associated with the occurrence of the disease . . . [including] sexual contact with large numbers of male partners [cases had an average number of partners double that of controls] . . . a history of syphilis and hepatitis other than Hepatitis B" [again cases were twice as likely to have had these infections], and the "use of various illicit substances" [relative to controls, AIDS cases had a greater lifetime exposure to inhalant drugs, known as "poppers"].[19]

Enabled by a midyear grant of $180,000 from Mayor Diane Feinstein,[20] Dr. Dritz and Carlos Rendon at the Department of Public Health continued surveillance in San Francisco throughout 1982, documenting suspected AIDS cases, reporting them to the CDC, and filing scant patient information on 3 × 5 index cards which were stored in shoe boxes in the department offices. Elsewhere in the United States, reports of AIDS in nonhomosexual IV drug users (13 percent of all reported cases) and among hemophiliacs and Haitians (both reported in July 1982) had already been published. This completed the categories commonly referred to as the "Four H's" who were at increased risk for the disease: homosexuals, heroin addicts, hemophiliacs, and Haitians. As of December 31, 1982, an additional 94 patients had been reported in San Francisco, including the first AIDS case in the nation that was associated with a blood transfusion.[21] Within a month a new category comprising female partners of IV drug using and bisexual men was added to the list as "heterosexual partners" of the aforementioned.

Mayor Feinstein subsequently authorized a supplementary grant of $4.3 million in 1983, enabling Dritz and Rendon to recruit additional staff to work in AIDS surveillance.[22] Tim Piland was the first AIDS disease control investigator hired, and he spoke with me in October 1994 about beginning surveillance work in San Francisco after receiving a master's degree in public Health from the University of California at Berkeley:

That was back in the late '70s, and in New York amebiasis was a big epidemic in those days . . . people were actually dying of it. . . . I did my internship for my MPH at the City Clinic [in San Francisco], and cases were beginning to show up there of amebiasis . . . 1978, 1979 . . . it was rampant on the East Coast . . . the same thing [as gay bowel disease]. . . . [We] treated it with Flagyl and lots of nasty chemicals. But we, "we" meaning the medical establishment here, wanted to prevent that from happening here in San Francisco. [So the city increased surveillance and hired me as a disease control investigator] to work at the City Clinic and . . . so I just sort of fell into working as a disease control investigator . . . tracing cases, doing interviews with people. . . . I don't think hepatitis was even the [largest epidemic in the city]. . . . There were huge amounts of syphilis and gonorrhea . . . those were the most rampant.

[I think] it was just the sheer numbers of people that elicited a response [from the PH Department]. . . . I think they were only as good to the gay community as they absolutely had to be. I don't think there was anything magnanimous about the response from the establishment, the medical establishment, or the Public Health establishment in terms of wanting to identify a problem and channel a lot of money into it and shut it down.

I remember the first time Selma Dritz came to the clinic and said, "You may start to see people who have these particular signs." She showed us pictures of people with KS, with wasting syndrome, and things like that, and we were just shocked. . . . That had to be 1981. . . . She came and presented it as if it were a murder mystery . . . like saying, "Here's this mysterious disease happening . . . and we don't know what's causing it . . . or how it's transmitted." She kept saying, "I just hope I'm around long enough to help figure this thing out." That's when I first became aware of it. . . . I was doing syphilis epidemiology at that point . . . there wasn't a lot of attention to it [AIDS].

February of 1983 was when I was picked to go over to work in the Bureau of Disease Control with Selma, and basically I was the surveillance unit. We had 273 cases at that point. . . . We used to take Polaroids. . . . Selma had a big blackboard in her office where we would identify cases in clusters and see if there were connections with LA clusters.

That's when AIDS was just . . . GRID . . . "gay cancer," KS. In February 1983 not many of us had friends yet who'd been affected by AIDS—it was all kind of abstract. . . . I had a friend who died in 1981 who was one of the first 100 cases in New York, and I knew it was there . . . but in San Francisco it seemed to have an abstract quality, it wasn't a real profound presence in our lives . . . it was pretty much business as usual.

Early that same year, shortly after Piland was hired, AIDS was officially declared a "disease worthy of note" in California. In a memo dated March 23, 1983, Dr. James Chin, chief of the Infectious Disease Section for the Department of Health Services of the State of California, notified local physicians that AIDS was now "a legally reportable condition under California Administrative Code Title 17, Section 2503, which pertains to the reporting of the occurrence of unusual diseases."[23] Chin elaborated in the memo on hypotheses regarding the etiology of the disease, observing that "up to now [AIDS] has been almost exclusively reported in population groups who may have some depression of their immune systems by virtue of high infection rates with disease agents which can temporarily depress certain immune factors . . . suggest[ing] that some pre-existing immunologic deficiency or depression in the host is necessary for the development of AIDS." Chin had expressed similar reservations about the alleged infectious nature of the disease six months previously, in an article promoting the safety of the recently licensed hepatitis B vaccine (HBV), which had been derived from the plasma of gay and bisexual men who participated in the national trials between 1978 and 1981: "Even if an agent transmissible by blood were found to be responsible for AIDS . . . a big 'if,' and if such an agent were present in some donors of the plasma for vaccine, it could not . . . survive . . . the chemical inactivation procedures required for the production of HBV vaccine in the U.S."[24]

That even the chief of the California Department of Health Services was skeptical that AIDS was infectious in the absence of predisposing host vulnerabilities attests to how widespread and credible this view was in light of the epidemiological evidence during the earliest years of the epidemic. As a gay man working as a disease control investigator in the midst of the epidemic in San Francisco, Tim Piland understood the disease similarly until late in the epidemic. It was "deep into the decade," perhaps as late as 1984 or 1985, that AIDS became personally relevant to men like him and precipitated changes in his own sexual behavior in response to it.

> I just think it's personal experience that makes people change their behavior and not Public Health campaigns. . . . I really think it was when people started going to their friend's funerals. Especially before there was a test for HIV, before there was some empirical evidence that you could actually find something in your blood, it was all basically anecdotal to me. It wasn't until 1984 . . .
>
> I mean, I knew one of the first people in New York to die, but it was an abstraction, there wasn't a significant change in my behavior or my friends' behaviors until deep into the '80s. . . . My friend [in New York who died] was into a lot of heavy-duty things [sexual things] and I know that he did drugs, the kinds of drugs I never touched. . . . I think there were a lot of those people getting it. If you do those kinds of things, those nasty things, you know you're going to put yourself at risk. . . . The whole thing of whether it was even sexually transmitted hadn't even been established yet. . . . [I thought] People like me don't get this disease. . . . I wasn't a fast-track city boy, you know.[25]

Chin's and Piland's views were neither atypical nor irrational at the time, as most anecdotal accounts and nearly all epidemiological studies of AIDS patients in the early years of the epidemic bore out this view that most persons who had acquired the disease had lived a "fast-track" lifestyle that might, in and of itself, suppress immunity. And despite the theoretical predisposition on the part of the CDC and prominent researchers that AIDS was a sexually transmitted disease, incongruously, little was done by the Health Department or anyone else to warn gay men in the early years of the epidemic. Safe-sex education did not begin in San Francisco until late 1983, and only then in the face of pressure from a minority of gay politicos in the Harvey Milk Club, and an exposé by local reporters charging that the Public Health Department was "attempting to suppress information about the spread of the disease." Thereafter, the San Francisco AIDS Foundation was established and began recommending the use of condoms for every sexual encounter between gay men. By late 1984, the Foundation's safe-sex guidelines were expanded to include recommendations that heterosexuals use condoms as well; and this despite the fact that less than 1 percent of all cumulatively reported AIDS cases in the country, and a grand total of four cases in San Francisco, were attributable to "heterosexual transmission."[26]

When a separate AIDS surveillance unit was established in 1984,[27] yet more staff were recruited and "active" surveillance began at San Francisco General Hospital and at the University of California at San Francisco replacing what heretofore had been "passive" AIDS case reporting by local physicians. Active surveillance relies on a cadre of disease control investigators who travel to Bay Area clinics and hospitals to capture and record AIDS cases by combing through medical charts and laboratory and pathology reports. Money began to flow into the city for AIDS services and prevention during this same time, augmenting resources available for surveillance. Lobbying Congress in the previous fiscal year, a California delegation of politicians and varied scientific researchers was instrumental in appropriating more than $26 million for research on the disease. A portion of this money sponsored several of the epidemiological and research studies in San Francisco discussed below.

Epidemiology—The San Francisco Cohort Studies

Before the blood test for detecting HIV antibodies became available in the United States in 1985, public health surveillance data were primarily used to "map" the evolution of the epidemic; in San Francisco, this meant literally counting AIDS cases by census tract and quantifying the impact of the disease on populations of homosexual/bisexual men, intravenous-drug users, and so on in the city. After the development of the HIV antibody test however, the surveillance department conducted research on HIV seroprevalence and prepared future projections of the city's AIDS caseload in collaboration with, and corroboration of, three seminal epidemiological studies in San Francisco. It is the powerful articulation of this epidemiological research with the historical narrative recounted above that produces such a coherent and credible account of the emergence and evolution of AIDS in San Francisco and throughout the United States.

AIDS cohort studies are the empirical evidence cited most often by public health professionals, patient advocates, researchers, and the media in order to educate the public about sexual risk factors for the disease, hypothesized cofactors for HIV infection and progression, and estimates of the incubation period from an HIV infection or AIDS diagnosis till death. These studies have been incorporated into public health policy and planning in San Francisco (and elsewhere in the United States) as they provide empirical evidence of risk factors associated with acquiring HIV or AIDS and demographic estimates for the size of the populations potentially at risk for developing the disease.

Three cohort studies which began in San Francisco in the early 1980s have played a seminal role in constructing and corroborating the following central premises of orthodox AIDS science:

1) HIV is a new virus recently introduced into the United States;
2) HIV is the sole cause of AIDS in the sense that it is the only salient marker for identifying those who are at risk for developing AIDS;
3) infection with HIV preceded the occurrence of AIDS in those populations at risk for the disease;
4) an exponential increase in the number of HIV-positive persons in the early 1980s was shadowed by an exponential increase in AIDS six to ten years later; during this time, those infected with HIV experienced a gradual but steady decline in immunity (as measured by declining numbers of CD4 T-cells);
5) progression to AIDS is primarily a function of the length of time one has been infected. Therefore the percent of HIV-positive persons who will progress to AIDS and death can be reliably estimated.

In support of these five claims and as a matter of internal consistency, it is incumbent upon these studies to demonstrate that HIV was present in the gay community in San Francisco in the late 1970s and preceded the outbreak of Kaposi's sarcoma (KS) and *Pneumocystis carinii* pneumonia in 1981 and 1982. Next, these studies must empirically demonstrate that HIV was being transmitted at sufficiently high levels between 1979 and 1983 to accelerate and sustain the AIDS epidemic throughout the decade. The cohort studies must also prove that unprotected receptive anal intercourse is the primary method of transmitting HIV among gay men, and that, ipso facto, those persons who engage in this behavior are highly likely to contract the virus and develop AIDS, while those men who have less sexual intercourse are less likely to contract the disease. Finally, in order to derive estimates for the trend of HIV infections and AIDS cases in the future, these researchers must reliably estimate current HIV transmission rates, sexual risk-taking behavior, the incubation period from HIV infection to AIDS, and the size of the gay male population at risk in San Francisco.

Although in aggregate the cohort studies corroborate orthodox constructions of AIDS historiography and epidemiology, a critical reading of these texts shows, at best, a messier picture of "science in the making." And when in key instances, data from the cohort studies either fail to confirm or explicitly refute central premises of orthodox AIDS science, accepted wisdom on risk factors for AIDS, or the proportion of HIV-infected gay men in San Francisco, and so on, these data are marginalized or wholly elided from subsequent scientific accounts.

The San Francisco General Hospital Cohort: 1982

Although it is the smallest and least known of all the cohort studies in San Francisco, the San Francisco General Hospital Cohort was the first epidemiological study in the city to look at the sexual and behavioral risks associated with developing AIDS. Established in late 1982 with money from the National Cancer Institute, the cohort study soon moved to San Francisco General Hospital, where it received funding from the California State University Wide Task Force on AIDS.[28] Researchers associated with this cohort are collectively referred to as the AIDS Epidemiology Group, and for their first studies on AIDS incidence and risk factors for the disease, principal investigator Dr. A. Moss and colleagues designed a case-control cohort study comprising 101 AIDS cases diagnosed in San Francisco between April 1983 and April 1984.[29] These cases were compared to HIV-negative homosexual controls, matched for age and race, and were randomly selected from the city's STD clinic as well as a neighborhood near the hospital. Moss acknowledges that "AIDS was generally believed to be caused by a sexually transmitted agent at the time of the study (April 1983)" because of the epidemic's "rapid spread . . . among homosexual men" early in the 1980s.[30] Therefore, interviewers focused on patterns of sexual behavior (sexual acts and numbers of partners) and drug use during the preceding year. After the HIV test was developed in 1985, it was used to evaluate blood samples from the cohort.

The AIDS Epidemiology Group estimated the size of San Francisco's male homosexual population at 43,650 persons and deduced that 4 percent of all homosexual/bisexual men in the city had already been reported as AIDS cases as of May 1986. By way of comparison, this estimate for the size of the population at risk for AIDS in San Francisco is less than one-half, or one-quarter, of previous estimates (100,000–200,000).

In a 1987 publication on risk factors for AIDS, Moss et al. found that "AIDS risk was strongly associated with number of sexual partners, [the risk] doubling with every 30–40 partners." When their own data demonstrated that "a relatively high proportion of [HIV] sero-negative [STD] clinic controls"[31] also had high numbers of sexual partners yet remained uninfected, the authors speculated that perhaps this was an indication that these 'highly-risky' men were "resistant to [HIV] infection."[32]

Moss et al. also found that "rectal receptivity was clearly the primary sexual behavior leading to the transmission of HIV . . . independent of number of partners. . . . [O]ther exposures associated with risk . . . were prior parasitic and other sexually transmitted diseases."[33] They found "no significant associations with drug use in the case-control associations . . . except possibly nitrites ('poppers')."[34] In conclusion, the authors suggested that STD infections and drug use might compromise host immunity, increasing the likelihood of becoming HIV-infected. Their prevention recommendations fell somewhat short, however, by merely advocating "restricting [the] number [of one's] sexual partners and [avoiding] unprotected rectal sex."[35] The San Francisco General Hospital Cohort study was one of the first of its kind in San Francisco to affirm that an increased risk for HIV infection was associated with receptive anal intercourse and promiscuity and to argue that, other than "poppers," drug use was not associated with contracting AIDS.

As for progressing to AIDS, Moss et al. found that the only salient factor associated with more rapid death was the age of the patient.[36] Once infected with HIV, "drug users do better or at least as good as gay men—heroin, smokers, bad nutrition—their time to AIDS is no better [nor worse]."[37]

HIV Seroconversion Trends and AIDS Case Projections

When the General Hospital cohort was recruited in 1983–1984, 62 percent of the gay men enrolled in it were already HIV-positive. Within the following three years, one out of every five of these men developed AIDS. The authors estimated that half of the cohort would be similarly diagnosed by 1988, with the caveat that "the likelihood" of an HIV-positive person developing AIDS was unclear, given the widely divergent three-year estimates from studies elsewhere: New York (34 percent); Washington, D.C. (17 percent).

By 1989, Moss and Bacchetti had extended to 10 years, the median incubation period from HIV infection to AIDS among gay men, although once again concluding that "the incubation period of AIDS is difficult to study," and more difficult to accurately predict, because instances of people seroconverting and becoming HIV-positive while in a study "are rare [thus] estimates based on them are highly uncertain."[38] As Moss and Bacchetti explained, the cohort studies were unable to actually document many men as they acquired antibodies to HIV because of "the dramatic drop in [HIV] seroconversion by 1984" when most cohort studies began. This "dramatic drop" in HIV infection was never observed, of course, but instead logically deduced from the fact that 62 percent of the cohort was already infected when enrolled in the study in 1984 and that few of those remaining became infected while under study. As HIV was presumed to be a *new* virus in San Francisco, quite obviously these men became infected in the years immediately prior to 1984. Although the reason for the swift decline in the rate of HIV transmission after this time is unknown, it seemed logical to conclude that it had something to do with less frequent unprotected sexual intercourse among gay men in the city, because the reported cases of rectal gonorrhea also declined at this same time in San Francisco.[39] The authors therefore projected that future AIDS cases in the city should reflect this 1984 peak in HIV transmission via a gradual decline in AIDS cases between 1988 and 1990. And all of the San Francisco cohort studies have similarly cited this period of declining male STD infections in the early 1980s as proof of the efficacy of AIDS prevention policies based on "risk reduction" (fewer partners, less receptive intercourse, and using condoms during sex).

The San Francisco Men's Health Study: 1984–1993

Beginning in 1984 and continuing though 1993, the San Francisco Men's Health Study is one of the longest studies in the world of AIDS in homosexual men,[40] and its import is enormous for the production of knowledge on AIDS both in San Francisco and globally. As of September 1993 more than 113 papers had been published by researchers in the study, and an additional 15 papers had been published by "non-key investigators" using its database.[41] Because many of these papers were produced in collaboration with the research staff at San Francisco's AIDS Office Seroepidemiology and Surveillance Branch, the study's research findings have been disseminated by Public Health officials in the pages of the *San Francisco Epidemiologic Bulletin*[42] and in presentations at international AIDS conferences. Here I focus on three key contributions of the San Francisco Men's Health Study in providing evidence (1) for the theory that HIV is the sole cause of AIDS, (2) for the role of particular sexual practices in transmitting HIV/AIDS, and (3) to enable researchers to estimate the incidence and prevalence of HIV in the city.[43]

The SFMHS, also known as "A Prospective Sero-Epidemiological Study of Acquired Immune Deficiency Syndrome (AIDS) in Homosexual Males Residing in San Francisco,"[44] is one of the principal sources of data for the arguments that HIV is the sole cause of AIDS, and that blood and body fluids (primarily sperm) transmit the disease among gay men. The study was funded by the National Institutes of Health (NIH) in 1984, and its principal investigator was Dr. Warren Winkelstein Jr., a professor of epidemiology at the University of California at Berkeley. Winkelstein began his proposal to study a cohort of gay men in San Francisco with the following statement of what was and was not known about AIDS at the time:

> AIDS has become epidemic in San Francisco since it was first identified here in 1979. By June 1983 a total of 201 cases had been reported . . . 69 deaths have occurred among these cases. . . . As in other communities where AIDS has assumed epidemic status, incidence has been almost exclusively in homosexual males. The evidence that the causative agent is transmissible by exchange of blood or bodily secretions is now substantial. However, the natural history of AIDS is not well understood, the agent has not been identified, and host susceptibility factors other than sexual promiscuity have not been determined. These issues can be studied most effectively by means of a population based prospective epidemiological study. A probability sample of single males 25–54 years old living in 19 census tracts where most of the AIDS cases have occurred will be recruited. . . . Comparison of the characteristics of study subjects who develop AIDS with those who don't should yield important new knowledge.[45]

Referring to prior evidence for an agent transmitted in blood and body fluids, Winkelstein cited studies that purported to find human T-cell leukemia virus

(HTLV-I) in blood specimens from several AIDS patients. This was not a reference to the human immunodeficiency virus but instead to Robert Gallo's cancer-causing HTLV-I, the *first* retrovirus alleged as the cause of AIDS in 1983. That same year, Luc Montagnier in Paris was arguing that a second retrovirus, dubbed lymphadenopathy associated virus (LAV) was more consistently associated with the new disease syndrome. By the time the San Francisco Men's Health Study began in 1984, further evidence supporting Montagnier's retrovirus was provided by Don Francis at the CDC and by Jay Levy, who isolated a similar retrovirus (AIDS-related virus, aka ARV) at the University of California at San Francisco. Belatedly, even Robert Gallo concurred that a distinct retrovirus must be the cause of AIDS, albeit alleging that a new virus (HTLV-III) isolated at his own virology lab at the National Institutes of Health was the real agent for the disease.[46]

Regardless of which retrovirus you bet your money on, or which acronym you choose as its reference, the working theoretical assumption in the design of Winkelstein's health study was that a sexually transmitted or blood-borne infectious agent was the cause of the syndrome among gay men and intravenous drug users. Winkelstein acknowledges the immediate power of this hypothesis by noting that "within . . . months after the first cases of PCP were reported in homosexual men [June 1981], the basic pathophysiological defect [abnormal T-lymphocyte response] and the probable mode of transmission through sexual contact had been identified."[47] Thus, Winkelstein maintains that a sexually transmitted agent was assumed by most researchers soon after the discovery of the first five AIDS cases in Los Angeles in 1981. And this causal hypothesis necessarily circumscribed the design of Winkelstein's study and the interpretation of the data contained within it, as the theory of an infectious agent transmitted in semen led researchers to collect information primarily about numbers of sexual partners and the association of particular sexual acts with the likelihood that a gay or bisexual man would develop AIDS.

The San Francisco Men's Health Study comprised 1,034 single men between the ages of 25 and 54 years old at the time they were recruited into the cohort between June and December 1984. Initially selected by stratified, random household sampling from neighborhoods of San Francisco where the AIDS epidemic had been most intense, "the men were recruited without regard to sexual preference, lifestyle, or HIV sero-status, which was not known at the time" (as the HIV-antibody blood test did not exist in 1984).[48] Presumably a representative cross section of the gay community in San Francisco, this cohort study of more than a thousand men continued for eight years, during which time participants donated laboratory samples and underwent physical exams and intensive interviews at six-month intervals to gather evidence regarding their sexual behavior, nutrition, drug use, etc.[49] After the HIV antibody test was developed in 1985, all blood samples taken at the time of enrollment were retrospectively tested for the presence of the virus.

Risk Factors and Prevention

The Winkelstein study is an empirical touchstone for "safe sex" as a prevention tactic in San Francisco because it demonstrates a compelling correspondence between the "numbers of sexual contacts in the previous two years" and the likelihood that a member of the cohort would test positive for HIV antibodies. For instance, researchers found that those men with the largest number of partners (more than 50), were most likely to be seropositive (greater than 70 percent). Despite this evidence of increasing relative risk, however, 23 percent of the HIV-positive men in the study reported *no* sexual contact in the preceding two years [1982–1984]. The authors attributed the extraordinary level of infection in these celibate men to the "number of sexual partners" with whom these men "presumably" had intercourse prior to June 1982.[50]

The greatest seropositivity [83 percent] was among the 8 percent of all gay men in the cohort who "gave a history of needle sharing within the past five years," but because intravenous drug use was considered to be an independent risk for HIV infection, these men were subsequently excluded from any calculations of "sexually risky behaviors." As for other recreational drugs, the study found no relationship between the use of poppers, marijuana, or cocaine and the subsequent risk for developing AIDS. Confirming other national studies of HIV risk factors, Winkelstein et al. identified anal intercourse as the greatest relative risk for HIV infection. Men who were strictly receptive, however, were two to three times more likely to be antibody-positive than men who were solely insertive. While Winkelstein acknowledges that there are "low levels of HIV in seminal fluids," nonetheless he concluded that the study "confirms that receptive anal/genital contact is the major mode of transmission of HIV infection . . . in fact, there was no evidence of epidemic spread due to any other sexual [act]."[51]

Researchers in the Men's Health Study amended their conclusions in 1993, however, because after eight years of study several men in the cohort developed AIDS despite the fact that they reported abstaining from anal intercourse. Surmising that there was "some evidence" that being a recipient in oral sex was also a risk factor for HIV infection, Winkelstein et al. proposed two hypotheses for these anomalous data: (1) perhaps the effect of this "risk" had been "masked" earlier in the epidemic because of the overwhelming risks associated with anal intercourse; or (2) perhaps AIDS patients were more infectious in later stages of the disease and consequently more likely to transmit HIV to sexual partners in even relatively "low-risk" sexual activity such as oral sex.[52]

HIV Incidence and AIDS Case Projections

Because the San Francisco Men's Health Study was a population-based study, it was the first research in San Francisco to produce estimates of HIV prevalence (number of cases existing at one point in time) and incidence (number of new cases occurring in a specified time period, for instance, a year) that could be extrapolated to the entire population of gay men in the city and thus used to make projections about future caseloads by officials at the Department of Public Health.[53] As the cohort was designed as a representative sample of all single men residing in these 19 census tracts, and because nearly half of these men were HIV-positive when they entered the study (49 percent), this proportion was subsequently applied to the entire population of 18,000 gay men that Winkelstein et al. estimated were living in these neighborhoods and by inference to the entire male homosexual community in San Francisco.[54] This research is the source of the widespread belief that persists to this day that one out of every two gay men in San Francisco is infected with HIV.[55]

Although half of the cohort was already HIV-positive when they enrolled in the study in late 1984, from the time that these men were under observation the annual rate of HIV seroconversions was 4 percent or less.[56] As the researchers believed that HIV was a new virus and one only recently introduced into the San Francisco gay community, they deduced that the rate of HIV infection must have been considerably higher in preceding years in order to have infected half of the cohort by 1984. Thus, Winkelstein et al. argued that HIV transmission was at its highest level in 1982, with an estimated 8,000 new HIV infections in that single year (an annual HIV incidence of 18 percent), a rate that presumably remained constant until the cohort began monitoring seroconversions in 1985 and incidence plunged to the 4 percent annual HIV incidence rate that researchers actually observed.

In order to bridge the gap between their hypothesis that HIV transmission was explosive in the early 1980s but declined *fourfold* after they began documenting HIV infections in 1985, Winkelstein et al. propose three mutually exclusive explanations, one of which must be true to maintain their theory about the evolution of the AIDS epidemic in San Francisco and its temporal correspondence with HIV. First, there could have been a selection bias in the design of the study whereby those men who were at low risk for acquiring HIV chose to join the cohort. Following this explanation to its logical conclusion then means that the study *underestimates* the number of HIV-positive gay men and the number of future AIDS cases in San Francisco because it excludes data about men more likely to acquire the disease. Conversely, Winkelstein et al. raised the possibility that "susceptibles [men practicing "high-risk" sex] were infected early in the epidemic leaving only low-risk persons available for infection during the study."[57] Following this line of reasoning would produce an outcome the reverse of the first explanation, as it would imply that the peak years for HIV infection had already passed as of 1985 and that AIDS caseloads would dramatically peak and fall in future years in a mirror image of HIV-infection trends. The third and final hypothesis suggests that gay and bisexual men in San Francisco dramatically reduced both their number of sexual partners and the frequency with which they engaged in receptive anal intercourse without condoms after 1984. Winkelstein et al. corroborate this hypothesis with data from the study wherein members of the cohort reportedly reduced their "high-risk" sexual behavior by 60 percent between 1982 and 1984, and the proportion of HIV-negative men engaging in risky sex declined by half in 1984, albeit resisting any further reduction in risk after that time.[58] The authors shore up their argument by citing the "dramatic decline of new cases of rectal gonorrhea in San Francisco from 1982 (200–300 cases per month) to 1985 (50 cases per month), the same corroborating evidence that Moss and company used to support their estimates of declining HIV transmission rates in the San Francisco General Hospital Cohort.[59] However, while Winkelstein et al. theoretically assume a constant 18 percent annual incidence of HIV from 1982 through 1984, San Francisco Department of Health data demonstrate that cases of rectal gonorrhea (an epidemiological marker for "high risk" anal intercourse) declined by 300 percent during this same time period.[60]

After eight years enrolled in this cohort, half (51 percent) of the men who were HIV-positive upon entering the study had developed AIDS, and 80 percent of these men were dead. These results produce an estimate of an eight-year incubation or latency period from HIV infection to AIDS that correlates well with other cohort estimates of six to ten years.[61] In tandem with the study's conclusion that 1982 was the peak year for HIV transmission, Winkelstein et al. argue that their estimate of 8–10 years from HIV infection to AIDS diagnosis "predicts" the observed decline in new AIDS cases that began in the city in 1992.[62]

The San Francisco City Clinic Cohort: 1978–Present

- **The Hepatitis B Studies: 1978–1980**
- **The Hepatitis B Vaccine Trial: 1980–present**
- **Natural History of HIV Infection: 1983–present**

National studies of the hepatitis B virus in the late 1970s and early 1980s were critical for providing a storehouse of immunological and epidemiological knowledge for theoretically modeling the sexual transmission of HIV via blood and body fluids, and building credibility for HIV vaccine research and development. San Francisco was the location for one of the five hepatitis B studies in the United States, and is historically and epidemiologically significant because it substantiated the "viral hypothesis" of AIDS by establishing that the populations at risk for hepatitis B were similar, if not identical, to the populations at risk for AIDS, and because the study maintained a databank of blood specimens from hepatitis B cohort members, some of which dated to 1978. After the HIV antibody test was developed in 1985, these frozen blood samples were then instrumental in constructing knowledge about the initial emergence of HIV among gay and bisexual men in San Francisco and its subsequent diffusion throughout the cohort.

As a repository of serological evidence that empirically demonstrates the presence of HIV in this country in 1978, prior to the emergence of the AIDS epidemic, the San Francisco City Clinic Cohort is assured immortality for its seminal role in generating claims that are central to orthodox constructions of the epidemiology of the disease and providing empirical evidence for an official chronology of the disease, backdating the birth of the AIDS epidemic to 1978. This orthodox claim is then reified and continually reproduced in AIDS surveillance practices that identify the mode of the acquisition of AIDS according to the most likely risk for a patient's HIV infection subsequent to 1978. Data generated from the study, "the longest follow-up study of any group of people in the U.S. or anywhere in the world for AIDS," are fundamentally constitutive of the theory that HIV is the single viral cause of the epidemic.[63] Responding to a question about how HIV first entered the San Francisco gay community, an AIDS epidemiologist replied: "it came in with a *whoosh* . . . that's clear from the hepatitis B study."[64]

Between 1978 and 1980, approximately 6,700 homosexual or bisexual men[65] who sought treatment for sexually transmitted diseases at the San Francisco City Clinic were "enrolled in a series of studies of the prevalence, incidence, and prevention of Hepatitis B virus infections."[66] A subset of these men comprised the San Francisco City Clinic Cohort for a clinical trial of the safety and efficacy of a hepatitis B vaccine (HBV) licensed shortly before by Merck, Sharpe and Doehme Pharmaceuticals. An account in the *San Francisco Epidemiologic Bulletin* in November 1989 said that "as part of these studies, serum samples were collected from all cohort members and tested for serologic markers of Hepatitis B. 359 HBV sero-negative men were then randomized into a double-blind placebo controlled vaccine trial with multiple serum samples collected from each participant. All unused sera were frozen and stored."[67] In October 1981, shortly after the discovery of AIDS, the hepatitis B vaccine was determined to be safe and "efficacious" in preventing hepatitis B infections, the trial was unblinded, and all placebo recipients were offered the vaccine.[68] But the concurrent discovery of AIDS patients within the cohort of 6,697 men in San Francisco who had been screened for the hepatitis B studies between 1978 and 1980 immediately raised concern at the CDC and in San Francisco; medical personnel and the public alike feared that a vaccine which had been derived from the plasma of gay men at high risk for contracting AIDS might itself be transmitting AIDS or an infectious agent associated with the disease.[69] The CDC's renewed attention to the hepatitis B cohort was also driven by panic from within the gay community that something about the nature of the government trials or the vaccine had brought about the new disease syndrome; these studies had been conducted in gay men of the same age as those developing AIDS, and the epidemic appeared first and remained most severe in the very same cities (San Francisco, New York, Los Angeles, etc.) where hepatitis B studies had been conducted. In response to these various concerns, intensive study of HIV and AIDS among members of the San Francisco City Clinic Cohort (SFCCC) began in earnest in October 1983.

> In 1981, six of the first 10 men reported with AIDS in San Francisco were discovered to be members of the SFCC Cohort. [As speculation grew regarding an infectious agent as the cause of AIDS] . . . the Hepatitis B vaccine cohort became the San Francisco City Clinic Cohort (SFCCC). Subsequently, the Department of Public Health and CDC began a study of cohort members for AIDS and for infections with HTLV-III/LAV, the cause of AIDS.[70]

Variants of the "hepatitis B conspiracy theory" have persisted since the beginning of the AIDS epidemic and continue to be widely publicized in books, radio shows, and popular magazine articles; even making the *San Francisco Weekly*'s "Ten Tiniest Conspiracies" list on April 12, 1995:

> AIDS: From the Makers of Agent Orange? In 1978, the National Institutes of Health tested an experimental hepatitis-B vaccine on a very specific demographic in Los Angeles, New York, and San Francisco: nonmonagamous homosexual males. Within six years, 64% of the men had AIDS. Is it just a coincidence that the AIDS epidemic followed on the heels of these mass inoculations? Many fringe physicians believe Uncle Sam created the plague at the National Cancer Institute's facility at Fort Derrick, Maryland, which until 1969 was the Pentagon's biological warfare lab.[71]

Paul O'Malley, the program manager for the Hepatitis B Clinic Study in San Francisco, affirmed the continuing appeal of "fringe theories" about HBV studies, and he chose to begin my interview with him in October 1994 by "dealing with [it] right off the bat." But in the course of this interview, O'Malley addresses not only why the hepatitis B vaccine trials were wholly unrelated to the coincident emergence of AIDS, but also introduces some of the study's major knowledge claims: that HIV was present in San Francisco before AIDS and before the vaccine trials began; that there was an explosive diffusion of HIV in San Francisco's gay community between 1978 and 1984; and that the correspondence between "risk groups" for hepatitis B and AIDS was epistemologically central to constructing the theory that AIDS was caused by a sexually transmitted virus.

> It's unfortunate that there's a lot of misinformation. . . . We've actually been finally talking about maybe having someone on the staff actually just put something formally in writing about this, just to deal with it once and for all, because frankly it is getting kind of tiring, this theory that somehow the hepatitis B vaccine is implicated in the spread of HIV, for example. . . . I can just deal with that part right off the bat because part of it's based on misinformation. . . . Like in San Francisco, the vaccine trial started in the spring of 1980. And we know from stored blood samples that go back to 1978, which is a full two years before the vaccine trial even began, that of the men we screened in 1978, about 4 percent of them were HIV-positive. And of the men we screened in 1979, it jumped up to 12

percent, and then by 1980, the year the vaccine trial began, it was somewhere between 20 to 25 percent that were antibody-positive that were walking through the door at City Clinic at that time.

When the antibody test was officially licensed, the CDC [decided]—because the HIV/AIDS study started in late 1983 and our samples were part of the samples used—to actually look and see if they were finding HTLV-III in the blood specimens of these men that were coming down with AIDS in our cohort. Because obviously if they weren't [finding HTLV-III], then they were climbing up the wrong tree in looking for what the cause of this disease was. As subsequently more refined tests were developed, we went back and retested specimens [so there wasn't really any] problem with false positivity, [because] unfortunately [the hepatitis B cohort was comprised of] high-risk gay men using an STD clinic. We did have some specimens that tested positive, and then on repeats were negative, but a real small handful considering the number that were tested positive altogether. By 1984, when we started systematically trying to bring everybody back in for a blood draw, the seroprevalence of HIV by that time was up to like 66 percent, so you can see what happened between 1980 and 1984.

I think one of the reasons [for] the theories about the hepatitis B vaccine somehow being implicated in this is—I guess some people will hear [that] the vaccine trials started in 1980 and 1981, and then the first AIDS cases were in 1981 and 1982. Some people have gone "Well, isn't that interesting?" The only thing that you have to realize is you just don't get AIDS without first [being] preceded by HIV. And HIV had already been in the community, according to our stored blood samples, at least a full three years before the first cases came down in 1981. . . . It's like we could have put 1,000 people in a room in 1984, and say 500 were positive and 500 were negative. And we've never had a phenomenon where some of these men who I'm telling you were negative then subsequently came up with AIDS—unless [you know] because of sero-specimens they got infected with HIV at some point in between, then yeah.

It's not like this [the idea of HIV-negative cases of AIDS] hasn't been bantered around. . . . I mean we looked for it. . . . I mean OK, if someone got diagnosed with AIDS in late 1981 or early 1982, and the only blood specimen we had on them was 1978, and the blood specimen came back negative, uh, well that could be a lot of things—you know, they may have been a rapid progressor, because there were several years there, you know, where we know some people got infected and progressed rather rapidly. But the only thing that I can say that we witnessed a couple of times, which would help to explain sometimes why there doesn't seem to be a documented history of being positive before somebody comes down with AIDS, is we now know . . . because it's been shown . . . there's this phenomenon that some people get an acute viral syndrome when they first become infected with HIV, [and] their T-cells plummet dramatically; now we realize there may have been some people who have gotten *Pneumocystis* as part of their acute viral syndrome. . . . And there is also the [same] suspicion [regarding] some of the Kaposi's sarcoma we saw early on, where people have lived for many years after that point with KS. . . . Matter of fact, I was talking to someone just last week that had KS "come and go," without treatment. And so there's also a possibility that some of the KS we saw maybe in the early years too might have [been that] . . . [because] there were only so many people [who] were getting infected with HIV at that point.

[Anyway] why would it be unusual that [Dr. Marcus Conant of the KS Clinic at UCSF] has got HIV-negative KS [patients]? I mean, I know people who got toxoplasmosis from their dog in 1975. You know, all these opportunistic infections have been around in our populations, rarely manifesting themselves—there's a history of people having *Pneumocystis* long before AIDS or HIV whatever you want to call it, showed up on the scene. So, I'm not surprised. If there's something associated with quote unquote "immune suppression" in manifesting some of these things, which in gay men again, I think HIV plays . . . I mean . . . I don't feel like I have anything invested in saying it's HIV more than anyone else, or even [in] the hepatitis B vaccine trial not having anything [to do with AIDS]. Well, you know some people think there was a government plot and that the hepatitis vaccine trial might be an instance of that. And as more and more stuff comes out about radiation experiments and everything else, you know. . . . But I think we're barking up the wrong tree with the hepatitis B vaccine because it's too late. If you believe that HIV is the cause of AIDS, then HIV was already all over the place in San Francisco and New York before their trials even began. I mean New York started a year before us, but still we're showing HIV showing up in the community in 1978. Obviously, we're not showing AIDS. . . .

But [another thing is that] . . . none of the first [AIDS] cases were in the [HBV vaccine] trial. You've got to remember that there were 6,700 men screened [for the presence of hepatitis B antibodies, and] only a quarter of those men had no markers for hepatitis B—so right away, there was only 25 percent of those men that were eligible for the vaccine. And of those quarter, 360 said, "Yes, I'll participate." So of 6,700, only 360 participated in the trial. And also, there's sort of a logic to why you wouldn't have expected any of the [AIDS] cases from [the hepatitis B vaccine recipients] anyway; I mean these men were hepatitis B virgins, that's why they were eligible for the trial: they were low-risk. And now we know the risk groups for hepatitis B, which became very apparent real quick, were the same as the risk groups for HIV: gay men, IV drug abusers, hemophiliacs, transfusion recipients. I mean, that was one of the reasons early on that people said, "Well hepatitis B is a blood-borne virus, maybe what we're talking about is another blood-borne virus" because the risk groups were so similar. That's why you would have expected [that] men who were hepatitis B virgins were probably more likely to be HIV virgins as well. Because whatever their sexual practices they were engaging in . . . or their own genetics, or immunology or biological factors, [all those things] may have made them more resistant to HIV infection. Matter of fact, we estimate that about 75 percent of the 6,700 men are [HIV]-positive, where with the vaccine trial recipients it's about 50 percent at this point [which is the same as the community estimate from the San Francisco Men's Health Study]. I mean we're gonna probably update these figures, but I think right now the progression rate [to AIDS] doesn't seem to be any different for the men that were in the trial.

O'Malley has a rather tortuous answer to the question, "Are there HIV-negative cases of AIDS?" He initially denies that there were any HIV-negative men in the SFCC cohort who subsequently developed AIDS, before acknowledging that there might be a few men in the study for whom "the only blood specimen we had on them . . . came back negative." O'Malley then speculates about the many things that could explain this and invokes an "acute viral syndrome" that presumably resolves any ambiguity about HIV's role in causing AIDS. By the conclusion of his explanation, however, this "acute viral syndrome" has been employed only peripherally as an explanation for "rapid progression to AIDS," and is instead used to bolster speculative explanations for the phenomenon of "long-term survivors"—people who are HIV-infected yet have episodes of Kaposi's sarcoma that "come and go without treatment."

This is rather like hedging one's bet vis-à-vis whether HIV and HIV alone is the single sufficient and necessary cause of AIDS among the gay men in this cohort. If there is no documentation of an HIV-antibody positive test and yet a man developed AIDS, then he is a "rapid progressor" who was diagnosed and died from the disease during "an acute viral syndrome." Incomprehensibly, this same "syndrome" also explains how a patient survives an AIDS diagnosis for 14 years—he was prematurely diagnosed with AIDS during an "acute viral syndrome," and for reasons unknown his immune system subsequently rebounded. Any additional HIV-negative cases of AIDS not covered by these explanations are relegated to the normal background incidence for these opportunistic infections, as with toxoplasmosis you get from your dog. It is by rhetorical elisions such as these that theoretical integrity is maintained and orthodox AIDS science resists the challenge of anomalous data to the hypothesis that HIV is the sole cause of AIDS. This issue of HIV-negative cases of AIDS, central to some dissident critiques, is similarly subsumed in a 1986 follow-up article on the SFCC cohort wherein the authors report that out of a total of 360 men who were initially HIV-negative, "of [those] who sero-converted, 41% developed the syndrome or related conditions as compared with 8% of those who did not sero-convert."[72] In other words, by the CDC's own admission, eight percent of those who developed the "syndrome of immune deficiency" or related conditions in this cohort did not test positive for HIV antibodies.

As for O'Malley's argument about "rapid progressors," in point of fact, none of the SFCCC data published thus far credibly documents any gay men in the cohort progressing from HIV infection to AIDS in less than two years. And whatever estimates for progression to AIDS that do exist are based on uncertain "best guesses" for the date of HIV seroconversion. Even with these guesstimates, only 2 of 41 reported AIDS cases among San Francisco hepatitis B vaccine recipients progressed to AIDS in the third year following infection with HIV; in a parallel study among members of the HBV trial in New York City, researchers stated that "none of the men known to be antibody positive for less than four years has yet developed AIDS," belying the existence of "rapid progressors" in that cohort as well.[73]

These estimates from various hepatitis B cohort studies of the theoretical speed with which HIV-infected men progress to AIDS imply that if HIV is the sole cause of AIDS, and infection with the virus requires a minimum of three years to result in an AIDS diagnosis (and only very rarely does it progress that quickly), then HIV must have been present in 1975 in New York City in order to have caused a case of AIDS in 1978. Similarly, HIV must have been present in the heterosexual intravenous drug-using community in San Francisco before 1978 in order to precipitate the earliest AIDS diagnoses (maternal transmission to two infants) retrospectively discovered among that city's residents in 1978 and 1979. As it is impossible to prove this point, it must be theoretically assumed.

The explanation for the CDC's interest in the San Francisco hepatitis B cohort after the vaccine trials were terminated is also turned on its head by Mr. O'Malley as he attributes the initial impetus for intensive study of the San Francisco City Clinic Cohort to an open theoretical inquiry into the causal role of HTLV-III (HIV), whose absence in frozen blood specimens would be "an indication they were barking up the wrong tree" in searching for the cause of the AIDS epidemic. Not only does the remainder of O'Malley's interview illustrate why the absence of HIV in some of these blood samples would not have dissuaded these researchers from their theory that HIV was the cause of AIDS, but we also know that fears on the part of the CDC, the public, and the medical and gay communities regarding the incredibly high "cumulative incidence of AIDS in the entire SFCC Cohort . . . the highest of any reported population (3,825 [cases] per 100,000 in 1985)" first catalyzed further study of this group of men.[74] O'Malley acknowledged this when discussing the hepatitis project in 1987, stating that his personal interest intensified when "many of the first AIDS cases in San Francisco—11 of the first 24 in 1981 [46 percent]—turned out to be participants in the hepatitis B vaccine project."[75]

Most of these questions regarding the hepatitis B vaccine trials were impossible for me to empirically document as I had no access to SFCCC data. However, I did try to verify when the first vaccine recipient was reported with AIDS in San Francisco, as this is central to O'Malley's argument absolving the hepatitis B vaccine from harm, as he stated that no vaccine recipients were among the earliest AIDS cases in the city. Despite 15 years of controversy and proliferating "conspiracy theories" regarding the HBV hepatitis B virus vaccine study, empirical documentation for his claim initially proved difficult to pin down. In the process of researching my inquiry, O'Malley discovered, contrary to his initial assertion, that a hepatitis B vaccine recipient was diagnosed with AIDS in the summer of 1981, making him one of the first San Francisco patients with the disease. Upon further research, however, including a call to the former doctor of the now deceased patient, O'Malley discovered that this vaccine recipient had been incorrectly reported to the city Public Health Department as a patient with Kaposi's sarcoma in 1981—in fact, he was not truly an AIDS case until he developed lymphoma in 1986. At the end of the day, this serendipitous reclassification of diagnoses absolved the vaccine trials of any direct association with the earliest AIDS cases in the city, albeit raising doubts about the reliability of early AIDS case reports and diagnoses at the Department of Public Health.

To resolve ambiguity about members of the HBV trial among early AIDS cases, O'Malley provided me with "corrected numbers" for the SFCCC, which indicated that 36 percent of all AIDS cases reported in 1981 were men who had been *screened* for the trials but did not receive the hepatitis B vaccine. Similarly, in 1982, 30 percent of the reported AIDS cases came from the entire cohort of 6,705 men, but again none of these men had received the HBV.[76] However, these "official" figures were contradicted by articles on the SFCCC that had appeared in well-respected medical journals years before. Hessol's analysis in 1989, based on AIDS surveillance reports written at the time that cases were initially reported, stated that "six of the first ten AIDS cases [in San Francisco] and nearly half of the [AIDS] cases reported in 1981 . . . were among the 6,697 cohort members originally screened for Hepatitis B studies (in this city alone)."[77] And George Rutherford, former supervisor for the AIDS Office, wrote that as of 1982, "41% of all reported AIDS cases in San Francisco were among members of the original Hepatitis B cohort."[78] I now had four widely divergent answers to a single question—How many men enrolled in this cohort developed AIDS in the early years of the epidemic in San Francisco?—36 percent, 41 percent, "nearly half" of the cases in 1981, and six of the first ten cases in the city.

Which answer is correct? Remarkably, all are, because of a peculiarity in the way AIDS cases were counted and recounted at different points in time. It is a policy of the AIDS Seroepidemiology and Surveillance Branch to backdate new AIDS cases to the earliest date at which the patient first met the CDC's surveillance definition for the disease. So when the official AIDS surveillance definition changes (as it did in 1985, 1987, and 1993), the date of a patient's diagnosis may also change, as symptoms which were previously unrecognized now qualify as determinants for an AIDS diagnosis. So just as the first vaccine recipient who developed AIDS was reclassified from 1981 to 1986 with a recently reported diagnosis of lymphoma (thereby reducing by one the number of cases reported in 1981), likewise AIDS cases reported in 1986 can be reclassified to 1981 (thereby increasing the numbers reported in that year) if a revision in the definition of AIDS now recognizes one of their prior symptoms as indicative of the disease or if a review of their medical charts uncovers an earlier diagnosis. As a result of this policy AIDS surveillance statistics are constantly in flux, and the original total of 24 reported AIDS cases in 1981 has now been adjusted to 36. Obviously, this policy minimizes the proportion of AIDS cases attributable to hepatitis B cohort members over time, as it holds the numerator constant (the number of SFCCC members diagnosed with AIDS) while increasing the denominator (the number of cases reported with an AIDS diagnosis in a given year). For these reasons, over time the number of AIDS cases reported in the first year of the epidemic has risen by approximately 30 percent, thereby decreasing the proportion of hepatitis B trial participants in the annual AIDS caseload and obfuscating what role, if any, these trials had on the health of gay men in the city.

Although published research from the early 1980s consistently denies any association whatsoever between hepatitis B infection, HBV vaccination, and the risk of developing AIDS, more contemporary publications by SFCCC investigators themselves have raised the possibility that perhaps the HBV vaccine contributed indirectly to disease in this community. This could have happened, they say, under the following circumstances: (1) when administered to an HIV-infected individual, the vaccine may have accelerated the replication of the virus, or (2) when administered to a man recently exposed to HBV, the vaccine may have increased the likelihood that he would become a chronic carrier of the hepatitis B virus. "The reasons for [this additional risk] are not known [as] the immunology of T cell response to hepatitis B vaccine is poorly understood."[79]

The Rapid Peak and Decline of HIV Transmission in San Francisco

"The AIDS incidence curve MUST look much like the HIV sero-incidence curve, but displaced in time by an appropriate incubation period, or it's all over for the HIV/AIDS theory."[80] In support of this point, SFCCC researchers observed that "the annual incidence of HIV infection [in the entire cohort of 6,705] was greatest between 1980 and 1982 [10–20 percent], and [thereafter] declined to 3% in 1988."[81] As illustrated in Tables 1a and 1b, below, however, there are important differences in estimated annual HIV infections among varying subsets of the SFCC cohort; between the SFCCC and other cohort

TABLE 1a   Annual HIV Incidence among Gay Men in San Francisco Cohort Studies

Annual HIV Incidence	'78	'79	'80	'81	'82	'83	'84	'85	'86	'87	'88
SFMHS gay men in SF (n=799) SFCC cohort	—	—	—	—	18%	18%	18%	≈4%	4%		1%
SFCC cohort*				10–20%		—	—	—	—	—	3%
SFCC/HBV vac. (n=320)**	0.3%	4%	10%	17%	20%	7%	3%	0.7%	2%	0%	3%

*From "Update: The SF City Clinic Cohort Study," *San Francisco Epidemiologic Bulletin*, November 1989, p. 47.
**Figures are from Hessol et al., "Incidence and Prevalence of HIV Infection among Homosexual and Bisexual Men, 1978–1988."

TABLE 1b Annual Incidence of Hepatitis B and Rectal Gonorrhea (1978–1988): San Francisco Data versus New York City Data

STD Data: SF vs. NYC	'78	'79	'80	'81	'82	'83	'84	'85	'86	'87	'88
(SF) Hepatitis B cases	NA	NA	NA	NA	NA	232	206	148	106	125	81
(SF) Rectal gonorrhea	4,975	4,874	5,098	4,833	4,008	2,109	1,299	708	379	197	169
(SF) Rectal gonorrhea*	5,000	4,500	5,100	4,800	4,000	2,100	1,300	691	373	195	166
(NY) Rectal gonorrhea**								934	464	211	
(NY) Rectal gonorrhea***		940	1,025	1,062	930	529					

*Numbers for years before 1985 are rounded to the nearest thousand. Figures are from the Division of STD Control, City and County of San Francisco, 1995. Unpublished report.
**T. J. Coates et al., "Does HIV Prevention Work for Men Who Have Sex with Men."
***Morbidity and Mortality Weekly Report 33, 21: 396–97.

studies; and between cohort studies and data on other sexually transmitted infections that are transmitted in the same body fluids and by the same risk factors as HIV is transmitted among gay men in San Francisco (i.e., hepatitis B and rectal gonorrhea).

It is with these estimates of the number of new HIV infections that occurred each year in each cohort (annual HIV incidence) that the most declarative statements derive from the most methodologically questionable data. For instance, the hepatitis B AIDS prospective cohort did not even begin until late 1983, and the HIV test was not developed until 1984 (and not commercially available until 1985). Therefore, most HIV infections among these men had already occurred before HIV antibody testing existed. Yet in one study examining a subset of SFCC cohort HIV positives written after 11 years of follow-up, the authors concluded that a full 81 percent of these positive men "had been infected between 1977 and 1980."[82] In fact, these dates for HIV infection are either probability calculations that derive the date of HIV infection from some time midway between a man's last negative and first positive blood test, or alternatively, they are best "guesstimates" deduced by backdating HIV infection to a time when a given man *recalled* "engaging in risk behavior (e.g., anal sex)" or was presumed to have done so.[83]

Public health authorities and epidemiologists have used data from the cohort studies as evidence that HIV was present only at negligible levels in San Francisco as of 1978, disseminated explosively until transmission crested in 1982, and thereafter declined rapidly until it stabilized at a low but consistent level of infection from 1984 until the present day. They argue that the trend in reports of new AIDS cases has followed a similar exponential increase and a gradual decline, rising approximately 10 years after the peak in HIV infection and declining after 1992. Tables 1a and 1b examine this alleged correspondence between the decline of HIV transmission and the "dramatic declines" in gay male sexually transmitted diseases (hepatitis B and rectal gonorrhea), especially between 1982 and 1984, and juxtapose data from the Departments of Public Health in San Francisco and New York City against the cohort estimates for coincident annual HIV infections. The data demonstrates that HIV incidence theoretically rose exponentially in these cohorts between 1980 and 1982 (and in the SFMHS through 1984) *despite* citywide declines in cases of rectal gonorrhea during those same years.

Some AIDS dissidents have challenged this representation of a rapid peak and contraction in HIV transmission as an artifact constructed by researchers. They argue that these methods are tautological, as cohort researchers employ estimates of AIDS progression rates and/or the current number of AIDS cases as baseline data for retrospectively calculating HIV infections during a time period for which there are no data. The method assumes as its premise the very association it is seeking to prove. Documenting a cohort member seroconverting to HIV-positive status while actively enrolled in a study would obviously be a more credible way of gauging the risk factors for HIV infection and the incubation period from HIV infection to AIDS, but this is difficult to do as so few HIV infections have taken place in these cohorts since 1984 when the studies began.

Precisely because "the numbers of sero-converters available for analysis (in individual cohort studies) are generally small," epidemiologists from the General Hospital Cohort, the Men's Health Study, and the City Clinic Cohort pooled all their seroconversion data in 1993 to analyze risk factors for contracting the virus.[84] From 1984 to 1989, only 84 HIV seroconversions occurred in a sample from all three cohorts out of a total of 1,393 susceptible HIV-antibody-negative men under observation, including some who were extraordinarily "high-risk" men who were sexual partners of AIDS patients (e.g., General Hospital Cohort seronegatives). Yet this metastudy of "sexual risk factors" for seroconversion affirmed, again, the increased risk for persons with multiple sexual partners, and for persons engaging in "receptive anal intercourse (RAI)"—and this despite the fact that 34 percent of all men who became HIV-positive did not report receptive anal sex during the study period. Therefore, the authors extended the study period backward in time in an attempt to adjust this number downward, reasoning that "some infections could have occurred shortly before the last HIV negative test and been due to behavior in the interval before (the one analyzed)."[85] This correction of the data reduced to 25 percent the proportion of men who became HIV-positive without engaging in the singular sexual act that is alleged to carry the greatest risk for contracting the virus.

Therefore the data still presented a conundrum to researchers, leading the authors to tentatively conclude that their analysis "provides some evidence [that] receptive ORAL intercourse is a risk factor for HIV infection . . . [a conclusion supported by] biological rationale and logistic modeling."[86] Just as Warren Winkelstein Jr. et al. had previously reasoned, they suggested that the lack of corroborative evidence in other cohort studies for a risk of HIV infection via oral sex could be explained by one of two factors: (1) a "masking" of the risk from oral sex by the overwhelming risks associated with anal intercourse; or (2) the "more infectious" nature of long-term survivors who may be "more apt to transmit infection through the less efficient route of oral intercourse."[87] This is really an extraordinary leap of logic, as the authors' data in this study show no increased risk for HIV infection with ejaculation versus without ejaculation—either way, oral sex was equally "risky."

A second disconcerting discovery in this study was that a higher risk for HIV seroconversion existed among men who sometimes used condoms versus men who never used condoms. As this result remained consistent "regardless of the total number of partners," the authors once again resorted to speculation: perhaps "some individuals who engage in receptive anal intercourse without condoms know that their partners are sero-negative and therefore do not require condoms to reduce their risk . . . there must be some confounder leading to a spurious association."[88]

The fact that condoms prevent the transmission of infectious agents and that most epidemiological studies of AIDS have consistently shown lower rates for HIV and sexually transmitted infections for individuals who always use condoms—is, for the moment, beside the point. Rather, what I am attempting to illustrate by these examples is the ease with which a sexual act (oral sex in the example above) is asserted to be risky on the basis of data from two men who became HIV-positive, while conversely, the finding that some condom use or abstention from receptive anal intercourse has not prevented 34 percent of the men under study from contracting HIV becomes data that are dismissed by "spurious associations" and the caveat that "reporting of specific sexual practices is not always accurate and may well be influenced by the use of recreational drugs and the strong social norms of sexual behavior which have emerged recently."[89] When orthodox AIDS researchers seek to bolster the hypothesis that there was a dramatic reduction of HIV transmission subsequent to 1984, they uncritically accept self-reported reductions in sexual activity by gay men; but when HIV seroconverters similarly self-report abstaining from hypothesized risk behavior prior to their infections, the subjects' credibility is questioned.

Studies promulgating leaps of logic such as these have led the psychologist Dr. Walt Odets to write about the way in which *all* sex between gay men is deemed "superfluous" in prevention discourse that fails to differentiate between empirically well-documented "high-risk" activities (e.g., anal inter-course with an HIV-positive person without a condom) and "low-risk/no-risk" activities (e.g., oral sex, or intercourse between HIV-negative partners). Odets argues that messages like these are cavalier about the intrinsic value of sexual expression for gay men and deliver an untenable prevention message to the community ("abstain from all exchange of body fluids with everyone for-ever") versus a message that gay men can live with ("use a condom during in-tercourse with a partner who is, or may be, HIV-positive"). Odets argues that as a result, a number of gay men have renounced all prevention strategies in despair and accepted the inevitability of HIV infection.[90]

Knowledge on AIDS in San Francisco has been reciprocally produced and ex-changed between the CDC, the AIDS surveillance branch of the Department of Public Health, the San Francisco Bureau of Disease Control, and university researchers with long-standing epidemiological cohort studies of gay men re-siding in San Francisco. As this knowledge is further disseminated in medical publications and at international AIDS conferences it is incorporated into an orthodox canon of knowledge comprising "AIDS science and discourse." By a process of reciprocal citation, each locus of AIDS science corroborates the other in the aggregate, reinforcing the coherence and credibility of the main themes of official AIDS knowledge and historiography while eliding the signif-icance of any discrepancy in data or conclusions that these studies may indi-vidually produce.

All of this research was theoretically premised upon the idea that a sexually transmitted virus is the cause of this disease, and that sexual promiscuity by gay men in the early 1980s enabled the epidemic spread of HIV. The theory ex-plicitly guides all of the accounts in this chapter; leading Shilts to demographic and sociological explanations of gay male sexuality, Selma Dritz to discourse on the medical and political contexts facilitating this behavior, surveillance of-ficers to marginalize any behavior other than homosexuality when reporting AIDS cases, and epidemiologists to design their studies primarily to elicit in-formation about sexual acts and sexual frequency. But even if the AIDS cohort estimates about the rapid "peak" and "dramatic reduction" in HIV transmis-sion are taken at face value, the period of the epidemic's greatest intensity had already ended by late 1982—well before the San Francisco AIDS Foundation's prevention campaigns gained momentum (late 1983), *before* the discovery of HIV as "the virus that causes AIDS" (April 1984), *before* large grants had been allocated for widespread public health educational campaigns, *before* sex was banned in the gay bathhouses in San Francisco (April 1984),[91] and even before the AIDS epidemic became personally relevant to many gay men in San Fran-cisco such as disease control investigator Tim Piland.

It is disingenuous for cohort researchers to infer that sexual behavior was the only change among gay men in response to the emergence of the AIDS epidemic. In May 1983, psychotherapists Leon McKusick et al. reported on a study of 600 gay men in San Francisco that demonstrated that there was a substantial "social revolution" in the "gay [male] lifestyle" during these same years: "drinking and drug use" declined dramatically, cocaine use was either reduced or eliminated altogether, and "[the use of] poppers had dropped by two-thirds." Increased anxiety about health had also led "88 percent [of the respondents to visit] their physician within the last nine months."[92] This constellation of immunosuppressive factors in "the gay lifestyle" of the early 1980s and the contradictions or lacuna of the cohort studies have sustained critiques by dissident organizations and individuals who advance a multifactorial theory of AIDS. They see AIDS not as a devastating disease caused by a single virus transmitted during a single sexual act but as an outcome of the synergistic and cumulative effect of a number of insults to host immunity over time.

Multifactorial views as espoused by Dr. Joseph Sonnabend and others were summarized succinctly by Michael Callen, editor, and Richard Berkowitz in 1982 in an article for the *New York Native* titled "We Know How We Are": "There is no mutant virus and there will be no vaccine. We must accept that we have overloaded our immune systems with common viruses and other sexually transmitted infections. Our lifestyle has created the present epidemic of AIDS among gay men."[93] Though two of these men are still living after 20 years

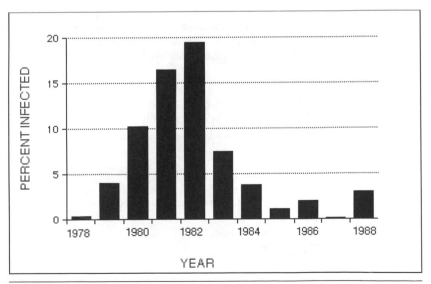

FIGURE 5   Incidence of HIV Infection among Hepatitis B Vaccine Trial Participants by Year, San Francisco City Clinic Cohort Study, 1978–1988
Source: Hessol et al., "Prevalence, Incidence, and Progression of Human Immunodeficiency Virus Infection in Homosexual and Bisexual Men in Hepatitis B Vaccine Trials, 1978–1988."

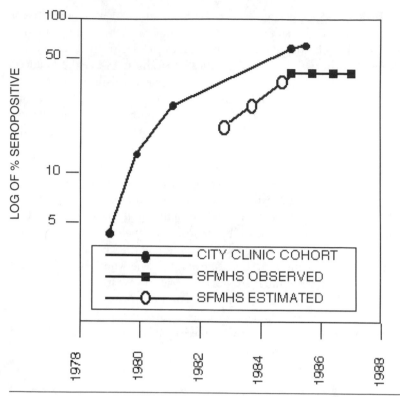

FIGURE 6 HIV Seropositivity in the Men's Health Study and City Clinic Cohorts, 1978–1986
Source: Winkelstein Jr. et al., "The San Francisco Men's Health Study: III. Reduction in Human Immunodeficiency Virus Transmission among Homosexual/Bisexual Men, 1982–1986."

of the AIDS epidemic, tragically, Michael Callen died at dusk on December 27, 1993, at the age of 38. In an article written shortly before his death, he bemoaned the abridgment of debate about the cause or causes of the disease that would soon take his life: "My only theory is [that] AIDS is a disease that requires the daily management of massive amounts of uncertainty . . . and people cling to any certainty they can find. Even if it's false. Once HIV was declared to be the cause of AIDS it became impossible to debate whether it was or not. It was settled by semantic fiat."[94]

III

The Early Demographics of AIDS
Case Studies of the First Nine
Gay Male AIDS Cases in San Francisco

AIDS Cases Reported in July 1981

Beginning in 1979 the San Francisco Department of Public Health intensified surveillance of gay men's health, most notably evidenced by recruiting approximately 6,700 "high-risk" gay men to participate in the city's hepatitis B epidemiology and vaccine trial cohort. In spite of this trial and greater vigilance for gay bowel syndrome, STDs, and infectious disease in the gay community, the department did not receive one single report from area hospitals or physicians of any emergent epidemic or cluster of unusual infections among gay men in the city.[1] Although San Francisco had the largest population of gay men (per capita) in the entire United States,[2] no emergent health problems were noted among these men until the CDC catalyzed surveillance efforts in the city in the summer of 1981. As I noted earlier, the AIDS epidemic arrived in San Francisco from the top down.

The CDC's alarming report on June 5, 1981, describing a handful of homosexual/bisexual men with *Pneumocystis carinii* pneumonia and Kaposi's sarcoma in Los Angeles prompted the San Francisco Department of Public Health to contact area physicians and hospitals and ferret out a number of suspicious diagnoses among gay men in recent months. Immediately thereafter, the CDC and the SFDPH contacted Bay Area physicians, dermatologists, and reviewed death certificates in the city and discovered evidence of exactly nine homosexual/bisexual men in the previous year who had developed clinical symptoms or died of conditions suggestive of AIDS. These nine men were reported in July 1981 as the first gay AIDS cases in San Francisco.

A review of primary source material such as medical charts and SFDPH AIDS case report files makes a compelling case for seeing the health department's records and the subsequent characterization of these patients in the press and in popular narratives as flawed in several respects. First, risk factors were reported inaccurately for one-third of the initial cohort; for example, although three of the nine were intravenous drug users, none was initially reported with that risk. It took five years for the SFDPH to properly reclassify Case #0004 as a gay IV drug user; the other two gay IV drug users were captured as a result of my review of their medical charts (15 years after the fact).

This finding is consistent with an argument I have developed throughout this text, namely that the social construction of AIDS as a sexually transmitted disease meant that drug use (and all other HIV/AIDS risks) among gay male AIDS cases has always been, and continues to be, significantly underreported in official AIDS surveillance statistics as homosexual and bisexual orientation preempts all other modes of HIV transmission in surveillance practice. Though my focus in the material reviewed below is on individual case histories for the earliest gay and bisexual men reported with AIDS in San Francisco in 1981, the same general argument could be made for the misattribution of HIV risk for heterosexual patients. Using a methodology similar to my own and cross-referencing various sources of patient data, researchers Murphy, Mueller, and Whitman found in a retrospective review that nearly 85 percent of a sample of 395 patients, originally reported as heterosexually transmitted cases in Chicago, between 1989 and 1994, were "reclassified into different transmission categories." As a result, "the cumulative percentage of cases attributable to heterosexual contact declined from 8% to 5%."[3]

Second, census tract data used by the city's Department of Public Health for reporting these patients were inaccurate for five of these men (55 percent of the total) and demonstrated a consistent bias toward overemphasizing the "gayness" of the disease. For example, when an AIDS case had no address, had an outdated address, or had several places of residence reported (even several cities of residence), then the department captured the case as a San Francisco resident (thus increasing the per capita incidence of the disease) and assigned the census tract that correlated best to a gay bathhouse or a predominantly gay neighborhood in the city. This social construction of the gay geography of AIDS diagnoses again overemphasized the correlation of the epidemic with homosexual identity and sexual behavior and elided the contribution of homelessness or drug abuse to the epidemic. Moreover, these census tract data were then used as the basis for geographical analyses of AIDS by the San Francisco Public Health Department and methodologically, for identifying city blocks for sampling the incidence of HIV and AIDS in subsequent epidemiological research and cohort studies.

As a third and related point, contrary to popular characterizations of patients in the early years of the epidemic, my review of primary source materials indicates that the socioeconomic status of the majority of these early AIDS cases was very tenuous. For instance, two of these early AIDS patients were homeless with no means of support (#1005, #1008), a third (#1004) had no known occupation and was known to inject drugs. Two other patients were employed in low-end administrative or service positions (#1003, #1001), and another two had only vague occupational information reported: one was "retired," one disabled (#1006, #1009). In summary, that leaves just two men of nine who were presumably middle-class individuals with a guaranteed source of income (#1002, #1007). The marginal socioeconomic status of these cases is also borne out by the fact that apparently only one of these nine men (#1007) had private health care in the city; and of this patient only minimal information is available because he was captured as an AIDS case following his death.

In other words, empirical evidence regarding the previous medical history and material well-being of these early AIDS cases in San Francisco is barely consonant with the oft-quoted characterizations of these patients in various popular publications. According to Shilts's *And The Band Played On*, AIDS first emerged among moderately wealthy Guppies who summered on Fire Island and lived the high and fast night life in New York City and San Francisco. They were politically well-connected individuals who were often engaged in long-term relationships and enjoyed access to social and medical support systems. In Shilts's narrative, it was only as the epidemic evolved out of this core group of moderately affluent gay men that AIDS appeared in the "corridors of poverty" associated with marginalized populations in urban centers on the East Coast.[4] I am suggesting, to the contrary, that the epidemic began, and to a large extent remains to this day, overwhelmingly (although not exclusively) concentrated among impoverished, politically disenfranchised, marginalized inner-city populations, a population that does not ipso facto exclude homosexual/bisexual men.[5]

But Shilts is not alone in his characterization of the privileged socioeconomic status of early gay male AIDS cases. In *Sentinel for Health: A History of the Centers for Disease Control*, Elizabeth Etheridge reviewed the CDC's initial case-control study of AIDS patients from the early 1980s. She described the various epidemiological investigations launched by CDC investigators throughout the country and gave an account of a trip to San Francisco by Dr. Harold Jaffe, one of the key members of the Kaposi's Sarcoma/Opportunistic Infections Task Force. Jaffe's comments regarding early AIDS patients in general, were as follows:

> We were struck by how sick these men really were. Many were obviously dying and were just wasting away. . . . Secondly, we were struck that these men did lead a particular kind of life style. These were not gay men who were in long-term monogamous relationships. These were highly sexually active gay men. Often they were well-to-do, had good jobs, traveled a lot. They tended to have sexual partners in many parts of the country, often anonymously. . . . They tended to use a lot of drugs along with this . . . [in the] fast track life style.[6]

Although my own research and early epidemiological research on AIDS patients supports Jaffe's characterization of heavy drug use among early cases, his socioeconomic characterization applies to just two of the nine gay men whose cases are documented in this chapter. While, it is possible that my case study is significantly biased or that San Francisco AIDS patients are atypical in this regard, Jaffe's own contemporaneous research and academic publications on early AIDS patients (1982–1984) also fails to empirically support his representation of socioeconomic privilege.

In 1983, Jaffe et al. at the CDC summarized their research of the various ways in which AIDS cases differed from matched homosexual controls in an article titled "National Case-Control Study of Kaposi's Sarcoma and *Pneumocystis carinii* Pneumonia in Homosexual Men."[7] The authors concluded that AIDS cases were more likely to have had a greater lifetime consumption of specific drugs, greater numbers of sexual partners, and more frequent exposure to several sexually transmitted infections. But the authors also noted that among all of the men in the study (both cases and controls), only one-third had an "income over $20,000 in [the] past year." So, although these data cannot be used to argue that AIDS was more likely to be associated with poverty, they certainly do not support an argument that homosexual men in general, or AIDS cases in particular, were "well-to-do and had good jobs." Instead it appears that the majority of these men, who resided in two of the most expensive cities in the United States (New York City and San Francisco), were barely getting by. And because the CDC's case-control income data were never disaggregated or presented with a high/low range for each category it is impossible to determine whether the 64 percent of the *AIDS cases* who earned less than $20,000/year had significantly lower incomes than the 63 percent of the *controls* who earned less than $20,000/year.[8] This would be my provisional argument given that three of the first nine cases reported with AIDS in San Francisco were homeless and unemployed. But again, the CDC's explicit a priori focus was on the "fast-track" promiscuous gay lifestyle and not the political-economic correlates of this disease.

Of the 24 AIDS cases that San Francisco reported between June and December 1981, all were ultimately designated as gay/bisexual men. Although a diagnosis can be deconstructed, risk(s) interrogated, and the cause or causes of debilitating disease and immune suppression debated, the acute suffering of these individuals and of those who loved them was profound and remains unmitigated by argument or inquiry. I did not review these early AIDS case histories to add insult to injury by victimizing the dead, nor was it my intent to demonize any health-care professional who participated in their diagnosis or care or the public health officials who conducted surveillance in an effort to understand and contain the epidemic. Rather, my purpose is to examine the process by which a previously unrecognized constellation of clinical phenomena came to be characterized as a single disease syndrome; in other words, how did health-care providers arrive at an individual AIDS diagnosis for given patients in the first months of the epidemic, and how did specific individuals become case numbers in the San Francisco AIDS Registry?

Although I deconstruct individual diagnoses and problematize the investigation and attribution of risk factors associated with disease and death for these men, there can be no doubt that all the men (with rare exceptions) had certain attributes associated with the nascent syndrome of immune deficiency that came to be known as AIDS. First, these San Francisco men (with one notable exception) self-identified as homosexual or bisexual, as did the first five men discovered with immune deficiency in Los Angeles in June 1981. While each of these men developed one or another of the signature opportunistic infections associated with the disease syndrome (primarily Kaposi's sarcoma or *Pneumocystis carinii* pneumonia)[9] the signal correlates of vulnerability to the disease were framed in terms of self-proclaimed sexual orientation and/or community of affiliation. These men are known to us as AIDS patients and recorded in epidemiological logbooks as some of the earliest AIDS patients in the country for one reason that owes as much to the social construction of this disease as to the biological correlates and risk factors for acquiring immune deficiency: they were homosexual men. The very essence of AIDS is the observation of increasing numbers of homosexual and bisexual men in major metropolitan centers, primarily in their thirties and forties, who clinically presented with aggressive skin cancer (Kaposi's sarcoma) and/or advanced respiratory infections (PCP or disseminated cytomegalovirus infections) that did not respond to medical treatment. The majority of these men died eight months after their initial diagnosis with an AIDS-defining opportunistic infection.[10]

The Earliest AIDS Diagnosis in a Homosexual/ Bisexual Man in San Francisco (November 1980)

The city's Public Health Department began AIDS surveillance in earnest after the June 5, 1981, *Morbidity and Mortality Weekly Report* was published, and as of July 1981, disease control investigators with the city and the CDC had discovered exactly nine homosexual/bisexual men in San Francisco with immune-deficiency.[11] At this time, the SFDPH began a chronological logbook of probable AIDS cases, entering identifying information and diagnoses for patients as they received reports.[12] The logbook contains the SF case number; patient name; initial (A1) opportunistic infection and the month/year it was definitively diagnosed; sex, and patient's age at diagnosis; race (W-White; B-Black) and risk categories (1-gay; 2-gay intravenous drug user, identified by the acronym "GIVDU"; 3-heterosexual intravenous drugs user, "IVDU"; 4-hemophiliac; 5-heterosexual, etc.);[13] and the date of death.

The final column, confirming the date of the patient's death, was filled in upon receipt of a published obituary in the local press, a death certificate, or a

TABLE 2 Sample ASSB Logbook for Reporting AIDS Patients in San Francisco

SF Case No.	Pt. Name	OI/ Date of Dx.	Sex-Age at Dx.	Race (Risk)	Date-of-Death
1011	Doe, J.	KS/7-81	M39	W (1)	1-8-83
1004	Smith, F.	KS-OI/8-81	M34	B (3)	6-12-82
1006	Johnson, M.	KS/4-81	M41	W (2)	—

physician's notification. At the time of my internship at the ASSB (1995), there was only one man still living from among 118 men reported with the disease between 1981 and 1982. Although I reviewed the AIDS case reports for each of these 118 patients, often they contained just the barest of facts. To better understand the prior medical history and demography of risk for these cases, I sought to examine either the patient's medical chart (if available), or the CDC's 25-page interview with each of these men. Unfortunately the majority of these interviews no longer exist within the files at the Department of Public Health; presumably they were commandeered by CDC investigators and taken to Atlanta.[14] In reconstructing how the disease syndrome was understood when it was first discovered in San Francisco I concentrated on case data for the very earliest patients for whom I had detailed records, the 24 men reported as AIDS cases in 1981; my account here deals with case data for patients #1001 through #1009.

Entries in the ASSB's logbook indicate that the first AIDS diagnosis in a gay man in San Francisco occurred in November 1980, nearly eight months before the "newly recognized, complex, medical syndrome"[15] of immune suppression was reported in the *Morbidity and Mortality Weekly Report*.[16] Apparently, neither the SFDPH nor the CDC was informed about this case of Kaposi's sarcoma in a homosexual man at the time, however, as data on case #1001[17] were not formally relayed to the SFDPH until July 1981, one month after publication of the CDC's groundbreaking article on the new syndrome. Patient #1001 voluntarily agreed to participate in a lengthy (20- to 25-page) CDC interview shortly after he was reported to the SFDPH as an AIDS case.[18]

Technically, patient #1001 was not the first, nor even the second, AIDS patient in San Francisco (as two pediatric AIDS cases retrospectively diagnosed in 1978 and 1979 bear that distinction).[19] Nor was this patient the individual that Randy Shilts identified as the first gay man in San Francisco with the disease, or even the first AIDS patient that Dr. Volberding, chief oncologist at San Francisco General Hospital spoke about so movingly in his lecture. In other words, no apparent distinction was ever given to this gay man with Kaposi's sarcoma, either at the time of his diagnosis (prior to the discovery of "AIDS"), nor when he was reported to the SFDPH after the CDC's seminal publication on the syndrome. He was simply one of a handful of gay men with Kaposi's sarcoma who were discovered retrospectively in San Francisco as of July 1981. As I had no access to this patient's medical chart, any information that I have gleaned about this case comes from notes within his ACR file, and the lengthy interview he completed with CDC officials, which remains behind in his case file.[20]

Case #1001: This was a 39-year-old man who had worked as a hairdresser for almost all of the 18 years he lived in San Francisco. Although he had been married briefly during the early 1970s, in the year immediately before his KS diagnosis he met most of his sexual partners (all male) at a local bathhouse. Although patient #1001 neither smoked nor drank, his consumption of recreational drugs paralleled the pattern reported for other early AIDS patients;[21] he told CDC investigators that in the five years preceding his KS diagnosis, he had smoked marijuana almost every other day, used oral amphetamines at least once a month, experimented with Quaaludes in 1979, cocaine in 1980, and had routinely used butyl nitrites ("poppers") "more than 10 times per month" from 1976 right up until the summer of 1981.

The CDC interviewer reported that the patient "felt that he could not talk about his sexual behavior comfortably" and thus declined to answer the four pages of questions quantifying his sexual partners in the previous year.[22] In other words, no one at the CDC or the SFDPH ever knew how many sexual partners this man may have had nor what sexual activities he may have engaged in. Patient #1001 did have a history of hepatitis (twice) and sexually transmitted infections, however, including gonorrhea once a year for the previous five years and a diagnosis of secondary syphilis in the early 1970s. During the five years preceding his KS diagnosis he had also used corticosteroid creams several times every month and various antibiotics (tetracycline, erythromycin) daily.

The patient first realized that he was ill in the summer of 1980 when he noticed a single enlarged lymph node and a single "bluish" spot on his leg. Although his physician initially diagnosed a "skin reaction," the diagnosis was changed to Kaposi's sarcoma (a form of skin cancer usually seen among elderly Jewish and Mediterranean men) after a positive biopsy in November 1980.[23] Chemotherapy with vinblastine was prescribed; within six months patient #1001 developed *Pneumocystis carinii* pneumonia.[24] He died shortly thereafter at the age of 40, 16 months after first noticing a blue spot on his leg.

Case #1002: According to the ASSB's logbook the second gay man to develop AIDS in San Francisco was diagnosed with PCP and KS in February 1981 (thus five months before the famous *Morbidity and Mortality Weekly Report* of June 5, 1981). The patient's medical chart indicates that this entry is in error, however, and that he was not definitively diagnosed with *Pneumocystis carinii* pneumonia until one and a half months after the June 5 alert by the CDC.[25] As for his Kaposi's sarcoma diagnosis, the ASSB's records documented a definitive diagnosis almost two years before the pathologist who biopsied this man's leg tentatively concluded the following: "although (displaying a) pattern not that of a classical Kaposi's sarcoma, the histologic findings are consistent with that diagnosis."

The SFDPH case file for patient #1002 is brief and notes only the following information (comments in brackets are my own): This 47-year-old white man was reported as an AIDS case to the SFDPH in July 1981 by Dr. Jaffe at the CDC; the patient was diagnosed simultaneously with PCP and KS in February

1981, both of which were definitively established by biopsy. He was treated with prednisone for two months, and "expired February 1983 with oral candida, systemic herpes simplex virus (HSV), Kaposi's sarcoma (KS), mycobacterium avium, and pancytopenia [i.e., anemia]."[26] Patient #1002's medical chart relates an infinitely more ambiguous story of the evolution of knowledge on how to diagnose and treat the disease however; and these records provide an unparalleled opportunity to examine the process by which a diagnosis of "gay related immune deficiency (GRID) and/or "acquired immune deficiency" was socially constructed for one specific gay man in the summer months of 1981 before the disease had even been named.

In May 1981, this "47 year old white male [with] a 60 pack-year" history of smoking tobacco complained of a cough that had gone on for several months and a recent onset of shortness of breath upon exertion (DOE). The patient explained that during the previous week he was "unable to work out in the gym like he used to," but he reported "no fever, chills, sweats, . . . chest pain . . . pets, pneumonia," and so on. His recent travel destinations included central California and Connecticut. Because an emerging epidemic of immune deficiency among gay men was unknown at this time, under social history the physician merely noted that the patient "lives with someone." Patient #1002 had no history of allergies and was not on any medication; as for habits, he acknowledged smoking two packs of cigarettes a day for the previous 30 years, social drinking, and the use of LSD. Concluding his physical examination of this "anxious, curious male," the physician found his chest to be clear, prescribed the patient an anti-inflammatory steroid (prednisone), and sent him on his way.

Patient #1002 was seen two weeks later as a "follow-up for interstitial pneumonitis—uncertain etiology," treated with prednisone and seen for follow-up on several occasions in the coming weeks. On his fifth consultation, the physician noted that the patient was slowly "improving on Prednisone . . . [and] his chest x-ray was clinically improved"; the patient's steroid dose was gradually reduced. Shortly after this appointment, the CDC published its report on the mysterious new syndrome among five gay men in Los Angeles.

When patient #1002 was seen in early July 1981 he had been taking prednisone for seven weeks and had gained 10 pounds. In addition, he now had a fever and was "anxious because he was called back to the clinic." While not overly distressed, his doctor suggested that it would be prudent to "rule out opportunistic infection . . . may be nothing more than a viral flu-like syndrome," and continued to wean the patient off of steroids. When seen again a week later, patient #1002 had continued to decline and now suffered with "low grade temperatures, sweats and chills, and candida [a yeast infection] times one [week]," and had reportedly stopped smoking.

The medical chart for patient #1002 documents a shift in perception about his illness by the end of July 1981, one and a half months after the CDC report first alerted physicians that "the possibility of *P. carinii* infection must be carefully considered in a differential diagnosis for previously healthy homosexual males with dyspnea [i.e., shortness of breath on exertion] and pneumonia" and three weeks after a second *MMWR* article on Kaposi's sarcoma and PCP in gay men.[27] His medical history was reviewed and a transbronchial biopsy "showed non-necrotizing granuloma and stains for acid fast bacteria but [was negative] for bacilli and fungi."[28] Elaborating upon the patient's travel history, his physician now noted prior travel "to the Far East in past, recently . . . to Central Valley, Chicago, and New York [albeit with] no contact with others with same disease." While the doctor refrained from specifying exactly what "contact" and "same disease" might refer to, the language in patient #1002's medical chart is most likely a paraphrase from the CDC's first report on the syndrome: "the patients did not know each other and had no known common contacts or knowledge of sexual partners who had had similar illnesses."

His health-care providers now elicit an in-depth medical history for patient #1002 that disclosed an "episode of jaundice eight years ago which went undiagnosed," an allergy to pollen, and the habit of "amyl nitrate [*sic*] heavy use."[29] His physician now also finds it relevant to note that the patient "lives with a roommate Gay." Patient #1002 became one of the earliest AIDS cases in the United States and the second gay man to be diagnosed with the disease in San Francisco when an open lung biopsy on July 31, 1981, confirmed the presence of *Pneumocystis carinii* organisms.[30] Although that PCP diagnosis was irreversible once reified as an AIDS diagnosis in CDC and SFDPH surveillance records, the diagnosis and its clinical sequelae were riddled with ambiguity and collective negotiation at the level of the patient's primary care. When the PCP infection responded rapidly to treatment his physician concluded: "Superimposed alveolar process[31] cleared promptly in response to antibiotics—negative PCP stain. . . . PCP represented a superimposed [infection] over his interstitial pathology. Infectious Disease and pulmonary consultants were consulted concerning management of the patient's steroids and antibiotics since there was a question of his continued high steroid dosage interfering with the eradication of the *pneumocystis* organism." Nonetheless, health-care providers once again increased the patient's steroids to full dose and added an antibiotic TMP-SMX (a sulfa-based antibiotic marketed as Septra or Bactrim) to his treatment regimen as PCP prophylaxis.

By early August 1981 the patient had improved; his prednisone dose was reduced to half the level initially prescribed and the TMP-SMX was reduced to a prophylactic dose. Throughout the next several months he reportedly exercised more and returned to work, but during an exam in late September physicians noted that "interstitial lung disease and *pneumocystis* [were] still present on his chest x-ray." Within a month the patient had developed a candida infection in his throat and also suffered from rectal ulcers despite the fact that he had "no recent venereal disease or anal sex."

By November 1981 the patient was diagnosed with "gay bowel syndrome," and his prednisone dose was again halved. At a follow-up appointment later the same month his physician became concerned that the patient, despite a previous history of treatment for syphilis, had not been recently retested. Consequently his doctor ordered another test and considered treating him presumptively for "secondary syphilis." The patient's anal ulcers persisted throughout the holiday season and he complained of "feeling horrified this time of year with finals, sick friends, and other problems," but as he was being slowly weaned off prednisone he apparently continued to improve during the next three months. As of February 1982, he had "no shortness of breath, no fever, no chills" and was back to the gym. In his physician's assessment, patient #1002 was improved, and "his respiratory symptoms" were now deemed "probably as much due to obesity as . . . *pneumocystis.*" His prescriptions were refilled.

Another three months passed and it was now the spring of 1982. Although his doctor noted that "his weight was stable or decreasing," according to his medical chart the patient's weight was slightly higher than it had been seven months previously. His prednisone dose was now negligible, but he continued to take double-strength Septra (TMP/SMX) and had developed "dermatitis"; his physician concluded that this recent symptom was probably "secondary to Septra and doubts Kaposi's." The patient was prescribed a steroid cream for topical application. The following month his "candida had cleared, and his rash had improved" and the patient had even lost a couple of pounds. During this appointment he was seen by another physician who "discussed patient's sexual habits frankly with him, and pointed out relationship, although not all details are known, between promiscuity and *pneumocystous craniae* [*sic*] pneumonia in the gay population. He understands this and is dealing with it apparently effectively."

All of the patient's symptoms had apparently been resolved by the time of a follow-up appointment in June 1982, and although he continued to take prophylactic doses of Septra, he no longer needed steroids. But by the following week the physician wrote "patient told of diagnosis of ? Kaposi's. No fever/cough/DOE." Case #1002 was referred to a local dermatology clinic for a work-up to "rule out Kaposi's" although his doctor suggested that his skin problems were probably "allergic secondary to Septra." Within a week the patient reportedly said that he felt "better off Prednisone and has lost twenty pounds." His befuddled physician mused about this man's various polymorphous medical problems: "etiology now even more uncertain: first transbronchial biopsy showed non-necrotizing granuloma [non-specific inflammation]. PFT's [pulmonary function tests] respond to Prednisone. Now with skin biopsy suggestive of sarcoid."[32]

The following week his physician confirmed that patient #1002 had still not been retested for syphilis and ordered another VDRL test while noting with shock that he had not been tested since "10/81 ! [*sic*]." When that test came back positive in early July 1982 the patient immediately began treatment for secondary syphilis. In his checklist of the patient's symptoms this doctor wrote that there was "no evidence of Kaposi ! [*sic*] [and] rash secondary to granuloma was resolving with steroid cream"; later the same month the physician concluded that this man's skin condition was "consistent with chronic relapsing secondary lues [syphilis]."[33] When seen again in August 1982 the patient's rash was much improved, and he was quoted as saying that "his fever disappeared the day after his first [penicillin] injection," he also reported that he had modified his sexual behavior and was no longer being exposed to semen during intercourse. Assessing patient #1002's symptoms his physician wrote: "No fever !! Shortness of breath resolved. Skin rash improved. ? secondary syphilis with positive VDRL—no change in titers, treated in past—currently retreated."

The patient was taken off of Septra at the end of August and the following week reportedly felt "generally stronger"; nonetheless he apparently suffered a dramatic decline over the next two weeks and was subsequently hospitalized for a week in late September 1982 with diagnoses of "1) pancytopenia—etiology unknown; 2) recurrent fevers—35# weight loss in three months; 3) AIDS; 4) PCP; 5) oral candidiasis."

What is new regarding this patient's health is the diagnosis of pancytopenia, "etiology unknown," and the diagnosis of AIDS, the new name for the syndrome of acquired immune deficiency that had been codified by the CDC that very month. Health-care providers remained concerned that patient #1002 continued to have positive VDRL tests while in the hospital despite two additional penicillin injections. "Multiple skin biopsies were negative for Kaposi's sarcoma," however. Acknowledging that the patient had now become allergic to the antibiotic TMP-SMX his physician considered several differential diagnoses to explain his underlying pancytopenia: "multiple [possibilities] but in him need to rule out tuberculosis, and ? Septra induced." Despite the fact that several biopsies had proved negative for KS ("showing granulomas" instead), the physician continued to consider "Kaposi's ?" as one of the differential diagnoses to explain the patient's skin nodules; additional skin biopsies were ordered.

At the time of the patient's discharge from the hospital a doctor concluded that his "persistent oral candidiasis is probably secondary to Septra" and reviewed several possible explanations for the patient's low blood counts:

> The cause of his overall illness and pancytopenia, in combination with fevers and weight loss, is not definitely known, thus it is suspected that the patient's underlying immune-deficiency status or his Septra therapy are implicated as etiologic agents (Septra discontinued mid August due to rash, loose stool, weight loss, fever). Hospital course: Problem 1. Pancytopenia. The patient was felt to be a victim of AIDS, which could account for marrow suppression. Alternatively, long-term Septra R_X could lead to pancytopenia as well. However, the timing of

this seemed off, as the patient had stopped his Septra one month or so prior to observation. The patient was transfused.

At his next appointment the following week (early October 1982) the patient looked "terrible" and had lost weight. This weight loss was not linked to any covert infection, however, but instead was a result of the patient declining to eat because of "severe pain secondary to [anal] ulcers." Once again he was no longer able to work and had a low-grade fever, although no shortness of breath. The physician assessed his symptoms as follows:

1) aplastic anemia [anemia resulting from undeveloped stem cells] secondary to Septra versus secondary to GRID syndrome (most likely!) [sic]. Doing poorly. Currently on Folinic acid.[34] 2) weight secondary to above, not eating well; 3) rash and ulcerations, rule out candidiasis, herpes; 4) rash; 5) subsequent to presentation with PCP, off Septra. Now secondary to aplastic anemia. Differential diagnoses include: Septra toxicity, lymphoma, tuberculosis, fungal disease, hepatitis, cytomegalovirus or Kaposi's sarcoma. Question the possibility of bone marrow suppression due to AIDS alone.

Consequently, as of the autumn of 1982 a GRID/AIDS diagnosis became the preferred explanation for the majority of this man's clinical symptoms. The skin biopsy results were also now available. Although the first biopsy was "essentially unremarkable" and thus determined to be negative for KS the pathologist concluded the following about the second "0.5 cm . . . nodule: Although the pattern is not that of a classical Kaposi's sarcoma, the histologic findings are consistent with that diagnosis. The histology is reminiscent of the post mastectomy lymphangiosarcoma one sees after radiation." With the stroke of a pen, as of October 1982 (not February 1981 as noted in his ACR file) this patient gained a definitive diagnosis of Kaposi's sarcoma confirmed by biopsy; during his subsequent medical check-up a physician noted a single diagnosis—"GRID," gay related immune deficiency.

Later the same month the patient was administered acyclovir intravenously for his presumed herpes infection and within a week he was gaining weight and his skin showed "remarkable improvement. Cleared! Best in years!" However, he was still running a slight temperature. The following day a physician described the patient as a "very ill appearing male who has also been in hospital recently for anemia of unknown etiology. He has also lost half of his hearing; impression hearing loss—? relation to medications." A week later he was readmitted to the hospital, and in a pattern that would remain throughout all subsequent entries in his medical chart the patient was described first and foremost as a "Gay male with AIDS syndrome."

Patient #1002 reported a recurrence of shortness of breath and was prescribed triple drug therapy for "Tuberculosis; type mycobacterium unknown." He remained in the hospital for almost two months and received multiple transfusions for low blood counts. When discharged in January 1982, the patient's physician summarized his complicated medical history and hospitalization as follows:

> Atypical mycobacterium identified on bone marrow biopsy culture [taken September 1982]. [During his hospital stay] his oral lesions were felt to be consistent with Kaposi's sarcoma, and indeed upon biopsy, were proven to be so . . . [H]e continued to spike fevers, and have intermittent chills. He also was noted to have a fairly significant hearing loss which had its onset after intravenous Acyclovir treatment for his disseminated Herpes. . . . The patient's chest x-ray . . . deteriorated somewhat as he did clinically initially. It was felt that some of his lung disease might be due to the Mycobacterium rather than to the *Pneumocystis*. By the third week in November, the patient had taken a dramatic turn for the better . . . enormous difficulties were encountered with discharge planning for the patient, partly because of his apparent slight cognitive deterioration which made him dependent on the medical staff and social service staff for planning.

Patient #1002 was discharged from the hospital only to be readmitted one week later. Within a month he was dead of a heart attack, "secondary to KS, AIDS, PCP, and atypical Mycobacterium of bone marrow, severe pancytopenia, and dehydration." This second gay man reported with AIDS in San Francisco was 49 years old at the time of his death and lived 19 months after his initial diagnosis with pneumonia.

Case #1003: This 31-year-old office worker was diagnosed with PCP and CMV in April 1981 although he was reported by the San Francisco Department of Public Health with a June 1981 diagnosis. The patient's ACR file also included the comment that his roommate had similarly tested positive for cytomegalovirus and "presumptive PCP" and "expired [in September 1981] of histocytic lymphoma."[35] That roommate was never reported as an AIDS case in San Francisco, either as a resident or as an out-of-jurisdiction case, however, so one can only assume that his official cause of death was attributed to lymphoma.

The patient was a native Californian who had enlisted in the military and served in Vietnam. As for previous medical events he reportedly contracted hepatitis B in the early 1970s shortly after joining the military and was diagnosed with gonorrhea nearly a dozen times during the six years before his PCP diagnosis. Case #1003 was initially seen at an area hospital in March 1981 for "respiratory symptoms." According to laboratory tests conducted at that time he was antibody-positive for "influenza A, adenovirus, and cytomegalovirus" and CMV, and *pneumocystis carinii* were grown from cultures obtained during a subsequent open lung biopsy. According to a medical history taken by the SFDPH on June 5, 1981, the very day that the CDC's initial report on immune deficiency among gay men was published, this patient had a "severe case of the flu two to three weeks before" he presented to the hospital and tested positive for cytomegaloviral infection. His chest X ray was negative at the time, so he was prescribed tetracycline and released.

Consonant with the pattern that was reported for many gay AIDS cases in the early years of the epidemic, this patient reportedly had used various recreational drugs on a continual basis, including marijuana six times per day, "amyl nitrites once a week inhaled for six years," Quaaludes two months before his visit to the hospital in March, and cocaine ("inhaled") during the summer before his presentation with "chest pains" and "respiratory symptoms." His brief medical history noted that before the summer of 1980, the patient had "frequent anonymous sexual partners," exclusively in San Francisco, but after that date, the patient denied any "sexual contacts other than with current 'friend,' " the roommate noted above who died of lymphoma.

As I had no access to this patient's medical chart, and the complete text of his interview with the CDC is missing,[36] I know little about the subsequent course of this man's medical treatment or complications other than the information included in a death summary contained within his AIDS case report at the SFDPH. His medical history documented a definitive (A1) AIDS diagnosis of PCP by "open lung biopsy" as of April 1981, and CMV was also grown from these lung specimens.[37] Nonetheless, the patient's medical complications were apparently resolved during this initial hospitalization.

The patient's X ray resolved after treatment with the antibiotic TMP-SMX, and he was discharged. He was readmitted the following day, however, for a "prolonged hospital course" during which a "transbronchial biopsy again grew CMV but did not reveal *Pneumocystis carinii*." Nonetheless, he was treated again with TMP-SMX, and underwent a tracheostomy [a hole in the neck directly into the trachea] to aid in breathing. Patient #1003 eventually required a tube implanted into his chest to drain fluid out of his lungs. The physician noted in this report that "nutrition remained a problem . . . and his weight remained in the range of 100–105 pounds." As the patient had been ill for only one month at most and had no history of gastrointestinal problems before his initial diagnosis, one can deduce that he was extraordinarily thin when he first developed respiratory problems.

According to the death summary, the patient was hospitalized almost continuously after his initial (A1) PCP diagnosis and spent the last four months of his life in the hospital battling "multiple infections." Initially his diagnoses included "lethargy, fever, and a left-lobe pulmonary infiltrate." A subsequent transbronchial biopsy failed to show any evidence of PCP, however. Eventually, a spinal tap uncovered a "cryptococcal infection," and he was given antifungal treatment; then a staph infection developed at the site where a catheter had been placed to administer medication. Repeated evaluations throughout this hospital course found "no evidence of Kaposi's sarcoma." Concurrent laboratory tests documented that his total T-cells were 75 percent of normal, but the ratio of CD4 T-helper cells to CD8-suppressor cells was inverted from the ratio expected in "normal" patients.[38] Though the patient's multiple infections were resolved individually (for instance, the cryptococcal infection was successfully treated, and he subsequently tested negative for the organism), "primary immuno-incompetence" remained his "primary problem." His medical complications at the time of death included a primary diagnosis of a "syndrome of severe immunosuppression and multiple infections related to above," complicated by:

2) nutritional depletion
3) anemia of chronic disease
4) thrombocytopenia [a decrease in blood platelets responsible for coagulation]
5) an ulcer
6) an arteriovenous fistula [a hole in the artery]
7) congestive heart failure (treated)
8) endophthalmitis [inflammation of the eye], etiology unknown
9) an abnormal bone scan, etiology undetermined, [and]
10) hearing deficit, secondary to antibiotic administration.

Although the patient recovered to the extent that he could eat a little and walk unassisted, he "suddenly became cyanotic [blue from a lack of oxygen]" and dropped dead while walking in hospital corridors. Patient #1003 died in the spring of 1982, exactly one year after being diagnosed with *Pneumocystis carinii* pneumonia, at age 32.

Case #1004: The SFDPH initially designated this 38-year-old man's risk for immune suppression as "Sexual Preference: Gay," a risk belatedly changed to "intravenous drug abuse" in 1986 as the result of a physician's notification. Again, neither the medical chart nor the CDC interview of this patient were available for me to review or cross-reference against the ACR file. Therefore, the SFDPH never determined anything about the man's sexual behavior, although his ACR file noted that his travel history had included visits to "New York, Toronto, Miami, Los Angeles! [*sic*]"

In March 1981, patient #1004 had a biopsy that revealed Kaposi's sarcoma and a concurrent infection with cryptococcal meningitis "which was successfully treated" (subsequent spinal taps were negative). Within a month the patient developed PCP and received antibiotics intravenously to combat the pneumonia. As of September 1981 the patient had undergone several months of chemotherapy and radiation treatments for Kaposi's sarcoma, and healthcare providers noted that his skin lesions "were all flatter and smaller than . . . before chemotherapy," but as a consequence of therapy the patient now developed "mild pancytopenia [aplastic anemia]." Patient #1004 was readmitted to the hospital in October 1981 with fever, herpes, and a CMV infection.

While hospitalized, the patient developed "increasing blindness," but no specific diagnosis was ever confirmed; a lung biopsy showed a recrudescence of cryptococcal and *Pneumocystis carinii* infections. Patient #1004 suffered "respiratory arrest" in November 1981 and died four days later. His autopsy "revealed Kaposi's sarcoma involving numerous organs as well as pneumonia" due to the cryptococcal and PCP infections invading his lungs. Tissue from the patient's eyes showed cytomegalovirus and PCP organisms; the latter organism, according to his physician, "has not been previously reported to infect eyes." This gay intravenous drug user lived eight months after his initial (A1) diagnosis of skin cancer, the shortest survival of any San Francisco AIDS case reported thus far.

Case #1005: Up until now, with the exception of two black pediatric AIDS cases retrospectively diagnosed with AIDS in 1978 and 1979,[39] all of the early San Francisco AIDS cases have been white bisexual or homosexual adult men. However, the fifth man to be diagnosed in the city was reported as a 25-year old "Negro . . . who lived on the streets in San Francisco." It does not appear that the CDC ever interviewed patient #1005, but given the exceptional aspects of the patient's diagnosis it was fortunate that I had access to his medical history.

Despite the fact that this man was repeatedly noted to "live on the streets," the SFDPH designated census tract 228 as patient #1005's official residence, locating his domicile somewhere in the vicinity of lower Market Street (near Fox Plaza) and thereby belying his marginalized socioeconomic status.[40]

Like all of the previous patients discussed above, case #1005 was reported to the SFDPH during the month of July 1981 when the department began surveillance for the new syndrome of immune deficiency among gay men in San Francisco. The case file for this "bisexual" man noted that he "lived on the streets," was employed as a "waiter/clerk," and had a "positive PCP" diagnosis by transbronchial biopsy in March 1981. A brief summary of his medical history is excerpted in the clinical résumé below:

> [This] 25 year-old black male was brought in . . . to the Emergency room, after being found unconscious following seizure activity witnessed by the family. . . . The patient gives a history of having twitching and rhythmic jerking of the left lower extremity (and left side of his face) associated with pain on several occasions during the last days prior to admission. . . . The patient claims to be a bisexual and has had daily use of alcoholic beverage up to one glass of wine, occasional use of amphetamine and Valium, and LSD orally, but no IV drug abuse. He admits to recent weight loss of roughly 12 lbs. in the last two months, and has a history of mild chills, lack of sexual drive [impotence] since January. He also admits to some DOE over the last several months, associated with a mild dry cough. . . . There was no unusual foreign or local travel, exposure to animals or dietary abnormalities. He has been employed as a waiter and a clerk. Past Medical History: Unremarkable (no allergies nor medications). He smokes roughly half a pack of cigarettes per day for the last 10 years. Family History: Brother has seizure disorder. . . . Physical Examination On Admission: A young black male in no apparent distress.

The patient's neurological examination showed abnormalities on the left side of his body and a CAT scan of his brain revealed "multiple . . . lesions." Tests for syphilis and various microorganisms were negative, and patient #1005 began treatment for a presumed "central-nervous system process." Although the lesions continued to grow, a brain biopsy was negative for both cancer and opportunistic infections. Following treatment with steroids and antibiotics, "a repeat CAT scan . . . showed perhaps some decrease in size of the lesions . . . [and a week later] another CAT scan . . . revealed that the lesions were further decreasing in size and the steroids were tapered." At this point laboratory tests suggested that the patient had an infection with toxoplasma,[41] but subsequent blood tests failed to confirm this diagnosis. Patient #1005 then underwent a brain biopsy, which showed "no evidence of bacteria, neoplasm, fungi, or acid fast bacteria," although "two toxoplasmosis cysts were seen."

After three weeks in the hospital, a transbronchial biopsy revealed that the patient had *Pneumocystis carinii* pneumonia, and he was treated with the standard sulfa-based antibiotics (TMP-SMX). A second brain biopsy was negative for any abnormalities, except that "one possible *Pneumocystis* cyst was seen." Patient #1005 remained on antibiotic therapy until the following week when his chest X ray had cleared and the lesions had decreased. Although he now had a "rash" possibly indicative of an allergic reaction to the antibiotics, doctors continued treatment with TMP-SMX "because of the uncertainty of the diagnosis of the CNS lesions and the improvement on the CAT scan;" after five weeks of hospitalization, the patient was slowly weaned off of steroids although he continued to be maintained on TMP-SMX.

By April 1981, patient #1005 was beginning to walk again and preparing to move back home to the East Coast to live with his family after being discharged from the hospital. He still limped on his left leg and now had difficulty raising his "right eyebrow, probably secondary to the incision for brain biopsy." At the time of discharge, his physician reviewed the patient's diagnoses of "iron deficiency anemia," and elevated liver function tests and "Monilia pharyngitis [i.e., an oral fungal infection, Candida"][42] most probably related to treatment with Bactrim, before elaborating on this man's primary diagnoses as follows:

1) Brain lesions. As enumerated in the above hospital course, the etiology of this patient's lesions are undiagnosed. He has been on TMP-SMX . . . because of the uncertainty of his diagnosis and because of the possibility of *Pneumocystis* or toxoplasmosis in his brain. He has improved dramatically neurologically over the past three weeks, and there has been decreased size in the lesions . . . after two weeks of therapy. . . . It should be noted that in no way is the patient's intellectual function at all compromised by the CNS process.
2) PCP. It is unclear why patient, who is by all standards we can measure, immunologically noncompromised, why this patient should have developed PCP. He did develop this on two weeks of Decadron [steroids], however, in a normal

host, Decadron in and of itself, should not decrease immunologic status of a normal person to the extent of developing *Pneumocystis* pneumonia.[43] Work-up in the hospital . . . did not reveal any obvious underlying malignancy or immunodeficiency. At present, patient's pneumonia is completely resolved. . . . In retrospect, it may have been worthwhile obtaining a bone marrow and a liver biopsy to look for an occult lymphoma in this patient, but we chose not to at the present time.

This homeless young man, with a family history of seizures, was admitted to a hospital in San Francisco following a seizure in the spring of 1981 before AIDS was known. Despite the fact that his physicians noted that he did not appear to be immune compromised, because patient #1005 was bisexual and because he had been recently diagnosed with *Pneumocystis carinii* pneumonia (PCP), this patient was captured as an AIDS case when aggressive surveillance began in the city in July 1981.

This man appears to have little in common with the other eight AIDS cases reported in San Francisco during July 1981, however. He was much younger than the other patients with immune deficiency (anywhere from 7 to 22 years younger) and never developed Kaposi's sarcoma; moreover, laboratory tests indicated that patient #1005 was even negative for the ubiquitous cytomegalovirus, the herpes virus associated with blindness and pneumonia in many of the other AIDS patients previously reported. Even the PCP diagnosis was problematic, as the diagnosis followed, rather than preceded, treatment with corticosteroids, and because the patient did not seem otherwise to be immunologically compromised.[44]

Once again, the patient's medical chart provides a richer and broader context for understanding his illness. And although case #1005 differed from previous patients in critical ways, what he had in common with other reported AIDS cases was an early death (he died in another state only eight months after his emergency-room visit), and a more complicated medical history than was alluded to in his ACR file at the SFDPH.

At the time the patient was admitted to the hospital, physicians responsible for his care noted that he had "no address and lives on the street or lives with girlfriend. History of gonorrhea. Bisexual?" They also documented that the patient's alcohol consumption pattern was considerably greater than that indicated in his clinical résumé, as he "claims to consume > two drinks [per day] and up to a half of bottle of wine; claims to have reduced consumption over past few days. Dropped LSD on Saturday [his first seizure was on Monday]; history of amphetamine and Valium use although none in past week." After being evaluated by Neurology, the physician noted "over the last month [the patient] has noted increasing irritability, headaches, a 10 lb. weight loss, [and] a cough. . . . Four days prior to being admitted he had onset of [seizures]." The patient's laboratory results at this time were also mildly reactive for syphilis. In the following week, while being evaluated "pre-op" in anesthesiology, the patient was described as having a "history of IV and oral use of Diazepam, amphetamines, LSD etc." (contradicting his characterization as a non-intravenous drug user in the clinical resume used as the basis for reporting this case at SFDPH). From this point forward throughout his chart patient #1005 was described as a "25 year-old gay black male unemployed waiter currently living in San Francisco," and his bisexuality was elided from this and all subsequent accounts.

Within four days of being admitted to the hospital, patient #1005 underwent a psychiatric evaluation and was diagnosed with histrionic personality disorder. Shortly therafter, a medical intern conducted a thorough review of the man's medical history and noted that the "patient was basically well until one month ago when he received a blow to his head with a stick. No apparent sequelae. Two weeks [before admission] patient was seen [at another clinic where he] claims he was diagnosed as having an "infection of cords going into the testicles," for which he was prescribed penicillin but "took only partially." The intern concluded that the leading diagnosis at this time was "carcinoma . . . the fact that the patient's lesions have increased with steroids and antibiotics indicates either a tumor or non-bacterial abscess [although] the infectious category is also appealing." The fact that "the patient was not taking his medicine religiously . . . may have predisposed to abscess formation." Concurrent with his steroid and antibiotic therapies, the patient was prescribed Dilantin, presumably in the belief that his seizures were epileptic in nature like those of his brother. *Pneumocystis carinii* pneumonia had yet to enter the picture as a differential diagnosis.

During his third week in the hospital the patient was described as a "28 year-old with a complicated disease process begun three to six months ago—now consisting of multi-system problems," including the continued growth of lesions and lung infiltrates. *Pneumocystis carinii* pneumonia now arose as a possible diagnosis "but the diagnosis is not yet confirmed." Writing an assessment and treatment plan for a presumptive PCP diagnosis, the physician noted "PCP, probably secondary to steroids (?) [*sic*]." His brain lesions continued to be poorly understood; a second brain biopsy showed a single toxoplasmus gondii cyst—a third biopsy showed nothing definitive. The patient was given TMP-SMX when a bronchial washing revealed *pneumocystis* organisms.

After one month in the hospital and several weeks of treatment with TMP-SMX, the patient's lungs and lesions improved, and plans were made for his release from the hospital. As he "has no funds and no housing in San Francisco" it was necessary to secure social service funds and a medical exception that would allow him to travel by air back to the East Coast where his family could care for him. At the time of his discharge, nearly six weeks after his admission to the hospital, a medical summary concluded that "to date the etiology of [the patient's] brain lesions is undiagnosed" although his symptoms were improved. And in a portion of this text that was inserted verbatim into the clinical résumé quoted above, the physician wrote that "it [was] unclear why an immunologically noncompromised host developed PCP . . . as work-up did not reveal underlying malignancy or immuno-deficiency." With the pneumonia "resolved" this patient left San Francisco in the spring of 1981, and nothing more was documented regarding the case until notice of the patient's death arrived in December 1981.

Looking back from the vantage point of the 1990s, we know that patient #1005 was either 25 or 28 years old and either bisexual or homosexual when he was diagnosed with AIDS in March 1981. In either event, no one appears to know anything definitive about his sexual behavior or previous medical history before the onset of seizures. He was reportedly a recent migrant to San Francisco, and it is unlikely that he could have been exposed to HIV in his hometown as he came from a state with no reported incidence of AIDS in the early years of the epidemic. Theoretically, he could have been exposed to HIV via injection-drug use while in San Francisco, but according to orthodox HIV/AIDS science that would imply that he was a rapid progressor, more rapid than any AIDS case documented in the city's cohort studies. In addition, his diagnoses were uncertain both at the time of admission and a month later upon discharge; even his physician concluded that PCP in this patient was "probably secondary" to his treatment with immunosuppressive steroids. According to his death certificate he died of "probable toxoplasmosis." In short, little was known of this man when he lived in San Francisco and even less can be intuited about him now, 20 years after his death. Apparently his only epidemiological significance was his membership in the first cohort of nine homosexual/bisexual men in San Francisco who were captured by the CDC or SFDPH surveillance staff in July 1981 following a diagnosis of Kaposi's sarcoma or *Pneumocystis carinii* pneumonia; it is unlikely that patient #1005 would have shared even that infamous distinction had he been exclusively heterosexual.

Case #1006: Although his medical problems began six months previously, this 44-year-old "retired" man was captured as an AIDS case just three days after the CDC's June 5, 1981, article on PCP among homosexual/bisexual men in Los Angeles was published in the *Morbidity and Mortality Weekly Report.* Because the patient's current address was unknown, the SFDPH assigned him to a census tract corresponding to his "old address," placing this AIDS case in one of few neighborhoods of the city densely populated by gay men.

During Christmas 1980 patient #1006 had a bout with intestinal parasites and was treated aggressively with antibiotics. As I was unable to access a medical chart for this patient, all of the following information derives from a review of his SFDPH case file and whatever medical history is contained within an April 1981 hospital discharge summary after being treated for *Pneumocystis carinii* pneumonia. At that time his physician noted that patient #1006 was a "44 year old gay man with an extensive travel history, who presented with a confusing and complex history of intermittent fevers, chills, diarrhea, abdominal discomfort, [and] malaise, since November 1980." For those symptoms he was diagnosed with multiple intestinal parasites and treated with a cocktail of antibiotics. Despite abbreviating therapy after ten days due to stomach upsets, the patient subsequently tested negative for all but one kind of parasite. Within one week he was readmitted to the hospital with "night sweats [and] head-ache," but because all of the test results were once again negative, patient #1006 was soon discharged. Five days later, and approximately one week after that, he was again thoroughly evaluated for fever and other symptoms, presumptively treated with additional antibiotics, and then sent home.

In early April 1981 the patient entered the hospital again with "nausea, vomiting, diarrhea, weakness, fevers, chills, muscular aches," and so on. Al-though a medical student believed that he saw "small white plaques on the [pa-tient's] soft palate," the SFDPH noted that these plaques were never seen or confirmed by any other physician throughout the course of his initial hospital-ization, which lasted one month. During this time, patient #1006 tested nega-tive for virtually every infectious disease imaginable including tuberculosis, malaria, and parasites, but within the first week of hospitalization a physician noted the following worrisome diagnosis: "A bronchoscopy was performed . . . results . . . were significant for 4+ *Pneumocystis* seen on silver . . . stain [and the patient was treated intravenously with Septra] . . . Because of the high as-sociation of *Pneumocystis carinii* pneumonia in immuno-compromised pa-tients, a work-up for that possibility was undertaken." The patient slowly improved although he began to develop additional medical complications from treatment, including "a decrease in his white blood cells, as well as return of fevers and a diffuse . . . rash. This was felt consistent with a drug reaction to the Septra [and it] was discontinued after ten days of therapy." Patient #1006 improved even more after he stopped taking antibiotics and shortly before dis-charge his "chest x-ray . . . showed no new evidence of infiltration." He was scheduled to be followed as an out-patient and was "also being evaluated by Rheumatology, who feel that, at present, there is no evidence for an immuno-deficient state. Rheumatology plan to run quantitative T cells . . . and lympho-cyte function tests." The patient was discharged on schedule "in good condition" approximately one month before he was reported to the SFDPH as the sixth AIDS case in the city. Reiterating the physician's comments that the patient ap-peared to have normal immune function, an SFDPH surveillance officer noted that the patient had "no history now of immuno-deficiency." All the same, within the next eight weeks this patient's *Pneumocystis carinii* pneumonia re-portedly "reactivated," and he was dead within a month. This 44-year-old man lived six months following his initial AIDS diagnosis of PCP.

Case #1007: Little is known about this patient beyond the sparse notes contained within his SFDPH case file documenting his identity, residence, and date of diagnosis and death. Presumably, this is so because the seventh gay man with AIDS in the city had already died when the SFDPH reported the case in July 1981. The SFDPH case file initially stated that the patient had a single diagnosis of PCP in July 1981 and died the same day: "Laboratory and Pathology [reports] pending." However, sometime after that date a diagnosis of Kaposi's sarcoma was subsequently amended to his AIDS case report, although material evidence of such a diagnosis was not included in his abbreviated medical history that listed concurrent infections with "disseminated herpes in the brain, lungs, chest," *Pneumocystis carinii* pneumonia, and Candida. Kaposi's sarcoma was also not included on his death certificate, which listed the causes of death as: "a) *Pneumocystis*, acute [1 day]; b) immunosuppressed state [2 1/2 months]." Patient #1007 was 40 years old at the time of his sudden death from pneumonia.

Case #1008 was diagnosed with Kaposi's sarcoma just weeks after the CDC's report was published in June 1981. Although the CDC interview with patient #1008 is long gone, a consent form remains behind in his case file as evidence that he participated in the CDC's extensive epidemiological investigation of the outbreak of Kaposi's sarcoma and *Pneumocystis carinii* pneumonia among urban gay men. Given this absence of crucial ethnographic data, it was fortunate that I was able to review the patient's medical chart, as it contradicts the SFDPH's case file regarding the patient's risk factors for acquiring the disease, his recent medical history, and even his age.

Once again the SFDPH arbitrarily assigned a census tract for patient #1008 when he was reported as an AIDS case in July 1981, despite the fact that the surveillance officer investigating the case stated that the "patient was not reliable for contact," and a CDC investigator noted the patient's comments to the effect that he "says he lives on [the] 'street' " on the signed consent form completed during an interview three months later. Also, according to the SFDPH, patient #1008's "risk factor" for the new disease syndrome was "Sexual Preference: Gay." However, even a cursory examination of his medical chart reveals that the patient's disease symptoms began subsequent to intravenous injections of amphetamines.

The medical chart for patient #1008 is especially valuable as historical source material for two reasons. First, it documents the way in which some gay men in the city (at least this particular gay man) were differentially diagnosed and treated during the period immediately preceding the discovery of a new "gay related immune deficiency" syndrome. Second, the medical history for this patient is relatively uninterrupted for a long period of time preceding his initial diagnosis with Kaposi's sarcoma. Such a deep medical record (relatively speaking) provides additional context for understanding this patient's specific health problems prior to AIDS and his multiple risk factors for disability and death.

The medical history for patient #1008 begins late in 1978 when a physician in San Francisco examined him for rectal pain subsequent to intercourse several days previously; diagnosing this "29 year old gay male" with "probable rectal gonorrhea," a condition for which he had apparently been treated for elsewhere in the previous month. The presumptive diagnosis for patient #1008 was deemed "uncomplicated," and he was prescribed antibiotics and sent home. When the lab results were subsequently analyzed they showed no evidence of "GC," (gonococcus, the cause of gonorrhea) a determination of little clinical relevance since the patient had already received treatment and did not return for follow-up care.

Eight months later (in the summer of 1979), the patient, who had undergone "chest surgery" a year and a half before, was admitted to the emergency room with chest pain "secondary to being kicked last night in the head and chest." A chest X ray was negative, and again the patient was sent home, this time with a palliative hot pack. Several weeks later he returned to the hospital for treatment of "alkali burns" in his eyes caused by an accident with cleaning solutions used at work. Patient #1008 was now described as a "20 year-old," which would make him nearly 10 years younger than he was reported to be when he first sought treatment in 1978. Because he complained of a "pruritic rash on chest, back, [and] hands times 11 days" the attending physician referred the patient for VDRL testing [for syphilis], although the doctor surmised that it was more likely that this was a case of common "heat rash." During the summer of 1980 (yet another year later) an entry made in this patient's chart confirmed that the syphilis test (taken in 1979) had been "reactive." The patient, however, had been lost once again to further follow-up, and thus his syphilis presumably remained untreated for more than two years.

After AIDS was discovered in the summer of 1981, the entries in this patient's medical chart begin to portend a more worrisome diagnosis as his health-care providers slowly become aware of a new syndrome of immune deficiency among young gay men much like him. In early June 1981, patient #1008 was characterized as a "treated case of VDRL—now negative," but with multiple differential diagnoses: "Diagnosis: metastic lymphoma with positive stool; enlarged spleen. Differential diagnosis: lymphoma, hemorrhage, leukemia, amyloidosis [various conditions "characterized by the accumulation of . . . insoluble proteins in various organs and tissues of the body"],[45] [among others]. Addendum: probably calcified gallstones." When seen again in mid-June for "probable gallstones," no particular significance was yet attached to the patient's sexual orientation as predictive for his medical condition, nor was any dire concern or mystery evoked by his current health. But an extensive medical history for patient #1008 was taken at this time, wherein he was described as a "22 year-old gay white male admitted for evaluation of cutaneous nodules."[46] As the June 1981 entry begins, the patient's "current complaint: is 'dark bumps on skin'":

This is the first admission for . . . [this] 22 year-old gay male with a history of IV drug abuse (speed & MDA) times four months. He first noted a raised red lesion on his left leg two months prior to admission which became darker and violaceous over time. Over the past two months, more lesions have appeared on his arms and trunk. Generally, they are initially small and red and become darker and larger over time.

Patient states that he has been sickly from birth and now complains of [increasing] fatigue, weight loss, occasional pruritus and occasional night sweats . . . he also complains of fullness in his neck associated with mild dysphagia.

Prior Medical History: Infectious disease—[positive for] multiple VD including genital herpes, and GC in 1979 and secondary lues [syphilis] with mild rash in 1980 . . . Medications: none except street drugs. Habits: Tobacco one pack per day times seven years = seven pack years. ETOH [alcohol]—seldom. Drugs: LSD @ two times/year; MDA rarely; Speed two times/week, last shot speed two weeks prior to admission.

Social History: Moved to San Francisco three years prior to admission. Education: quit school in ninth grade. Employment: . . . Currently does odd jobs, sleeps in bath houses. . . . Sexual History: gay male involved in SM [sado-masochism], lives in bath houses, history of multiple VD's. Financial: no significant income other than odd jobs—poor nutrition with plus [or] minus one meal/day.

The very same day, a second medical intern characterized the patient as a "Marfanoid white male in mild distress:" an assessment indicating that Marfan's syndrome, a congenital disorder, was the most likely explanation for this man's "gangly" body, his double-jointedness, his visual problems, his prior need for chest surgery, and his potential risk for cardiovascular problems. The intern's "overwhelming impression is that this man has multisystem disease involving skin, GI tract, bone marrow and plus (or) minus chest cavity. In his age group, with normal white blood cells, this is most suggestive of lymphoma, and I feel that this is the probable diagnosis." The patient was admitted to the hospital for further evaluation and testing. A consultation report filed at the same time reported that "the patient, shortly before development of nodules, started IV speed use. Consult re: numerous social problems and IV drug use (shares needles with lover)."

Several days later, the Department of Medicine referred patient #1008 to the Department of Dermatology for evaluation. The consultation report:

> Attending note:
> Several local dermatologists have recently seen young gay males with 1) *Pneumocystis Carinii;* 2) CMV infection; 3) Kaposi sarcoma type lesions. I was unable to see this patient today . . . but a biopsy from yesterday should be available in pathology later. For more information on this syndrome call [two local doctors were named, both of whom had reported previous AIDS cases].

Several days later, the patient was referred to the cardiology department for evaluation. The attending physician noted the following under "History of Present Illness":

First . . . admission for this 22 year-old gay male who has a 3–4 month history of raised, purplish lesions non-pruritic, night sweats, chills and weight loss. He came for evaluation because his lover noticed the same type of lesion on his lower leg. The lesions came on after patient began using I.V. amphetamines and MDA (he and his lover share needles) . . .

Past Medical History: . . . ETOH: four years of one case beer/day; past 2–3 months 1–2 beers/day. Drugs: LSD two times/month; Amphetamine I.V., MDA I.V., Quaaludes.

The next day a consultation was arranged with one of the two local dermatologists who had previously reported AIDS cases to the SFDPH. This physician noted that the patient had engaged in "fisting" five months previously and concluded that the skin biopsy was "possible Kaposi's sarcoma":

These lesions are absolutely consistent with those on a patient I have recently treated, with Kaposi's sarcoma, *pneumocystis carinii*, cryptococcal meningitis and cytomegalovirus positive cultures from blood and urine. . . . There are now over 40 such cases known. I have discussed this with [the attending physician] and he has obtained the appropriate biopsies. It is my impression that this patient does have the syndrome of Kaposi's sarcoma with cytomegalovirus infection with other opportunistic infections occurring in young gay males, particularly "fisters."

Patient #1008 was subsequently discussed at the Tumor Conference held at the San Francisco Department of Public Health on July 1, 1981: "Bone marrow biopsy was non-diagnostic. Subsequent biopsies of one of the skin lesions and an axillary lymph node was reported as Kaposi's sarcoma." It was recommended that the patient "be seen in the Hematology-Oncology Clinic for multi-drug chemotherapy." On the same day, a pathology report confirmed that the patient's biopsy was positive for "Kaposi's sarcoma involving a lymph node." Yet despite the evidence of KS, a diagnosis of "lymphoma [was] not ruled out" and concurrent entries dating from July also noted that the patient was anemic when admitted to the hospital and "had been emaciated previous to present illness." In a six-page summary of the patient's past medical history and record of symptoms, a medical student elaborated on additional social circumstances that contributed to patient #1008's ill health and distress:

Is currently unemployed and is living more-or-less on the streets with his last residence being a bathhouse[47] where he was allowed to stay when doing some janitorial work. A typical day was spent walking the streets. [He] apparently has no resources and no place of residence or plans upon discharge. He is gay and has had the same lover for the last few months, but indicated a loss in libido since his illness and some ill-defined problems with the relationship. His lover has a lesion on his leg similar to [the] patient's and was urged to come to [the hospital] to have it checked.[48]

Under "drug abuse" the intern also noted that the patient used greater quantities of recreational drugs than had previously been reported: "speed 3–4 times/week; LSD 3–4 times/month, occasional Quaaludes and occasionally snorting amyl nitrite." Within several days the patient was released from the hospital and referred to an oncology clinic where he received weekly chemo-therapeutic treatments with vinblastine.

Clinical entries resumed once again in early July 1981. The patient was now reportedly "a 28 year-old homosexual with KS, on chemotherapy with Vin-blastine. Last seen last week, feels better, injected 'speed' IV two days ago. Has noted a sore throat times several days. Throat—Candida albicans." Thus the patient is now reportedly six years older than the 22 years cited in his AIDS case file reported by the SFDPH this same month. Although his medical chart is ambiguous, I believe there is greater material evidence in support of the older age (28–29 years old) given that the earliest medical entries from 1978 indicated that this was an older patient and at least one imprinted hospital ID bears an earlier birthdate (case #1008 had several IDs). All derivative sources that I have reviewed, however, refer to this patient as 22 years old. And because of this, case #1008 has been consistently (mis)represented as the youngest of 118 AIDS patients reported in San Francisco during the first two years of the epidemic (1981–1982).

Chemotherapy continued throughout July 1981; the patient developed nausea, and his anemia persisted. By the end of July the physician noted that "the lesions are improving on R_x though [the patient] is quite depressed over personal problems." At this point he began to complain of "difficulty walking, painful gums," and an inability to eat because of "vomiting which has gotten worse." The physician concluded his assessment: "Kaposi's sarcoma; Subjec-tively improved but objectively?" SFGH's Medical Social Services confirmed that "the patient has [been given] a hotel room and is receiving food stamps. He is angry and fearful." Physicians responsible for his care determined that the patient was not responding to treatment and summarized their conclu-sions: "Extremely unfortunate young gay male who seems to fit the recently described syndrome of KS and other Opportunistic Infections [with PCP, can-didiasis] and has very virulent form of KS. Unresponsive to Vinblastine. More aggressive chemotherapy is obviously necessary." A second form of intra-venous chemotherapy was added to his treatment regimen.

Another attending physician noted that the patient was continuing to use drugs: "Last week prior to admission—I.V. speed. Impression: unfortunate young man with KS . . . Possible relationship to his sexual preference/gay life-style." The physician stapled a typed bibliography of references into the patent's chart listing citations (*MMWR, Lancet* et al.) on the recent syndrome of immune deficiency among gay men in the United States. Thus in a signifi-cant material way, national publications, like those of the CDC's *MMWR* and several other medical journals, guided the differential diagnoses of gay men being evaluated and treated at hospitals in the Bay Area. The social construc-tion of AIDS was also materially reproduced when health-care providers consulted with physicians (primarily out of state but occasionally local) who had previously reported gay men with similar symptoms of immune deficiency, or diagnoses of Kaposi's sarcoma and *Pneumocystis carinii* pneumonia.

By the following month the patient was receiving three forms of chemotherapy to stem the spread of Kaposi's sarcoma. He developed thrombocytopenia (a low platelet count), and his white blood cell count and hematocrit level dropped; he began receiving transfusions. He developed shortness of breath and was evaluated for *Pneumocystis carinii* pneumonia. The patient briefly refused weekly infusions of chemotherapy and insisted on being admitted to the hospital. Once admitted, he was again evaluated by Medical Social Services: "Since patient's cancer was diagnosed, he has been constantly in crisis—changing living situations, getting evicted from hotels, living with various friends. He recently received SSI and just spent $700–1000 on drugs, stereo, etc. He states he has *no* money for food or rent until his October check comes."

The patient went back on chemotherapy while hospitalized, and a psychiatric consultation was obtained: "Patient (has) long history of many sexual contacts. Low on $. Seeks lover partially for place to stay. . . . Patient states he doesn't really care that he is so gravely ill, adding there's nothing she [*sic*] can do anyway. Acknowledges he's angry at his unfortunate fate but quickly adds that there is no point in getting angry—it won't help." After reviewing the major tenets of E. Kübler-Ross's book *Death and Dying*, the consultant concluded that the patient's "illness, loneliness and isolation only add to the anger he must be feeling in what I think is an aborted second stage."[49] Patient #1008 was briefly discharged from the hospital only to be readmitted shortly thereafter.

Back in the hospital, another consultation was obtained to evaluate the patient's pulmonary function. The physician noted that the patient "denied a history of pulmonary disease, but smokes 3–4 packs per day times six years [thus four times as many cigarettes as was initially reported when he was evaluated only four months previously] and has a cough times one month. Denies chest pain." A clinical summary was stapled into his medical chart acknowledging that the patient's first indications of illness were associated with "decreased libido, anorexia and painful muscle spasms which he [the patient] attributed to concurrent I.V. amphetamine use." The physician went on to characterize the patient's "lifestyle" risks for disease as "significant in that he was a gay male who had worked as a male prostitute since the age of fifteen years." Although it is theoretically possible that whoever dictated this clinical summary had access to personal information that I was not privy to, there was no mention of anything in either the patient's medical chart or in SFDPH case files to support such a characterization of this man's sexual behavior.

As the patient continued to deteriorate in the hospital, "laboratory tests came back negative for CMV,"[50] and a lung biopsy proved positive for "multiple foci of Kaposi's sarcoma" albeit "negative for PCP." Within 24 hours case

#1008 was dead. An evaluation of lung tissue by the pathology department reportedly uncovered *Pneumocystis carinii* pneumonia, but only minimal evidence of the organism was found during an autopsy conducted several days postmortem. While the patient's death certificate listed the sole diagnosis of Kaposi's sarcoma, nonetheless, the SFDPH amended his case file to reflect the postmortem PCP diagnosis as well.

Before I leave this case, I would like to take a moment to reflect on the role of IV drug use in exacerbating this man's illnesses. Regardless of one's opinion of the role of HIV in his illness, intravenous drug use is central to understanding this man's debilitated medical condition; he was already emaciated at the time of diagnosis and spent the bulk of his social security insurance payments on drugs, which left him unable to buy food or pay rent. Many AIDS dissidents would indict injecting drug use as the precipitating cause of this man's physical deterioration; even the patient himself said that IV drug use preceded and caused the bumps on his skin. And while orthodox AIDS researchers would argue that drugs don't cause AIDS, they would still acknowledge that intravenous drug use exacerbated this man's risk for contracting HIV infection/ AIDS, either by sharing needles, or because the patient's drug use contributed significantly to poor judgment vis-à-vis high-risk sexual practices.

Yet despite the central role of drugs in precipitating and perpetuating this man's multiple medical and social problems there is no evidence in his medical chart to suggest that any of the health-care providers for patient #1008 ever sought to arrange treatment or counseling for his addiction—and he reportedly continued to inject "speed" while receiving aggressive chemotherapy for Kaposi's sarcoma. In my opinion, this is yet more evidence of the danger of the immediate myopic construction of AIDS as solely a sexually transmitted disease, an a priori theoretical bias evident in medical charts for the very earliest patients reported in 1981. With respect to case #1008, health-care providers appeared to be more interested in his lover (who was never reported as an AIDS case) and his alleged sexual practices (prostitution and fisting) and bathhouse residency than they were in that fact that patient #1008 was emaciated, lived on the streets, could afford neither food nor rent, had belated and incompletely treated infections such as syphilis, and injected drugs every 48 hours. And yet it is only these latter facts that were materially evident from his medical record, and only these latter facts of malnutrition and drug abuse that were historically recognized as correlates of immune dysfunction, premature disability, and death.

Case #1009 was the final AIDS case reported to the SFDPH during the month of July 1981. The patient was a 47-year-old paraplegic that the CDC discovered at the city's veteran's hospital. As the patient did not reside in San Francisco he was reported as an out-of-jurisdiction case, and thus the SFDPH conducted no investigation of the patient's past medical history or risk factors for the disease. For instance, although the AIDS surveillance officers report-edly knew that this patient had "sex with a male," they did not investigate whether case #1009 ever injected drugs, donated blood, or received a transfu-sion. According to the minimal notes recorded in his case file at the ASSB, case #1009 developed "skin nodules" subsequent to a "trauma" that left him a para-plegic several years previously. These nodules were subsequently diagnosed as angiosarcoma (tumors of the blood vessels) which disseminated to the bladder and lymph nodes and led to multiple amputations. Although the patient un-derwent chemotherapy, he died of hemorrhaging and "angiosarcoma, multi-centric" the same month that he was reported to the SFDPH as an AIDS case.

Why was patient #1009 captured as an AIDS case? An ambiguous comment on the patient's case form noted that "Histopathology: doesn't fit K(S)? Anaplastic variant clinically does fit K(S) in internal organs and lower extrem-ities." In other words, while the pathological examination of this man's tissues was ambiguous for a diagnosis of Kaposi's sarcoma, his clinical presentation as a homosexual male with cancer disseminated throughout his internal organs and on his legs was sufficient evidence for the CDC and the SFDPH to capture and report case #1009 as yet another "previously healthy" gay male inexplica-bly suffering from immune deficiency. Again, the patient's sexual orientation seemingly overdetermined his membership in the initial cohort of AIDS cases reported in San Francisco during the first month of surveillance for the disease in 1981.

More Gay Men Reported with AIDS in San Francisco

Fifteen Case Studies from 1981

AIDS Cases Reported from August 1981 through December 31, 1981

As early as August 1981, Dr. Conant (a dermatologist at UCSF) and Dr. Volberding (an oncologist at SFGH) established a specialty clinic in anticipation on an onslaught of gay AIDS cases in San Francisco. Beginning in the late summer of 1981, it was now common for any gay man with suspect "spots" and/or respiratory difficulties to be immediately referred to the small coterie of overnight AIDS specialists in the city and subsequently treated at the Kaposi's Sarcoma/Opportunistic Infections Clinic that was established at San Francisco General Hospital (SFGH). Consequently, within just one month of the CDC's discovery of the disease, a bureaucracy for AIDS health care and social services began to form in San Francisco concomitant with a centralization of "expert knowledge" in the city. A standardized protocol for diagnosing and treating these men emerged simultaneously; first, a biopsy of skin or lung tissue, then treatment with an antibiotic such as TMP-SMX (for *Pneumocystis carinii* pneumonia) or aggressive experimental chemotherapy with vinblastine and vincristine (for Kaposi's sarcoma).

Fifteen homosexual/bisexual AIDS cases were reported in San Francisco between August 1 and December 31, 1981, at a rate of several men each month, except for November, when neither the SFDPH nor the CDC reported a single case of immune deficiency among gay men in the city. My review of ASSB case files and medical charts for the 15 patients captured between August and December 1981 suggests that the major tenets of orthodox AIDS discourse (an infectious sexually transmitted disease, transmitted via homosexual intercourse and associated with promiscuity and bathhouses) had been well-assimilated by clinicians, public health officials, and other medical professionals in the city within the first 30–60 days of the epidemic's discovery. The theory that the emergent disease syndrome was caused by a single, new, sexually transmitted virus was readily assumed from the moment that the disease appeared in San Francisco residents. It doesn't appear that this hypothesis was ever seriously interrogated; it was, from the outset, the very premise by which surveillance officers and physicians operationalized their surveillance and documentation of AIDS patients. This theoretical predisposition led public health officials to disregard any rigorous investigation of other hypothesized risk factors for the disease (e.g., poppers, or such well-established viruses as CMV).[1]

Public health officials and historians of the epidemic have also minimized the significance of the observation that half of the AIDS cases reported in San Francisco in 1981 were members of the hepatitis B study (a subset of whom became the San Francisco City Clinic Cohort). Nine of the 15 AIDS cases reported after August 1981 were members of that cohort study, and from early publications by the SFDPH and the CDC we know that two additional gay male AIDS cases reported in 1981 belonged to the HBV study (11 of the 24 AIDS cases reported in San Francisco in 1981 were current or former members of the HBV study).[2] It is difficult to know what to make of this correlation between AIDS and membership in the hepatitis B study and vaccine trials. Perhaps these men received greater scrutiny for symptoms of immune deficiency after GRID was discovered because they were already enrolled in a CDC-sponsored epidemiological project. Or perhaps exposure to the hepatitis B virus itself made one more physiologically vulnerable for contracting AIDS or contributed to the disease's progression. However, this specific hypothesis is discounted by research publications from the early 1980s, such as the CDC's national case-control study on AIDS (which failed to find any significant clinical or pathological association between hepatitis B infection and AIDS). Instead, the striking observation that so many of the early AIDS patients had participated in a national HBV vaccine study was relevant for most AIDS epidemiologists only because it demonstrated that the two diseases, coincident in the same "high risk" populations, were transmitted by similar "risk factors." Ipso facto, AIDS must also be caused by a virus present in body fluids such as semen and blood.

With these thoughts in mind and an eye to brevity I now turn to a review of the 15 homosexual/bisexual AIDS cases reported in San Francisco between August and December 1981. The discussion of these patients is followed by my concluding remarks on the accuracy of narrative accounts and AIDS surveillance case information regarding these men and their risk factors for debilitating disease.

Case #1010: This 49-year-old divorced man was initially captured in July 1981 by CDC investigator Harold Jaffe, albeit not officially reported as a San Francisco AIDS case until August. The ASSB files did not retain the interview for patient #1010 although a consent form remains behind as evidence that he participated in the CDC's initial round of AIDS case studies. The patient lived in San Francisco but was being treated for Kaposi's sarcoma at Stanford as of July 1981 when he first came to the attention of the CDC. According to SFDPH notes at the time, "No other information was given" regarding the case, although notes in his case file indicate that the patient tested positive for Kaposi's sarcoma and cytomegalovirus, and his risk factor for the disease was coded as "Sexual Preference: Gay." As the sole reference to this man's sexual life was the notation "divorced" on his death certificate, I can only presume that his homosexual "preference" was information relayed to the SFDPH after the CDC interview. A death certificate dated Christmas 1981 was the only additional information available in the patient's ACR file. He died of "1) pneumonia (four days) and b) complications of KS (11 months)" five months after he was reported to the SFDPH as an AIDS case. And although there was no subsequent medical documentation amended to this patient's file, his KS diagnosis was later backdated to the summer of 1980; on the basis of what evidence this was done is unclear.[3]

Case #1011: Because the CDC interview of this patient still exists within his ACR file it was possible for me to glean something of the past medical history of this 42-year-old gay male diagnosed with Kaposi's sarcoma. The interview also provided a cross-reference for the accuracy of the SFDPH's reporting. In this regard, the SFDPH erred by reporting patient #1011 with an occupation somewhat more prestigious than the garden-variety office position that this high school graduate claimed during his CDC interview, implying that the patient had a higher socioeconomic status than can be supported given the patient's self-characterization. Once again there were also problems with the census tract designation for this case. In August 1981 the SFDPH reported one particular address for the patient despite the fact that the physician who informed the SFDPH of the patient's diagnosis the very same month used a different address. It was this second address that the patient claimed as his residence at the time of his interview with the CDC one month later. Again, this is not an insignificant observation, because the address the SFDPH used for reporting the case was in the heart of the Castro district, the area of the city most associated with gay male residency. Meanwhile in contrast, the area of the city where the patient himself claimed to live was in a district that was not known for a large homosexual population. As was true for homeless patients that I've discussed previously, the SFDPH's method of designating census tracts demonstrates a bias in the direction of overemphasizing the geographical correlation of AIDS cases with homosexual sites of business and residence.

Patient #1011 fits the profile of AIDS patients that many clinicians reported early in the epidemic as he shared many of the same risk factors for immune deficiency that we saw among patients in the previous chapter. He had smoked 1–2 packs of cigarettes a day for the preceding 20 years and had used various antibiotics and sleeping pills on a daily basis in the five years preceding his recent illness. The patient also acknowledged that he had used recreational drugs heavily during the previous five years and continued to do so even after his diagnosis with Kaposi's sarcoma. His drug use habits included the use of marijuana more than 10 times per month; amphetamines "rarely"; Quaaludes less than once a month "until present"; LSD and MDA one to 10 times per month "until present"; and unlabeled bottles of nitrites (poppers) "more than ten times per month from 1976 until present."

As for his past medical history, case #1011 reported that he had experienced multiple bouts of sexually transmitted infections including at least six episodes of gonorrhea and three diagnoses of tertiary syphilis (1978, 1979, and 1981). He was also positive for cytomegalovirus (CMV), hepatitis B antibodies, and had belonged to the city's HBV cohort study. According to his extensive interview with CDC investigators, patient #1011 had engaged in sex with approximately "1,844" contacts during the 16 years that he had lived in the city; I was unable to reconstruct how this number was arrived at, as there was no quantitative data provided in response to the CDC's questions of lifetime sexual behavior.[4] Almost all of his 192 sexual contacts in the previous year were reportedly with men that he met at the city's bathhouses.

The patient said that he initially became concerned about his health in January 1981, when he developed fatigue, fever, and skin abnormalities (eczema). Concurrently he was diagnosed with tertiary syphilis for the third time in four years. Meanwhile AIDS was discovered in June 1981, and by August 1981 the patient's physician had ordered a skin biopsy, which revealed Kaposi's sarcoma. At the time, officials at the SFDPH noted that he tested positive for high titers of CMV and herpes simplex virus, and within a month the patient was additionally diagnosed as suffering from "diffuse lymphoma." Curiously, on that same day the SFDPH wrote in patient #1011's file "T and B cells [were of] normal quantity;" which seems to indicate that this AIDS case was not absolutely deficient in CD4 T-helper cells and therefore did not manifest the peculiar surrogate marker of immunodeficiency that essentially defined the clinical syndrome. There was no additional documentation of the patient's further medical complications or of any treatment(s) that he may have received for these multiple opportunistic infections. Patient #1011 died at the age of 44, two years after his initial Kaposi's sarcoma diagnosis.

Case #1012: Once again, Dr. Jaffe of the CDC initially informed the SFDPH about this patient in August 1981, at which time this 34-year-old man had just recently been diagnosed with Kaposi's sarcoma and tested positive for high titers of Epstein-Barr virus (the cause of mononucleosis). Despite the fact that an interview still remains in this patient's chart, very little can be intuited about this man's previous medical history or sexual behavior as he declined to answer many questions in detail. He told investigators nothing about his sexual life.

The patient's past medical history included six to seven episodes of gonorrhea, one diagnosis of syphilis, numerous bouts of amebiasis, and a diagnosis of hepatitis A in 1979. In addition, during the previous five years the patient had used cocaine, amphetamines, and barbituates. He had also used unlabeled ampules of amyl nitrite 1–10 times per month for the preceding 15 years. Soon after his diagnosis, this patient left for New York City, where he reportedly experienced two successive bouts of *Pneumocystis carinii* pneumonia (PCP). Patient #1012 died at the age of 37, 26 months after he was initially reported with Kaposi's sarcoma in San Francisco.

Case #1013: A member of the hepatitis B vaccine study, this 45-year-old man was diagnosed with Kaposi's sarcoma in September 1981 shortly after returning from work in New York City. According to his interview with CDC representatives, he had been diagnosed with polio as a child, and his prior medical history was also significant for an infection with hepatitis A in 1971. The patient said he had been treated with numerous antibiotics in recent years (e.g., ampicillin, tetracycline, Flagyl) for repeated bouts of intestinal parasites and gonorrhea. In a striking departure from accounts of early AIDS cases, this man reportedly neither smoked nor drank, and replied that he had never taken any recreational drugs or used poppers during the five years preceding his illness. The patient also reported that he had traveled out of the country several times in the previous decade, most recently (1979) to Mexico.

In 1981, before being diagnosed with Kaposi's sarcoma, patient #1013 had also acquired hepatitis B and been diagnosed with gonorrhea and genital herpes. He first noticed lesions indicative of Kaposi's sarcoma while in New York City the previous month; he developed a lingering cough and various "skin abnormalities" at the same time. Soon he broke out with herpes, and his throat became infested with Candida.

During his interview the patient estimated that he had had sex with approximately 100 men in the previous year, and met half of his sexual partners on the street. Although he acknowledged that this was "typical behavior for the preceding five years" he was unable to estimate how many sexual partners he had had in his lifetime. Despite the fact that patient #1013 denied knowledge of any friends who had been hospitalized since 1979, diagnosed with cancer, experienced unexplained fevers, weight loss, or died from "natural causes," the SFDPH subsequently amended his interview by noting that one of the patient's former "sexual partners" had died of Kaposi's sarcoma.

As the CDC had revised the interview form administered to this patient in December 1981 to include disaggregated income data, I learned that this man reportedly earned between $10,000 and $20,000 the previous year—hardly evidence in support of the CDC's representation of "well-to-do" AIDS patients. Following his interview, the patient returned to New York City where he died of *Pneumocystis carinii* pneumonia and a disseminated cytomegalovirus infection at the age of 46; patient #1013 had lived 13 months following his initial Kaposi's sarcoma diagnosis in San Francisco.

Case #1014: Much like the previous patient, this was a 45-year-old waiter diagnosed with Kaposi's sarcoma in September 1981 and also a member of the hepatitis B study in San Francisco. As his CDC interview was absent from his case file, however, nothing can be intuited about his sexual behavior, his past medical history, or his recreational drug habits. Patient #1014 died within 10 months of his initial KS diagnosis, and although he was a San Francisco resident, his file does not contain an official death certificate.

Case #1015: The final AIDS case reported during the month of September 1981 is exceptional in several respects. Although this 35-year-old man was similarly diagnosed with Kaposi's sarcoma the same month as the men above, his course of treatment differed significantly from many of the other AIDS patients discussed thus far. His ACR file was silent for a period of two years following his diagnosis, and then he began treatment with interferon for "early lesions—?K(S)?" The following year he was reportedly "in remission."

Although case #1015 was a San Francisco resident, he was frequently lost to follow-up by the SFDPH because he also maintained apartments in New York City and Los Angeles. Nonetheless, the AIDS Seroepidemiology and Surveillance Branch continued to track his health on an annual basis, noting that he left San Francisco following the death of his lover in 1984. He was treated after that for several years with radiation in New York City. After surviving for seven years with AIDS, the CDC tried to enroll the patient #1015 in a study of long-term survivors, but were informed that he "refused to participate" when the SFDPH contacted his New York physician. As of the time of my internship at the ASSB in San Francisco in 1994–1995, case #1015 was reportedly still living, 14 years after being diagnosed with AIDS.

Case #1016: Although this 35-year-old member of the hepatitis B study was originally diagnosed with Kaposi's sarcoma of the "palate" in June 1981, he was not reported as an AIDS case in San Francisco until nearly four months later; this latter date was erroneously used by the SFDPH in reporting his diagnosis, thus officially abbreviating the duration of his survival with AIDS. According to notes in his ACR file, the patient's KS symptoms began the moment he stopped a six-month course of treatment with the sulfa-based antibiotic Flagyl for treatment of intestinal parasites.

Patient #1016 also tested positive for CMV at the time he was diagnosed with KS; several months later he then developed an acute infection with Epstein-Barr virus. Although the CDC interviewed this man for its national AIDS case-control study, the interview itself no longer remains in his file. The only additional documentation regarding the case was his death certificate;

patient #1016 died "accidentally" due to an "overdose of morphine and barbit-uates. Other conditions contributing but not related to the immediate cause of death [were diagnoses of] AIDS, Kaposi's sarcoma and cytomegalovirus." And because official AIDS mortality and survival reports do not eliminate patients who die of natural or accidental causes from their cumulative statistical totals, patient #1016's death was officially attributed to AIDS (after a survival period of 17 months with the disease); he was 36 years old.

Case #1017: This 38-year-old man with Kaposi's sarcoma was also a member of the San Francisco City Clinic study on hepatitis B. Though it seems redundant to observe that the census tract that the SFDPH used in reporting this patient appears somewhat arbitrary (one address was designated from among three possible residences), in this particular case all of the San Francisco addresses roughly correspond to the same geographical vicinity and are traditionally identified as gay male neighborhoods, thus making any critique irrelevant.

It does not appear that patient #1017 received any immediate therapy for Kaposi's sarcoma, although approximately 14 months after he was captured as an AIDS case the SFDPH reported that he had undergone "six courses of chemotherapy and then relapsed." His ACR file also noted an alternate diagno-sis of "squamous cell cancer of the tongue." In 1984, and again in early 1985, the patient was being seen for "recurrent KS," but initially appeared to be "doing well with no R_x [no additional chemotherapy or medication] and no additional diagnoses." Nonetheless, case #1017 died in the spring of 1985 at the age of 42. A SFDPH investigator commented that the patient's lungs had eventually "filled up" with Kaposi's sarcoma; his death certificate listed KS and AIDS as the official causes of death. Patient #1017 lived 42 months following his initial (A1) AIDS diagnosis.

Case #1018: As was true of the previous two patients, this man was diag-nosed with Kaposi's sarcoma of the mouth (specifically the tonsils) and was also a member of the city's hepatitis B study. He was a veteran of the U.S. military, as were several of the early AIDS cases in San Francisco. Supporting my contention that "homosexual preference" informed the methodology by which SFDPH assigned census tracts, patient #1018 was reported with a resi-dence placing him in the vicinity of the Castro district despite the fact that he was twice documented with different addresses in the Fillmore district.

Though the distinction between the Fillmore and the Castro areas may be seen as small, given that both neighborhoods had significant concentrations of gay men, I would argue that the emphasis on sexuality masks important differ-ences: the Fillmore has historically been associated with more indigent popu-lations, more sex workers, and more intravenous drug users. And in other case data that I have reviewed, the SFDPH's designation of residence for a given AIDS patient has skewed the representation of the medical geography of the disease in the city to a greater degree, resulting in the publication of official data such as those presented in the figure below, which identifies the census tracts associated with the greatest prevalence of the disease (the current number of AIDS cases) in San Francisco as of 1985 (Figure 7). This consistent trend in the early case files I reviewed supports my contention that the geographical analyses of AIDS incidence per census tract as published by the San Francisco Department of Public Health were, in the early years of the epidemic, biased toward locating reported AIDS cases near the Castro and other neighborhoods traditionally perceived as meccas for gay life in the city.[5]

Shortly after an honorable discharge from the military in 1979 at the age of 21, Patient #1018 was seen at the hospital for a "small lesion over his hard palate," but apparently nothing was made of this observation. A month later the patient complained of a "sore throat" and a "rash on his face." Again, there is no indication that the patient was ever definitively diagnosed nor treated for these symptoms. Four months later (now early 1980), he was seen for "chills

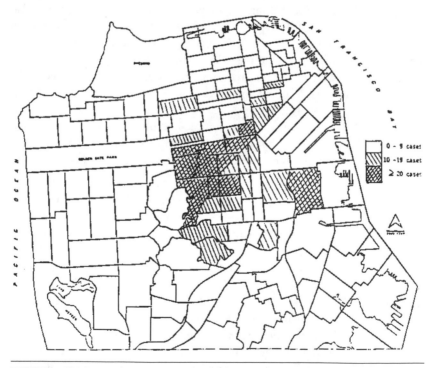

FIGURE 7   AIDS Cases by Census Tract of Residence: First 1,000 Cases, San Francisco, 1981–1985
Source: City and County of San Francisco, Department of Public Health, Bureau of Communicable Disease Control, "Update: Acquired Immunodeficiency Syndrome—The Tenderloin, San Francisco." *San Francisco Epidemiologic Bulletin* 4, no. 9 (September 1988): 37, fig. 2.

and nausea" and diagnosed with a hepatitis B infection. When seen for follow-up shortly thereafter, patient #1018 "stated [that he was] ill and unable to work"; he was placed on medical disability for a period of three months and changed residence at least twice. All told, case #1018 was documented with six different residences in the two years immediately preceding his diagnosis with Kaposi's sarcoma, thus confounding any reliable interpretation of his official census tract designation.

The patient apparently recovered from hepatitis and remained relatively well until the fall of 1980 when he had a bout of intestinal parasites. Approximately three months later (January 1981) he developed a sore throat and was treated with large quantities of penicillin. And at this time, coincident with his AIDS diagnosis, the medical chart for patient #1018 goes silent for a period of three years; whatever I have gleaned about his medical history during that time has been reconstructed from comments made retrospectively as of 1984.

These subsequent entries assert that the patient underwent a "routine tonsillectomy" in October 1981 and was diagnosed with Kaposi's sarcoma after these tissues were biopsied. Additional lymph node biopsies were also positive for KS in 1982 and again in 1983, and patient #1018 had "three KS lesions removed from his nasopharynx [the membranes lining the passage between the mouth, the larynx and the esophagus]." I haven't a clue about any treatments that he may have received thereafter.

The SFDPH reported the man as an AIDS case in October 1981 but did not rigorously update his health until 1983, when they noted that he had donated blood in the Bay Area on numerous occasions in 1978 and 1979, and had sexual contact with a "known AIDS case" approximately "a dozen times" between the summer of 1980 and 1982. Given that the patient had already been documented with a "lesion" on his palate in 1979, this reputed "sexual contact" could not have been the origin of this man's presumed HIV infection.[6] And in fact, the information about his reported sexual contacts was irrelevant unless one was convinced that Kaposi's sarcoma or AIDS was caused by an infectious disease organism transmitted sexually among gay men. If it was true that health-care providers were theoretically open to a range of possible explanations for immune deficiency in 1981 and 1982, as is often asserted, then this information could have led investigators to consider that there were multiple common factors in the social and sexual lives of AIDS patients that independently conferred health risks (poppers, recreational drug abuse, intravenous drug use, multiple bouts of sexually transmitted diseases, viral and parasitic infections, etc.) quite apart from sexual intercourse.

In late 1983, the SFDPH received information that the patient "seems to be in 'spontaneous remission;' . . . no new signs of illness—very healthy. Has been on Vitamin therapy." According to his case file, patient #1018 remained in "great shape" on "Vitamin C therapy" until the summer of 1984; at which time his medical chart resumed once again in San Francisco. The patient was now 26 years old and had recently been hired as a clerk. His pre-employment physical noted a prior medical history of a positive PPD test (exposure to tuberculosis), a "Grade II/VI early systolic click," and a hepatitis infection in 1980. Remarkably the physician described the patient as a "healthy adult male" with no history of "chronic or recent acute disease," suggesting one possible explanation for the three-year gap in his medical chart (the patient's tonsillectomy and Kaposi's sarcoma diagnosis occurred at a different medical facility).

Two months after this 1984 physical the patient was hospitalized for *Pneumocystis carinii* pneumonia and treated with the antibiotic TMP-SMX. After breaking out in an allergic rash he was successfully treated with aerosolized pentamidine for two weeks and recovered. At the same time, the patient was found to be culture positive for herpes, and acknowledged a recent 15-pound weight loss. Throughout the next six months the patient was successively diagnosed with bronchitis, herpes, and a Candida yeast infection (for which he was treated with acyclovir and ketoconazole respectively). Nonetheless, the SFDPH noted that the patient was "doing well" one year after coming down with "gay pneumonia," and almost four years to the day after his initial diagnosis with Kaposi's sarcoma.

Five months later (in late 1985) the patient began to decline, and by the spring of 1986 he had "stopped working." Although his chest X ray remained clear, and his doctor stated that he was negative for both a recurrence of *Pneumocystis carinii* pneumonia and Kaposi's sarcoma, within weeks patient #1018 took to his bed "secondary to fatigue and pain in his right leg." His physician diagnosed his impression of "muskoskeletal atrophy" and recommended an "exercise schedule." The patient briefly pursued daily exercise and grew stronger but by the summer of 1986 he had developed "progressive leg weakness and an unsteady gait." He was prescribed an antidepressant and died five months later of "a) cardio-pulmonary arrest; b) KS; c) AIDS."[7] This 28-year-old man had survived 62 months following his initial AIDS-defining diagnosis.

Case #1019: This 34-year-old was a member of the city's hepatitis B study when he was diagnosed with Kaposi's sarcoma in December. As this man no longer lived in San Francisco, his AIDS case report form stated "from New York" and listed a local address in "care of" another resident in the city; predictably, this "in care of" residence was used to designate the census tract associated with his diagnosis. No medical records were available to review in San Francisco because all of the man's AIDS treatments took place out of state; therefore, I relied exclusively on the quite limited information contained in his ACR case file at the AIDS Seroepidemiology and Surveillance Branch.

Although patient #1019 was first diagnosed with Kaposi's sarcoma in December 1981, the SFDPH did not begin periodic updates on his health status until 1983, at which time he was reportedly being treated with interferon in

New York City. A year and a half later it was noted that patient #1019 remained on "Intravenous-Interferon with increasing lesions [but] no new diagnosis," and in 1985 his New York physician informed the SFDPH that he was "doing relatively well." Shortly thereafter however, the patient returned to San Francisco in search of a "new experimental R_x" and informed the health department that he planned to remain in the city. There was no additional documentation for case #1019 until his death certificate arrived from New York City; he passed away from "bronchopneumonia; AIDS; and cryptococcal meningitis" in 1987. The latter diagnosis was amended to this man's report form along with a diagnosis of PCP; the determination that patient #1019 suffered from *Pneumocystis carinii* pneumonia was presumably made post-mortem after an (undocumented) autopsy or was a presumptive diagnosis inferred from "bronchopneumonia."

Case #1020: This 31-year-old man was diagnosed with *Pneumocystis carinii* pneumonia in December 1981 while living out of state. Although his case file states that the patient had been "in New York from September 1980 . . . until October 1982" (shortly before his death), all the same the SFDPH recorded a San Francisco address for case #1020 and designated a census tract in the city to correspond to his diagnosis. In laboratory tests conducted several months before he died, the patient tested positive for infections with cytomegalovirus, herpes, adenovirus (one cause of respiratory disease), and an "atypical mycobacterium in his bone marrow." One month after returning to San Francisco, he died of "respiratory arrest; disseminated mycobacterium intracellulare; [and] AIDS" at the age of 32. "Cachexia" (physical wasting and malnutrition) was listed as yet "another condition contributing to but not related to the immediate cause of death."

Case #1021: This 40-year-old clerk was diagnosed with *Pneumocystis carinii* pneumonia in December 1981 and reported by the SFDPH with "Risk Factors: Sexual Preference Gay." Although the patient was too ill to endure the CDC's 25-page interview, his roommate agreed to assist in completing the questionnaire. This friend gave little information about the patient's past medical history or previous medications, and he volunteered nothing about the patient's sexual behavior. The roommate did seem to have intimate knowledge of the patient's use of recreational drugs, however, reporting that he smoked and drank on a daily basis until he was diagnosed with pneumonia, and that he used marijuana, cocaine, and unlabeled bottles of poppers on a monthly basis preceding his illness. The roommate also reported that the patient injected "speed" intravenously several times a month; in other words, the man's risk factor for AIDS should have been designated "Gay Intravenous Drug User," not "Sexual Preference: Gay."

Additional information volunteered about patient #1021 included the fact that he earned between $20,000 and $30,000 annually, and that he had recently traveled to "Australia and Brazil." A SFDPH surveillance officer subsequently amended this abbreviated travel history with the comment "New York, Fire

Island 1981?" citing a local doctor (not the patient's primary physician) for the tip. Moreover, for the first time thus far in a patient's ACR file, laboratory data included at the time of this patient's PCP diagnosis confirmed that patient #1021 "has a markedly decreased percentage of T-cells. The latter indicates severe cellular immunosuppression."

Patient #1021 never recovered subsequent to being diagnosed with AIDS and died approximately two months later from "septic shock; pulmonary failure; [and] immunodeficiency," complicated by other contributing conditions including "*pneumocystis* pneumonia and renal failure." In fact, according to the roommate's comments in the CDC interview, the patient had been diagnosed with glomerulonephritis (an acute inflammation of the kidneys) just two months before coming down with *Pneumocystis carinii* pneumonia.

Case #1022: This 48-year-old member of the hepatitis B study was diagnosed with Kaposi's sarcoma in December 1981. The AER form noted that his risk factor for the disease was that he was gay, and reported that he had "contact with a Los Angeles [AIDS] case?" Although the patient consented to be interviewed by the CDC, the questionnaire itself no longer remains in his file. Once again, I relied on medical records that begin well before AIDS was discovered for providing some context for this man's medical problems.

The first chart entry is dated in late 1977 at a time when the patient had "just quit heavy ETOH [alcohol]," and was noted to "smoke two packs per day times 35 years." Although he had no health complaints and his family history was unremarkable, the attending physician wrote "ETOH [alcohol] abuse; chronic smoker," and recommended that the patient continue to abstain from drinking and quit smoking.

During the next two and a half years the patient had few medical complaints other than an allergic reaction to a meal and a sore throat that went away. By the spring of 1980, however, he had developed a rather severe infection on his scalp and shoulders and was treated for the next six months with a variety of antibiotics. In the late summer of 1980, his physician noted that the patient's "back was clear except for one papule. . . . Will biopsy if no change in two weeks." A skin punch was taken the following month and, although nothing was documented regarding this biopsy, patient #1022 continued to receive treatment for a staph infection on his scalp; he remained heavily medicated with antibiotics throughout the remainder of 1980.

When seen again in January 1981, physicians noted that his VDRL (syphilis) test was "positive," and case #1022 acknowledged that he had the disease a "long time ago." Doctors concluded that it was most likely that the patient's positive VDRL test was attributable to this previous infection, and no treatment was prescribed. Somewhere around this same time, the patient completed a formal review of his prior medical history, and, contrary to the information documented during his first clinic visit, he reported a significant family history of cancer, kidney disease, and alcoholism. Moreover, both parents had died when they were just several years older than the patient was at this time.

Case #1022 reported a litany of medical problems during this review: a "chronic cough and shortness of breath," prior diagnoses of "liver disease [cirrhosis, hepatitis]" and "venereal disease," and a previous history of alcoholism and a "cancer or tumor." With respect to the latter event, the patient was apparently referring to an operation for a "benign breast tumor" some 15 years previously. Patient #1022 was also currently undergoing treatment for "emotional problems" and stated that he was "now having serious or disturbing problems with: financial matters." As a final note, the physician observed that this 48-year-old man had "clinically impaired hearing" on his left side.

Patient #1022 continued to be treated for bacterial infections of his skin and scalp throughout the spring of 1981. In May (1981) he was diagnosed with intestinal parasites and treated with antibiotics specific for giardia; within a month and a half the giardia infection was gone, but patient #1022 had returned to the hospital because he had contracted gonorrhea proctitis in the interim. He was treated with 5 million units of penicillin. It was now late June 1981, and the San Francisco Department of Public Health had just begun surveillance for AIDS subsequent to the publication of the CDC's *Morbidity and Mortality Report* on June 5.

When patient #1022 returned to the hospital in July for follow-up he was referred to for the first time as a "48 year-old Gay male," and his "multiple gastrointestinal infections over the past two months" were reclassified as "gay bowel syndrome." The physician prescribed Pepto-Bismal and Lomotil as palliative treatments, but noted that he would consider yet another antibiotic if the patient continued to test positive for giardia.

For the next four months there were no entries in this patient's medical chart, but a letter from his primary physician to another Bay Area doctor summarized patient #1022's recent medical problems. The letter is intriguing because it introduces the conundrum that the patient was *presumptively* diagnosed for intestinal parasites on multiple occasions and treated with extraordinarily potent antibiotics for six consecutive months without any evidence of a pathogen being present. During this time he lost approximately 20 pounds and the diarrhea resolved; but alas, shortly thereafter the patient developed additional complications. In December 1981, he was seen for a fever of 102° and found to have anemia, "adenopathy? [and] Hepatosplenomegaly [an enlarged spleen]." Differential diagnoses for patient #1022 included: "lues, cytomegalovirus, Kaposi's, tuberculosis [or] fungus, a liver abscess [and] lymphoma." The patient was immediately admitted to the hospital for a liver scan, a lymph node biopsy, and additional tests; the attending physician noted at the time that he was taking Tylenol with codeine "for fever," but "no other medications save occasional Quaaludes."

A week later, the lymph node biopsy returned positive for a diagnosis of Kaposi's sarcoma. And during a physical exam his physician observed that the patient had "sundamaged skin, especially on his face and chest," and described "two . . . red papules minimally infiltrating [the patient's] left chest; one above the nipple, one below." His assessment: "consistent with Kaposi's in young homosexuals." Though acknowledging that he had "no chart" to reference when he examined this "homosexual," had the physician reviewed said medical records he would have seen that these two red papules were located in the very site where the patient had undergone surgery in 1963 for a "benign [breast] tumor" and that the patient (and several family members) was predisposed to developing abnormal growths in this very tissue.

Patient #1022 was immediately admitted to the hospital and scheduled for intravenous chemotherapy that night for a diagnosis of "Kaposi's sarcoma; secondary diagnoses include: tachycardia, pancytopenia, diarrhea." In his discharge summary, his "habits [and] social history" were characterized as follows: "tobacco, two to three packs daily since age seven; ethanol—reformed alcoholic; no IV drug use . . . indeterminate history of recreational drug use . . . Gay. Has no steady partner. Frequents the baths about two times per week."

The patient underwent chemotherapy (and a transfusion due to problems with his red blood cell count) but developed an allergic reaction to bleomycin, one of the drugs used during the infusion. Subsequently readmitted to the hospital in late December 1981 complaining of a sore throat, weight loss, and difficulty swallowing, he was diagnosed with a Candida infection in his esophagus.

While hospitalized, patient #1022 began to suffer from bloody diarrhea, presumed to be a result of therapy; thus all "antibiotics were discontinued except for Septra and amphotericin." When the patient then developed pain in his abdomen, appendicitis was suspected. This latter event "spontaneously resolved" but further tests revealed that "the percentage of his T-cells appeared decreased." Following a brief rebound the patient was deemed healthy enough for a second course of chemotherapy; these infusions again contained bleomycin, the drug that precipitated an allergic "drug sensitivity" when used previously in the same patient. Patient #1022 was discharged to his home on the antibiotic TMP-SMX/Septra, a drug that his physician recommended the "patient needed to be on . . . for life as *Pneumocystis carinii* pneumonia prophylaxis."

Within a week of being released from the hospital the patient broke out with "peri-anal herpes." Concurrently, physicians noted a "secondary diagnosis" of "immuno-compromised secondary to chemotherapy for KS," and the patient was repeatedly transfused. Although suffering from fevers and a whole body rash, by March 1982 his doctors concluded that "it is clearly risky to treat this patient but it is obvious he will not survive unless we try." He received additional transfusions and infusions of chemotherapy "with much improvement" but by the following month the patient was again having "trouble swallowing" and "his platelets continued to drop."[8] This 49-year-old man died several weeks later with "widespread Kaposi's sarcoma"; he had survived slightly more than four months following his initial AIDS diagnosis.

Case #1023: This 30-year-old unemployed clerical worker was diagnosed with *Pneumocystis carinii* pneumonia in December 1981. Though the SFDPH stated on the patient's ACR form that patient #1023 had "no T-cell subset confirmation" at the time of his diagnosis and subsequent hospitalization, disease surveillance officers indicated that they had "multiple slide confirmations" of Kaposi's sarcoma; remarkably, this latter KS diagnosis was not annotated to the patient's AIDS case report form as a second AIDS diagnosis. However, SFDPH investigators did methodically amend his case file with notes indicating that the patient had engaged in "sexual contact" with another AIDS case two years previously, albeit acknowledging that he had maintained a "low sex profile ('Gay—denies in last six months')" and a "low drug profile ('some Coke, grass, amyl occasionally')" more recently. Patient #1023 was reported with "Risk Factors: Sexual Preference Gay [and] IV drug abuse positive for 'some Coke.'" This 30-year-old man died less than two months after his initial diagnosis with *Pneumocystis carinii* pneumonia; in the absence of medical records, I was unable to resolve the ambiguity surrounding his alleged diagnosis with Kaposi's sarcoma.

Case #1024: The final AIDS case reported in San Francisco during the first year of surveillance for the new syndrome of immune deficiency played a seminal role in confirming the theoretical hypothesis that AIDS was an infectious disease spread through body fluids and establishing that this was a disease with a singularly unique and extended latent asymptomatic phase. But the SFDPH knew remarkably little about patient #1024 given the extraordinary importance attached to this man, who was retrospectively identified as a blood donor for the first transfusion-associated AIDS case in the United States.

The ACR file for patient #1024 contained the following abbreviated information. This 47-year-old "heterosexual" was diagnosed with *Pneumocystis carinii* pneumonia in December 1981, and reported as an AIDS case in San Francisco the same month. He subsequently developed " 'cotton-wool' retinal patches," indicative of an eye infection caused by cytomegalovirus. Eight months after his initial PCP diagnosis, patient #1024 died of "encephalitis [and] severe Acquired Immunodeficiency." No special theoretical significance was attached to this case either at the offices of the San Francisco Department of Public Health or the Centers for Disease Control in Atlanta until almost four months after the patient's death.

It was then, in November of 1982, that Dr. Selma Dritz, the assistant director of the Bureau of Communicable Disease Control of the SFDPH, retrospectively identified Case #1024 as one of the blood donors linked to the first transfusion-associated AIDS case reported in the United States, a male infant with Rh factor disease.[9] This seminal transfusion-associated AIDS case associated with a baby diagnosed in San Francisco catalyzed public health interventions to protect the U.S. (and global) blood supply from further contamination and accelerated research for the specific virus that caused acquired immune deficiency syndrome.

In an oral history published by the Bancroft Library at the University of California at Berkeley in 1992, Dr. Dritz recalled this pivotal theoretical juncture in the search to find the cause of AIDS; the moment when public health officials dismissed rival hypotheses of immune-system overload and drug-induced immune suppression, and unanimously embraced the theory that a specific infectious virus was the cause of this disease:

Suspicions of a Transmissible Agent

Dritz: Now, when you have so many people in close contact, so easily visible to each other, and the police aren't bothering you, there's a lot of [sexual][10] activity. If you have a transmissible disease, that's where it's going to be transmitted. We had proved that gays transmit the enteric diseases, so we were beginning to be almost certain that with this, too, we had a transmissible disease.

Hughes: How early do you think you could say that?

Dritz: Well, by the end of '82 we had the case of the baby at UCSF infected through a blood transfusion. That was sort of the nail in the coffin, as far as we were concerned, as proof that AIDS was a blood-transmissible disease. We didn't know *what* was being transmitted yet, but we knew something was being transmitted. . . .

Hughes: You mentioned your diagrams of transmission. Was he [AIDS patient Gaetan Dugas][11] the first that reinforced the idea of a transmissible agent?

Dritz: I had a lot [of indication] that it looked like AIDS could be transmissible. There was all this contact among these men, and they all had the disease, one kind or another. On the other hand, all of these men were having other contacts, too, and we didn't know then that the incubation period was a long number of years in some cases.

Hughes: Right. And they were maybe using the same poppers or—

Dritz: Whatever, yes. And we didn't have the answer on the poppers yet, because CDC was still waiting for money for a statistician to run the computer analysis on the questionnaire. So the problem then was to test the rest of our theories about transmission, and that didn't happen until the end of '82 . . .

Hughes: With Art Ammann's baby. [UCSF doctor who reported the pediatric case]

Dritz: Let's go on to Art Ammann's baby, because that was where we knew we had an infectious disease. Well, we had the hemophiliacs, too—we knew something was being transmitted into the bloodstream.

Hughes: You have spoken of Art Ammann's baby as the nail that sealed the coffin. Tell me why it was so conclusive.

Dritz: Well, we had Gaetan Dugas, presumptive evidence. We had hemophiliacs, presumptive evidence, although they were not in direct contact with gay men. They were not in direct sexual contact with anybody, except their own wives. They were not getting blood transfusions, but they were using Factor VIII and Factor IX, which are made from pooled human plasma . . . The only thing that we, the scientific community, could see that was common with the hemophiliacs and the gay people who were apparently getting injected with the virus was that they must be getting it from plasma. So that was a presumptive, a very terrifying presumptive, suggestion that it was a virus in the bloodstream of infected persons.[12]

Now, Art Ammann had the idea . . .[12] He said, "I've checked this baby back and forth for combined immune deficiency," which is the congenital form. . . . Well, "this one," he said, "isn't characteristic. . . . And yet this kid is getting diseases one after the other. His immune system is down. Maybe it's like AIDS. He did have blood transfusions . . ."

Because Ammann thought it was AIDS and I was working the AIDS problem in the department, he called me. So I called the Irwin Memorial Blood Bank. Of course, they cooperated. . . . We got the thirteen donors' names, and right in the middle of them was number seven, an AIDS patient in San Francisco, already dead. I can still see it on that yellow page that Herb Perkins sent me. I won't use the patient's name that I recognized from my AIDS case file. And the same birthdate; there wasn't any question that the donor was our AIDS patient.

So I called Art Ammann and I told him that the blood donor was an HIV case. This was November of '82. The man had already died, vehemently denying that he was gay. That was not true. We proved it later from his medical records. . . .

I called Herb Perkins at the blood bank. He was medical director of the Irwin Memorial Blood Bank. I told him what we had. He must have had a heart attack. . . .

Hughes: Because the significance must have hit both of you: AIDS was transmitted by blood.

Dritz: Oh, yes. Well, it hit Art Ammann too, because at UCSF they were transfusing a lot of babies with Rh factor problems. And transfused adults also had to be considered at risk . . . So then I called CDC and told them this new development, and Harold Jaffe talked to me on the phone. He said, "Oh, Gads! We've been afraid of it . . ." Because with the hemophiliacs getting it, we'd already been afraid . . .[13]

Randy Shilts narrated Dritz's subsequent investigation of Case #1024, nearly one year after this self-identified heterosexual blood donor had been reported as an AIDS case in San Francisco [my comments in brackets]:

Dritz contacted the Irwin Memorial Blood Bank, which had supplied all of the baby's blood. In the early days of November [1982], the bank completed its records search. . . . Dritz's eyes froze on the name of one donor. She recognized it as the socially prominent international trade consultant who had died of encephalitis in August, the one who so vehemently had denied being gay . . .

Dritz . . . had the public health to worry about and there was still a troubling aspect to this case. The donor, the blue-blood who had died in August, insisted to the end that he was heterosexual. The case for blood transmission of AIDS had to be made as clearly as possible if health authorities were going to get about the business of saving lives, Dritz thought. The man's disputed sexual orientation only muddied the scenario. He certainly was not a prime suspect for sharing needles in some shooting gallery. He was probably gay, like 98% of the city's other AIDS cases. . . .[14]

Dr. Dave Auerback, one of the CDC's Epidemiological Intelligence Service officers, went to see the donor's brother. Like Dritz, Auerbach also had previously interviewed the recalcitrant AIDS sufferer who had so vehemently denied being gay during their various epidemiological investigations. The brother was more cooperative, . . . showing Auerbach a small black address book.

Back at Public Health, Dritz leafed through the pages eagerly, thankful once again that she was born so nosy. Under "B," Dritz saw a name she recognized. . . . Dr. Bud Boucher was one of the first local physicians to direct a practice specifically at gay men. . . . [Boucher] pulled that patient's files without hesitation. The donor only came to Boucher for those messy little troubles that he didn't want to tell the socially prominent physician handling his routine medical care. Among those problems was a case of rectal gonorrhea back in 1980. The mystery was solved.[15]

As a consequence of this investigation by the Centers of Disease Control and Dr. Dritz at the SFDPH, the ACR form for case #1024 was officially changed from "Heterosexual (male)" to "Risk Factors: Sexual Preference Gay." But what is intriguing to me is that a rigorous investigation of the patient's alleged sexual orientation never officially took place until he was reported as the source of the first transfusion-associated AIDS case in the city (and in the nation). Certainly, if the patient was as "vehemently heterosexual" as claimed, no investigation could have taken place until after his death; in point of fact however, patient #1024 died in August 1982 and presumably the SFDPH and the CDC could have ferreted out details of his sexual life at that time had they been so inclined. But per Dr. Dritz's comments, the patient's "disputed sexual orientation" became salient only when it "muddied the scenario" and unnecessarily complicated the search to prove that AIDS was in fact blood-borne and thus a looming threat to the integrity of the nation's blood supply.

It is equally curious to me that no historical narrative recounting these events brings attention to the fact that this donor's blood was also transfused into a second child in San Francisco, a little girl who received a transfusion at UCSF at roughly the same time as the male infant with Rh factor disease. This child, who was also identified by name on the AER/ACR of case #1024 as a "recipient" of the donor's blood, has never been reported as an AIDS case in San Francisco.[16] Apparently, none of the other recipients of these contaminated blood products ever developed the disease in San Francisco or elsewhere to the best of my knowledge.[17]

Given their theoretical premise that AIDS was being transmitted by an infectious agent, public health officials were by necessity overly vigilant and cautious given any evidence of the occurrence of transfusion-associated AIDS in 1982, and rightly so. But an argument based on the reliability of material evidence in San Francisco (as it existed of the fall of 1982) supporting such a mode of transmission for AIDS seems less than compelling in hindsight. In point of fact, the San Francisco Department of Public Health did not report any additional transfusion-associated AIDS cases among Bay Area recipients of blood products throughout the remainder of 1982, 1983, or 1984. And this is hard to reconcile with the following orthodox claims and representations about the epidemiology of HIV and AIDS, the progression to AIDS among transfusion recipients, and the frequency with which "high-risk" populations in San Francisco donated blood:

1) transfusion-associated AIDS cases reportedly progress to the disease more rapidly than other AIDS cases (median estimates of 28 months);[18]

2) generally speaking, pediatric AIDS cases progress very rapidly from HIV seroconversion to full-blown AIDS and death;

3) in the early 1980s, San Francisco's gay community reportedly contributed 5 percent to 9 percent of all blood donations at the Irwin Memorial Blood Bank alone;[19] researchers later estimated that "these [HIV-infected] donations resulted in over 5300 transfused HIV-1-positive components";[20]

4) many AIDS patients reported in San Francisco during 1981 had donated blood; this became clear to me as I reviewed the case histories of the first 24 patients, and Randy Shilts reported that 10 or 11 of these patients were known to have donated blood in the Bay Area on one or more occasions preceding their illness;[21]

5) Dr. Selma Dritz also confirmed that "the people who will come into a plasmarpheresis center—which were all in the drug-sex Tenderloin area or south of Market [in San Francisco] will be those who are

TABLE 3 Summary Statistics of 24 AIDS Cases among Gay Men in San Francisco, July–December 1981

Residence & Census Tract	CDC Interviews vs. Chart Reviews vs. ACR file	Hepatitis B Study and Military Service	Initial (A1) AIDS Diagnosis	Age at Time of (A1) AIDS Diagnosis	Risk Initially Reported by SFDPH in 1981	Risk Reported after Investigation
12 SF census track ambiguities	5 interviews	9 hepattis B participants (vs. 11 reported in literature)	15 KS	Range: 23 years to 49 years	22 'Gay or Bisexual' Men	19 'Gay or Bisexual' Men
2 homeless	5 charts	5 prior military service	9 PCP		1 'Gay IVDU'	5 'Gay IVDUs'
5 dual residences in NY and SF	15 ACR review only		5 additional PCP diagnoses after treatment for 'AIDS'		1 'Hetero-sexual Man'	0 'Hetero-sexual Men'
Median:				**38.5 years**		
TOTAL:					24 Men	24 Men

probably a high-risk population anyhow, if they sell their blood for money."[22]

6) And finally, as I have already noted, many of the early AIDS patients belonged to the "high-risk" population of gay men enrolled in San Francisco's hepatitis B study. Researchers have estimated that approximately 6 percent of this cohort was HIV-positive as early as 1978, which rose to 19 percent in 1979, 33 percent in 1980, 44 percent in 1981, and finally 53 percent by 1982.[23]

Yet despite all of these claims about the prevalence of HIV-infected blood donors in San Francisco and the ominous potential for an unfettered contamination of blood supplies during the seven years preceding the use of HIV-antibody screening tests (1978–1985), only one transfusion-associated AIDS case was reported in the city in the last months of 1982, a male infant born with Rh factor disease. No additional TA-AIDS cases were reported until well into 1985. Surely this is extraordinary. Moreover, although it is certainly true that new TA-AIDS cases dramatically declined throughout the United States after 1985 when an HIV-antibody test was deployed to screen blood products, to a significant degree this trend of declining TA-AIDS cases is an artifact of surveillance practice and policy. Since the blood supply was deemed "safe" after 1985, TA-AIDS patients reported after that date were rigorously scrutinized for additional risk factors or earlier dates of infection; in one study cited, fully three-quarters of all TA-AIDS cases reportedly infected after 1985 were

TABLE 4 Survival from (A1) AIDS Diagnosis to Death for 24 AIDS Cases among Gay Men in San Francisco, July–December 1981

AIDS Cases by Risk after Investigation		Range of Survival in Months	Range of Survival in Months (median)
'Gay or Bisexual' Men (GM)	17 GM	0–62 months	18.26 months
'Gay or Bisexual IVDU' Men (GIVDU)	5 GIVDU	1.5–8 months	4.7 months
Aggregate Subtotal:	**22 Men**	**0–62 months**	**15.8 months**
Data Eliminated:*	2 GM		
TOTAL COHORT	**24 Men**		

*Two patients eliminated from analysis: one committed suicide, and the other was still living as of 1995.

reclassified to other modes of transmission or earlier dates of transfusion following reinvestigation.[24] Meanwhile, in classic tautological fashion, all transfusion-associated AIDS cases reportedly infected *prior* to 1985 were assumed to be legitimate by default, and no similarly rigorous investigation was required when reporting these cases.

In sum, many of the AIDS patients reported in San Francisco during the first several years of this epidemic had preexisting health problems (whether congenital or chronic) and/or engaged in risk practices that independently elevated the likelihood that they would experience premature disability or death (e.g., high levels of recreational drug abuse, injecting drug use, alcoholism, repeated and/or unresolved systemic infections).[25] However, the majority of these contributing factors to disease were elided from official surveillance reports and historical narratives on the epidemic that were intended for the lay public and the representation of a mysterious epidemic striking down previously healthy and relatively wealthy gay men persisted. Tables 3 and 4 comprise my attempt to concisely summarize these risk factors and vital statistics for the 24 AIDS patients discussed at length in this and the previous chapter.[26]

V

The Mechanics
of AIDS Surveillance

An Historical Critique of the Demography of Risk

Many HIV/AIDS dissidents have vociferously criticized official public health quantitative and qualitative representations of the AIDS epidemic. Robert Root-Bernstein and social scientists such as Murray and Payne, for example, claim that the risk factors and co-factors for the disease have been deliberately misrepresented in HIV/AIDS surveillance statistics. Root-Bernstein's fundamental premise is that "people . . . identified as being a high-risk for AIDS have a multitude of recognized immunosuppressive factors at work on them long before they encounter HIV, and quite often in its complete absence."[1] According to this view, HIV infection and AIDS themselves are opportunistic infections in populations that are already immune compromised for other reasons. And Peter Duesberg and several organizations comprising persons with AIDS (PWA) and long-term survivors (LTS or LTNPS) have undermined the CDC's AIDS case definition as clinically and rhetorically tautological.[2] They note that, for example, an HIV-positive person with a diminished number of CD4 T-cells is clinically diagnosed as an AIDS patient, but an HIV-negative person of similar clinical status is categorized as an aberrant patient with "CD4 T-cell lymphocytopenia"—that is, a person with no T-cells for no known reason. Similarly, an HIV-positive person with tuberculosis has AIDS, but an HIV-negative person merely has TB.

Some dissidents have also argued, albeit from different vantage points, that the construction of HIV as an inevitably fatal infection is not only empirically false but the genesis for a self-fulfilling prophesy when iatrogenic treatments such as AZT and its sister nucleoside analogues (DDI, DDC, etc.) are aggressively marketed and commonly prescribed to HIV-positive patients.[3] Despite their vastly divergent theoretical positions vis-à-vis the etiology of AIDS and the contribution of the "homosexual lifestyle" or co-factors to disease progression, the dissidents are almost of one voice in their criticisms of U.S. public health officials and global institutions such as the World Health Organization (WHO) for their official consensus that AIDS portends a threat to heterosexuals worldwide. Duesberg, Root-Bernstein, Michael Fumento, and others maintain that there was never credible evidence to suggest that the AIDS epidemic would spread beyond high-risk populations and evolve a similar heterosexual dynamic in industrialized countries. On this point, dissidents cut no slack to public health officials for their good intentions or prudence in cautiously assessing the potential risk for widespread heterosexual transmission of the disease in the West. Instead, they posit that advocates of major AIDS research institutions and prevention organizations (the Gay Men's Health Crisis of New York City, the San Francisco AIDS Foundation, AMFAR, among others) have been disingenuous about the risk of heterosexual intercourse as a mode of AIDS transmission from the moment of their institutional inception. In the words of one anonymous informant, the construction of AIDS as an "equal-opportunity disease" was an empirically vacuous slogan which emerged sui generis in 1985 as the calculated invention of a publicist at a prominent nonprofit AIDS organization—expressly designed to enhance the power and appeal of fund-raising efforts.[4] In the spring of 1996, the *Wall Street Journal* published an article confirming this thesis but placed the onus for an heterosexual AIDS prevention campaign on the Centers for Disease Control.

> In the summer of 1987, federal health officials made the fateful decision to bombard the public with a terrifying message: Anyone could get AIDS. While the message was technically true, it was also highly misleading. Everyone certainly faced some danger, but for most heterosexuals, the risk from a single act of sex was smaller than the risk of ever getting hit by lightning. In the U.S., the disease was, and remains, largely the scourge of gay men, intravenous drug users, their sex partners and their newborn children. . . . But nine years after the America Responds to AIDS campaign first hit the airwaves, many scientists and doctors are raising new questions. Increasingly, they worry that the everyone-gets-AIDS message—still trumpeted not only by government agencies but by celebrities and the media—is more than just dishonest: It is also having a perverse, potentially deadly effect on funding for AIDS prevention. The emphasis on the broad reach of the disease has virtually ensured that precious funds won't go where they are most needed. For instance, though homosexuals and intravenous drug users now account for 83% of all AIDS cases reported in the U.S., the federal AIDS-prevention budget includes no specific allocation for programs for homosexual and bisexual men. . . . Much of the CDC's $584 million AIDS-prevention budget goes instead to programs to combat the disease among heterosexual women, college students and others who face a relatively low risk of becoming infected. And needle-exchange programs, widely seen as among the most effective methods available in fighting infection among drug users, are denied any federal funding.[5]

One must understand the way in which new AIDS cases are captured in order to understand the inherent biases in surveillance practices and policies that systematically tend to attribute risk for HIV infection predominantly to sexual intercourse thereby eliding multiple risk factors for AIDS from official publications and AIDS case reports. The process, practice, and politics of AIDS surveillance is illustrated below via an ethnography at San Francisco's AIDS Seroepidemiology and Surveillance Branch.

Fieldwork at the ASSB and SFGH, July 1994–May 1995

As of 1994, active surveillance for AIDS cases was being conducted at the following health facilities in San Francisco (with the initial year that surveillance began noted in parentheses). The list is not a comprehensive one of all hospitals and clinics in the region for two reasons: 1) the Department of Public Health must negotiate permission to report AIDS cases from each facility and, 2) because of budget and labor constraints, only those facilities that have historically reported a significant AIDS caseload merit the investment in active surveillance by a designated disease control investigator.

- San Francisco General Hospital (1984)
- The University of California at San Francisco (passive 1984; active 1989)
- Office of Vital Statistics (1984)
  Located at the San Francisco Department of Public Health at 101 Grove. Staff at Vital Statistics conducted passive surveillance for AIDS between 1984 and 1988—in other words, the office itself took on the responsibility for reviewing and reporting any death certificates that looked suspicious for an AIDS diagnosis. Active surveillance began in 1989, when the San Francisco Department of Health assigned a disease control investigator to review all death certificates at the end of each week. Data derived from vital statistics is always slightly out of date, as there is approximately a two-week reporting delay from the time an individual dies to the date at which a death certificate is available for review.
- Conant Center (1985)
  The city Department of Public Health performed active surveillance for AIDS cases at this location continuously for four years as part of its activities at the University of California at San Francisco. Surveillance was interrupted between 1989 and 1991 and then resumed; it has continued to the present.
- Kaiser Hospital (1985)
- Irwin Memorial Blood Bank (1987)
  The San Francisco Department of Public Health checks records at the blood bank to ascertain if reported AIDS cases have ever donated blood. Staff at the blood bank are responsible for identifying and arranging counseling (a process called "look-back") for any known recipients of blood products from a diagnosed AIDS patient.
- R.K. Davies Medical Center (1989)
- Children's Hospital, also known as California Pacific Medical (1989)

- Pacific Presbyterian Hospital (1989)
  This hospital's active surveillance continued even after the hospital merged with Children's Hospital in 1992 under the consolidated title of California Pacific Medical.
- Mt. Zion Hospital (1991)
- St. Mary's Hospital (1992)
- The Tom Waddell Clinic (1992)
  Disease control investigators assigned to San Francisco General Hospital captured new cases from this clinic prior to 1992.
- The Lyon-Martin Women's Health Center (1992)
  The ASSB receives lab results for patients attending this facility, then visits the center to review charts suspicious for AIDS diagnoses.
- Health Center 1 (1992)
  Prior to 1992, staff assigned to San Francisco General Hospital also conducted surveillance at this clinic on Seventeenth Street near Castro. Because of the large volume of cases reported from this location after 1992, the Health Department designated a paid staff member to conduct on-site active surveillance.
- City Clinic and various public health clinics
  This municipal clinic for sexually transmitted diseases in San Francisco is not technically an active surveillance site. Instead, the City Clinic sends the Department of Public Health all lab results (i.e., CD4 counts) for persons attending the clinic, and then SFDPH follows up on patients with CD4 t-cell counts meeting the surveillance case definition for AIDS.[6] Because the clinic does not have a sufficient caseload to justify on-site surveillance by a designated DCI, the City Clinic reports directly to SFDPH for any patients not captured by CD4 counts.[7]

AIDS cases are rarely reported from other health facilities in the city, and then only as a result of the personal initiative of staff or a physician; at the time of my research at ASSB the San Francisco Department of Public Health did not conduct active surveillance at any other locations. For instance, as of 1995, there had been only one reported AIDS patient from the Chinese Hospital; a transfusion recipient who was attended by a physician with staff privileges at the hospital. Any AIDS patients attending the Haight-Ashbury Free Clinic are usually captured when they seek treatment at San Francisco General Hospital. In the event that patients are diagnosed with AIDS at St. Lukes Hospital, St. Francis Hospital, or The Veterans Administration Hospital, a doctor or member of the hospital staff reports the patient directly to the AIDS Seroepidemiology and Surveillance Branch; in other words, these cases are reported by "passive surveillance." In total, the ASSB had attributed outpatient AIDS diagnoses to 165 private physicians in practice in San Francisco by the end of the first decade of the epidemic (1981–1992).[8]

Active AIDS Surveillance: Capturing Cases in the Field

As of 1995, national AIDS surveillance included AIDS cases reported from all 50 states, "the District of Columbia, and independent nations in association with the U.S." (Puerto Rico, the U.S. Virgin Islands, etc.) using a uniform surveillance case definition (Figure 8) and a standardized AIDS case report form.[9]

AIDS surveillance staff in San Francisco are legally prohibited from reporting or surveilling HIV-positive patients indiscriminately (as is true elsewhere in California and in states that prohibit mandatory HIV reporting by name).[10] Instead, the Public Health Department monitors only those patients who meet the CDC's definition for a clinical diagnosis of AIDS, a diagnosis delimited by three broad categories:

1) In the absence of all other causes of immunodeficiency (e.g., recent chemotherapy or a congenital immune defect), a person is considered to have AIDS by a definitive diagnosis of *Pneumocystis carinii* pneumonia, Kaposi's sarcoma, or nine other opportunistic infections, even in the absence of a positive HIV antibody test;[11]
2) Even in the presence of other causes for immunodeficiency, a person who has tested positive for the HIV antibody has AIDS if he or she is diagnosed with invasive cervical cancer, tuberculosis, HIV "dementia," lymphoma of the brain, HIV wasting syndrome, or one of nine other opportunistic infections;
3) Even in the presence of other causes for immunodeficiency, a person who has tested positive for the HIV antibody has AIDS if he or she has a single CD4 T-cell count with fewer than 200 T-cells/ul, or if CD4 T-cells comprise less than 14 percent of the person's total lymphocytes.[12]

While confirmation of HIV infection is arguably the most important laboratory documentation in a patient's medical chart, and the raison d'etre of current AIDS surveillance activities, due to the stigma of an AIDS diagnosis and early fears regarding patient confidentiality there is rarely hard evidence in a medical chart that a patient has in fact tested positive for the HIV antibody. Instead, this information is usually indirectly documented by citing patients' comments or doctors' notes to the effect that the patient is HIV-positive. Certainly in recent years it is more common for HIV tests to be enclosed in medical charts, but this is still true only for a minority of cases and more often seen at a county hospital like San Francisco General than at hospitals in the city where private physician care and health insurance is the norm. The unfortunate reality is that many AIDS patients at San Francisco General Hospital

I. **Without Laboratory Evidence Regarding HIV Infection**
   If laboratory tests for HIV were not performed or gave inconclusive results and the
   patient had no other cause of immunodeficiency listed in Section 1.A below, then any
   disease listed in Section 1.B indicates AIDS if it was diagnosed by a definitive method.
   A. **Causes of immunodeficiency that disqualify diseases as indicators of AIDS
      in the absence of laboratory evidence for HIV infection**
      1. high-dose or long-term systemic corticosteroid therapy or other immu-
         nosuppressive/cytotoxic therapy $\leq$ 3 months before the onset of the indi-
         cator disease
      2. any of the following diseases diagnosed $\leq$ 3 months after diagnosis of the
         indicator disease: Hodgkin's disease, non-Hodgkin's lymphoma (other
         than primary brain lymphoma), lymphocytic leukemia, multiple mye-
         loma, any other cancer of lymphorecticular or histiocytic tissue, or angio-
         immunoblastic lymphadenopathy
      3. a genetic (congenital) immunodeficiency syndrome or an acquired im-
         munodeficiency syndrome atypical of HIV infection, such as one involv-
         ing hypogammaglobulinemia
   B. **Indicator diseases diagnosed definitively**
      1. candidiasis of the esophagus, trachea, bronchi, or lungs
      2. cryptococcosis, extrapulmonary
      3. cryptosporidiosis with diarrhea persisting > 1 month
      4. cytomegalovirus disease of an organ other than liver, spleen, or lymph
         nodes in a patient > 1 month of age
      5. herpes simplex virus infection causing a mucocutaneous ulcer that per-
         sists longer than 1 month; or bronchitis, pneumonitis, or esophagitis for
         any duration affecting a patient > 1 month of age
      6. Kaposi's sarcoma affecting a patient < 60 years of age
      7. lymphoma of the brain (primary) affecting a patient < 60 years of age
      8. Mycobacterium avium complex or M. kansasii disease, disseminated (at a
         site other than or in addition to lungs, skin, or cervical or hilar lymph
         nodes)
      9. Pneumocystis carinii pneumonia
      10. progressive multifocal leukoencephalopathy
      11. toxoplasmosis of the brain affecting a patient >1 month of age
II. **With Laboratory Evidence for HIV Infection**
   *Regardless of the presence of other causes of immunodeficiency (I.A.), in the pres-
   ence of laboratory evidence of HIV infection, any disease listed above (I.B.) or
   below (II.A or II.B) indicates a diagnosis of AIDS.*
   A. **Indicator conditions diagnosed definitively**
      1. CD4 T-lymphocyte count < 200 cells/ul, or CD4 T-lymphocyte percent
         < 14
      2. recurrent pneumonia, more than 1 episode in a 1-year period
      3. cervical cancer, invasive
      4. coccidioidomycosis, disseminated (at a site other than or in addition to
         lungs or cervical or hilar lymph nodes)
      5. HIV encephalopathy (also called "HIV dementia," "AIDS dementia," or
         "subacute encephalitis due to HIV")
      6. histoplasmosis, disseminated (at a site other than or in addition to lungs
         or cervical or hilar lymph nodes)
      7. isosporiasis with diarrhea persisting >1 month

FIGURE 8   1993 AIDS Surveillance Definition

8. Kaposi's sarcoma at any age
9. lymphoma of the brain (primary) at any age
10. other non-Hodgkin's lymphoma of B-cell or unknown immunologic phenotype and the following histologic types:
    a: small noncleaved lymphoma (either Burkitt's or non-Burkitt's type)
    b: immunoblastic sarcoma (equivalent to any of the following, although not necessarily all in combination: immunoblastic lymphoma, large-cell lymphoma, diffuse histiocytic lymphoma, diffuse undifferentiated lymphoma, or high-grade lymphoma)
    Note: Lymphomas are not included here if they are of T-cell immunologic phenotype or their histologic type is not described or is described as "lymphocytic," "lymphoblastic," "small cleaved," or "plasmacytoid lymphocytic"
11. any mycobacterial disease caused by mycobacteria other than M. tuberculosis, disseminated (at a site other or in addition to lungs, skin, or cervical or hilar lymph nodes)
12. disease caused by M. tuberculosis, pulmonary or extrapulmonary
13. salmonella (nontyphoid) septicemia, recurrent
14. HIV wasting syndrome (emaciation, "slim disease")

B. **Indicator diseases diagnosed presumptively**
Note: Given the seriousness of diseases indicative of AIDS, it is generally important to diagnose them definitively, especially when therapy that would be used may have serious side effects or when definitive diagnosis is needed for eligibility for antiretroviral therapy. Nonetheless, in some situations, a patient's condition will not permit the performance of definitive tests. In other situations, accepted clinical practice may be to diagnose presumptively based on the presence of characteristic clinical and laboratory abnormalities.

1. recurrent pneumonia, more than 1 episode in a 1-year period
2. candidiasis of the esophagus
3. cytomegalovirus retinitis with loss of vision
4. Kaposi's sarcoma
5. M. tuberculosis, pulmonary
6. mycobacterial disease (acid-fast bacilli with species not identified by culture), disseminated (involving at least one site other than or in addition to lungs, skin, or cervical or hilar lymph nodes)
7. Pneumocystis carinii pneumonia
8. toxoplasmosis of the brain affecting a patient >1 month of age

III. **With Laboratory Evidence against HIV Infection**
With laboratory test results negative for HIV infection, a diagnosis of AIDS for surveillance purposes is ruled out unless:

A. **all the other causes of immunodeficiency listed in Section 1.A are excluded; AND**

B. **the patient has had either:**
1. Pneumocystis carinii pneumonia diagnosed by a definitive method; OR
2. a. any of the other diseases indicative of AIDS listed above in Section 1.B diagnosed by a definitive method; AND
   b. a T-helper/inducer (CD4) lymphocyte count <400/mm^3.

FIGURE 8 Continued
Source: Reprinted from San Francisco Department of Public Health, "1993 Revision of the HIV Infection Classification System and the AIDS Surveillance Definition," *San Francisco Epidemiologic Bulletin* 9, no. 1 (January 1993): 2–3.

(which has reported 35 percent of all AIDS cases in the city) are medically indigent, and the state requires that a person is verifiably/certifiably HIV-positive before they are eligible for coverage of certain medical expenses and/or disability claims. An individual with private health care may or may not need such documentation.

As the ELISA test for the detection of HIV antibodies was not commercially available until 1985, and not immediately in widespread use, none of the patients in the early years of the AIDS epidemic could have been documented as HIV-positive, unless of course they survived until 1986 or 1987. And in San Francisco several men diagnosed with AIDS in the early 1980s did just that. Consequently, the CDC enrolled a subset of these men into a national study on long-term survivors. Members of the cohort underwent an interview and extensive immunological tests, which included various tests for the HIV antibody and for the virus antigen itself. My access to these data was extraordinarily limited and haphazard; as was true for the 1981–1982 CDC study of the earliest AIDS patients in the country, all of the interview schedules and data have disappeared from San Francisco's files—a signed consent form is usually the only evidence that remains in a patient's file to indicate that he was enrolled in these studies. However, serendipitous exceptions to this general observation did occur. When I was reviewing the first 118 AIDS cases in the city, I even uncovered results of all the blood work for one individual enrolled in the long-term survivors study; imagine my surprise when the CDC's own documentation indicated that his culture was HIV-negative despite his AIDS diagnosis. Evidence that "HIV-negative AIDS" exists? Not necessarily, according to Kevin McKinney of the ASSB, whom I spoke with about the lab tests during my fieldwork:

McKinney: The CDC's lab probably screwed up the culture. What year was it done?
Author: 1987.
McKinney: I suppose you can regularly get HIV culture from venipuncture blood, and I think probably the virus techniques have improved over the years, but we regularly disregarded HIV-negative culture results, if you had an HIV antibody positive test. I received some training around that time from virologists at the Department of Public Health. I worked on some studies for them and . . . it's just the impression I got that you could expect to get an HIV-negative culture due to low levels of the virus in circulating blood.
Author: So it was significant if you got an HIV-positive culture but not that significant if you got an HIV-negative culture?
McKinney: Yeah.

Again, I reiterate that the veracity of this statement is not my concern here as Mr. McKinney's comments are reasonable and frequently echoed by other researchers in the field; it *is* hard to culture HIV from peripheral blood cells. What interests me is the way in which interpretive ambiguities are resolved during surveillance work always in favor of the theory that HIV, and HIV alone, is the cause of AIDS (and if we can't find it, it's because we don't have the right technology). Ambiguities are resolved in the direction of male-to-male sexual transmission of the disease and in the direction of aggrandizing the actual numbers of cases reported and the size of the populations at risk for the disease. Consistently during my fieldwork these trends appeared and reappeared.

I can best illustrate the process and practices of active surveillance for AIDS cases in San Francisco by detailing the procedures I followed as a disease control investigator at San Francisco General Hospital, which accounts for approximately 35 percent of all AIDS cases reported in the city (and half of those associated with intravenous drug use) since the beginning of the epidemic. An investigator assigned to SFGH discovers a patient who may have AIDS by one of four primary avenues: (1) by reviewing computer printouts of CD4 T-cell counts; (2) by reviewing the organisms cultured from patients at the hospital's Microbiology/*Pneumocystis carinii* pneumonia laboratories; (3) by reviewing surgical reports at the pathology laboratory; and (4) by cross-referencing the names of patients admitted to the AIDS Ward at San Francisco General Hospital against AIDS case files at the AIDS Seroepidemiology and Surveillance Branch. Each of these techniques for capturing new cases and updating the health status of reported AIDS patients is discussed in greater depth below.

1. CD4 Results: Since the discovery of AIDS in 1981, the preeminent clinical sign of the disease has been either a relative or an absolute loss of a type of white blood cell called a CD4 T-lymphocyte. CD4 T-cells are specialized white blood cells that signal the host's immune system to defend the body against a foreign pathogen. The fact that these cells are either absent or dysfunctional in the circulating bloodstream of an AIDS patient means that these individuals are "immune deficient," and their bodies no longer contain or resist invasive organisms—pathogens that would be vanquished in all likelihood by a person with a competent immune system. In sum, AIDS patients do not die from HIV or AIDS per se, but rather from one or more of the 27 different opportunistic infections that take advantage of a vulnerable host who is "compromised," and whose immune system cannot mount an adequate response.

As a disease control investigator in training I began my daily rounds at San Francisco General Hospital by retrieving a printout of CD4 results from the microbiology laboratory. The printout individually lists patients by name, medical record number, age, sex, and quantifies their CD4 T-cells, both in absolute numbers and as a percentage of total lymphocytes, e.g., Joe Smith MR# 032572 42 M CD4=180 [15%].

Mr. Joe Smith, a hypothetical patient, meets the current AIDS case definition because he has fewer than 200 CD4 T-cells per cubic milliliter of blood.

He is therefore registered as a potential AIDS case, pending further investigation to verify (a) whether his medical chart contains an HIV-positive test, and (b) whether this particular Joe Smith has already been reported as an AIDS cases in San Francisco.[13] For the moment, let me put aside any further investigation of the particularities of Mr. Smith or any other potential AIDS case as I finish my morning rounds at San Francisco General Hospital.

2. SFGH Microbiology: While in the lab I also pick up a sheaf of microbiology laboratory printouts to review later and then enter the cytology/parasitology laboratory to review logs for acid-fast bacteria, and results of cultures for tuberculosis, mycobacterium-avium, and *Pneumocystis carinii* pneumonia (PCP) produced from patient specimens obtained either by induced "spit" (sputum) or "swab" (bronchial lavage). All of the above are common opportunistic infections among AIDS patients; however, according to the disease control investigator training me, the reality is that "we rarely get new [AIDS] cases via the PCP lab these days unless it is someone who breaks through with PCP at a high CD4 count or someone who has never been in care before."[14] And as predicted, it was also my experience that the majority of these lab results were negative for the *Pneumocystis carinii* organism. For example, on a single day in July 1994 I noted that of five evaluations completed, only one culture was positive for PCP; the following day all six lab reports were negative. This seems to imply that the test is frequently requested by a physician on the basis of suspicious clinical symptoms and the fore-ordained expectation that a person with AIDS will develop this opportunistic infection; alternatively, physicians in San Francisco may be exceedingly cautious and run these tests as a matter of course to rule out latent infections.

An interesting example of the "construction" of an AIDS diagnosis occurred one day during my rounds in this laboratory. A sputum sample of "bloody pleural fluid" from a patient with a low CD4 count and no evidence of being HIV-positive was submitted to be cultured for *Pneumocystis carinii* pneumonia (PCP). As the lab technician was experiencing some difficulty in interpreting what was in this pleural fluid, she asked me whether this individual was known as an AIDS case at the Department of Public Health. I inquired, "So if you knew the patient was HIV-positive, would you be more inclined to think it was PCP?" And she responded, "Yeah, that would help, 'cause I don't personally think it is. But if he's an AIDS patient you know, that would be more evidence [for the diagnosis]." Due to confidentiality laws, I was unable to provide any information about our case files, and the matter was turned over to my supervisor. However, during my daily rounds later on that same week, the lab technician informed me that she had received the information she needed through alternative means, and that "it told me something, a little bit at least" to know that the patient had never been diagnosed with AIDS. Thus, *Pneumocystis carinii* pneumonia was dropped from the list of differential diagnoses for this patient, and the laboratory search for a culpable pathogen continued.

I do not mean to suggest that this incident is illustrative of how most, or indeed many, diagnoses of opportunistic infections are arrived at, but it does demonstrate how a conclusion about this particular ambiguous laboratory specimen was resolved tautologically. When a patient has been diagnosed with AIDS he is expected to develop pneumonia caused by the *Pneumocystis carinii* organism—in the event of an ambiguous lab sample, one diagnosis will be resolved by the other; PCP confirms an AIDS diagnosis, and an AIDS diagnosis confirms PCP. Moreover, if this patient belongs to a population perceived to be at high risk for contracting AIDS, the mere presumption of the presence of PCP in his sputum would be sufficient to confer an AIDS diagnosis on this man regardless of his HIV status and regardless of whether or not he was suffering from pneumonia caused by this particular organism.

3. SFGH Pathology: I continued on my rounds to the hospital's pathology lab, where the disease control investigator must review each and every pathology report for evidence suspicious for, or indicative of, an AIDS diagnosis: for example, cervical cancer in a young woman, or a biopsy report on Kaposi's sarcoma in a gay man. Again, very few of these pathology reports reveal previously undocumented AIDS cases; during rounds on a representative day in July 1994, I found that only one of 57 reports was even suggestive of an AIDS diagnosis.

4. The "AIDS Ward": The final stop on daily surveillance rounds at San Francisco General Hospital is a ward on the fifth floor, where I scan the inpatient tote board for names of AIDS patients that might have been missed via CD4 printouts, laboratory results, pathology reports, or reports from private physicians. This last stop completes the daily hospital circuit whereby a disease control investigator actively seeks information to update the health status of AIDS cases previously reported, and gleans sufficient information to begin follow-up on patients who may constitute new AIDS cases in San Francisco.

Follow-Up at the AIDS Seroepidemiology and Surveillance Branch

Once a pool of potential AIDS cases has been captured, the DCI returns to the AIDS Seroepidemiology and Surveillance Branch with a list of patient names and unique identifying information (e.g., corresponding medical record numbers and birthdate if known). This list of possible or probable AIDS patients is then cross-referenced against a set of files containing an AIDS case report for each of the 27,982 persons previously reported with the disease in San Francisco since the beginning of the epidemic (March 2002 data).[15]

The patient's identifying information from the pathology, PCP/microbiology labs and/or the CD4 printout (e.g., our hypothetical patient Mr. Joe Smith MR# 032572) is checked against these files to establish whether he has already been reported as an AIDS case. If a disease control investigator finds a matching file for the patient's name and date of birth, then relevant information such as the patient's CD4 count or diagnosis of an opportunistic infection is recorded in his/her file,[16] dated and encoded as an "health status update" (HSU), and recorded in a ledger to be entered into a computer database.[17] To protect patient confidentiality, by default, the computer software automatically assigns an AIDS case number (e.g., 01259) for each case entered and is thereby devoid of any identifiers, ensuring that it can never be used to search for, or collate, information on the basis of a patient's name.

If there is no AIDS case report for our hypothetical patient (Mr. Joe Smith with the low CD4 count), then the investigator checks a second set of files referred to as "out-of-jurisdiction" (OOJ) files which contain information on persons who were diagnosed with AIDS in another city or state before seeking treatment in San Francisco. Although these patients may in fact be current residents in the city, it is still the legal responsibility of the jurisdiction which initially reported him/her as an AIDS case to continue monitoring that patient's health status. So in the event that Joe Smith's name and birthdate does indeed match a case report in the OOJ files, then AIDS surveillance staff in San Francisco terminate any further follow-up.

Finally, if neither set of files yields an AIDS case report corresponding to this patient's name and birthdate, only then is this individual potentially a new San Francisco AIDS case. Under these circumstances, the DCI returns to SFGH (or the relevant diagnosing hospital) in order to obtain additional information needed to document a new AIDS case (e.g., evidence of an HIV antibody test; evidence of a diagnosis of an AIDS-associated opportunistic infection; evidence of risk factors for acquiring HIV).

Documenting and Reporting a New AIDS Case

Apropos the previous example cited, let us assume that after thorough investigation at the AIDS Seroepidemiology and Surveillance Branch we can find neither a previous AIDS case report nor an out-of-jurisdiction file corresponding to our hypothetical patient, Mr. Joe Smith (MR #032572), a 42-year-old male with fewer than 200 CD T-cells. This means that a disease control investigator must return to the diagnosing hospital to collect sufficient information for reporting Mr. Smith as a new AIDS case, resident in San Francisco. At SFGH, the DCI utilizes the hospital's computer database to search for Mr. Joe Smith's medical charts and verify his complete name, his address in the city (and a telephone number for "No Identified Risk [NIR] cases),[18] his date of birth, sex, age, race, and a record of the last date he was registered as a patient at the hospital. Armed with this electronic sketch of Mr. Smith and profiles for all other potential AIDS cases discovered during medical rounds, the disease control investigator now has sufficient identifying information to request the SFGH medical chart for each patient with an opportunistic infection or laboratory report suspicious for an AIDS diagnosis.

As medical charts are frequently signed out to treatment wards or clinicians on duty, there can be a reporting delay of new AIDS cases while a DCI waits a week or even several months for a chart to be located and returned to the medical records department. Once the chart arrives, at a bare minimum, the following questions must be answered to properly and thoroughly document an AIDS case in San Francisco:

- "(HIV Risk) How did this patient 'contract' AIDS?"[19]
- "What was the date and result of any HIV tests for this patient?"
- "What were the dates and results of all CD4 T-cell counts available for this patient?"
- "What was the date and nature of the initial AIDS diagnosis that this patient presented with?"
- "What treatments has this patient received to treat and prevent opportunistic infections associated with AIDS?"
- "What subsequent diagnoses of opportunistic infections or AIDS indicator conditions have been confirmed for this patient?"

As demonstrated in the example above from rounds in the microbiology lab, even relatively objective clinical diagnoses, such as a PCP culture, can be fraught with subjectivities; an organism in a petri dish is diagnosed as one pathogen if it was cultured from a known AIDS patient and diagnosed as another pathogen in the absence of an AIDS diagnosis. Even greater ambiguities attend the construction of AIDS surveillance knowledge from information abstracted from a patient's medical chart, however, as subjectivity is inherent to a process that abstracts data from the complexity of a patient's lived reality.

Establishing Risk for HIV Infection

Because a disease control investigator in AIDS surveillance is not granted hours or days on end to methodically comb through every page of a medical chart, the practice of documenting a patient's HIV risk usually means that the DCI officially reports the first explicit risk reported for the patient, or "the most likely risk" implied in the medical chart.[20] This is especially true for AIDS cases captured in 1992 and 1993, when the national caseload exploded as a result of the expanded surveillance definition and there was even less staff time available for DCIs to thoroughly research each case.[21]

These very real time constraints mean that multiple risk categories are not consistently researched and recorded for each AIDS case. For example, a hemophiliac who is also an intravenous drug user may be reported solely as a hemophiliac, or a heterosexual who had sexual intercourse with an IVDU may be reported solely as heterosexual contact. And even in the rare event that multiple risk categories are fortuitously captured during medical chart reviews, there are only limited and oblique mechanisms for systematically reporting this information.

As Kevin McKinney, San Francisco AIDS surveillance field unit coordinator, explains, "The CDC has a hierarchy of risk and it lists first the most likely mode of transmission: 'homosexual/bisexual' is classified as risk '1', a heterosexual intravenous drug user (IVDU) as '2,'[22] a gay intravenous drug user (GIVDU) as '3,' a hemophiliac as '4,' a heterosexual as '5,' et cetera." This hierarchy of risk is also encoded in the HIV-AIDS Reporting System (HARS) software, created by the CDC and used in-house at the AIDS Seroepidemiology and Surveillance Branch at SFDPH.

As there is no separate category for "hemophiliac and IVDU" I asked McKinney how an individual with these multiple risk factors would be classified, and he responded that this patient would be reported according to the CDC's hierarchy of risk; the primary risk factor is heterosexual intravenous drug use (Het IVDU), and secondarily the individual would be identified as an hemophiliac.[23] Also eliding any contribution of multiple risks to one's likelihood of contracting HIV/AIDS, there is no category of risk for "gay men who had sex with an IVDU," or "gay men who had transfusions," although sex with an injection-drug user is the second greatest risk for contracting AIDS among heterosexuals. Corresponding to this hierarchical pyramid of risk, the risk attributed to homosexual intercourse supersedes that of one or more blood transfusions, and, by default, only the highest priority risk for contracting HIV is recorded in the San Francisco database as the means by which a patient acquired AIDS.

Reducing a patient's HIV risk to one categorical variable in an arbitrary hierarchy of "less versus more risky" categories of behavior or identity obviously discounts the synergistic effect of a constellation of factors that can potentially compromise one's immunity to disease. Consequently, these surveillance practices explicitly construct official statistics that are systematically biased in the direction of overreporting male homosexual intercourse as a risk for HIV/AIDS. This reporting bias was even more explicit in the first five years of the epidemic, when the CDC did not even differentiate between gay and bisexual men who injected drugs and those who did not—the risk category for all male AIDS patients who engaged in homosexual intercourse even once after 1978 was homosexual/bisexual transmission. Not until 1985 was a separate category comprising "gay men who use intravenous drugs (GIVDU)" instituted to denote a distinct mode of transmitting AIDS; more evidence, as Lauritsen and Murray and Payne argue, supporting the thesis that from the very beginning of the AIDS epidemic the CDC defined male homosexuality as the most egregious threat to a man's health, to the exclusion of all other patient behaviors or clinical histories.[24]

TABLE 5 AIDS Cases by Hierarchical Risk Group and Probable Mode of HTLV-III/LAV Acquisition, First 1,000 Cases, San Francisco, 1981–1985

Acquisition	Risk Group	N	Total (%)
Sexual	Homosexual men	941	
	Bisexual men	41	
	Heterosexual contacts of persons in other risk groups	3	985 (99%)
Parenteral	Intravenous drug users	6	
	Blood transfusion recipients	3	9 (1%)
Perinatal	Children of mothers in risk groups	2	2 (<1%)
Unknown	No identified risk group*	4	4 (<1%)
			1,000

*Includes one Haitian
Source: City and County of San Francisco. Department of Public Health, Bureau of Communicable Disease Control, "AIDS in San Francisco: The First 1,000 Cases," *San Francisco Epidemiologic Bulletin* 1, 2 (October 1985).

I often heard that San Francisco's surveillance practices differed in this regard and that, from the very beginning of the epidemic, homosexual and bisexual men who injected drugs intravenously were consistently reported as gay IVDUs to distinguish them from other gay male AIDS cases. While this may be true theoretically, in practice many gay men who injected drugs were collated and reported within the generic male homosexual/bisexual transmission category, as exemplified by a report in the *San Francisco Epidemiologic Bulletin* updating information on the first 1,000 AIDS cases in the city. In the text of this summary on the first five years of the epidemic, the SFDPH reports that 13 percent (131) of the 982 homosexual/bisexual men reported in San Francisco as of October 1985 were gay men who had also injected drugs.[25] But all of the graphic representations used in the report attribute AIDS cases among gay IV drug users and gay transfusion recipients exclusively to "sexual acquisition," and tabulate them within the male "homosexual and bisexual" risk categories. In contrast, all six AIDS cases among heterosexual IV drug users are attributed to "parenteral acquisition" (Table 5).

Given the CDC's hierarchy of attributing risk whereby many surveillance departments did not count, and often do not consider, any other mode of viral transmission among homosexual/bisexual men, the San Francisco Public Health Department's contention "that sexual transmission is the primary mode of HTLV-III/LAV spread in the City" was a foregone and tautological conclusion.[26]

While it is theoretically possible for an astute DCI to capture multiple risk factors for an AIDS patient during a medical chart review and record these multiple risks in San Francisco's database by answering "yes" to questions such as "did this patient ever receive blood products" or "ever inject drugs," this is obviously an excessively cumbersome way to routinely enter and tabulate surveillance information and is therefore infrequently done. Nor does San Francisco's AIDS Seroepidemiology and Surveillance Branch publish any statistics of aggregate or multiple risks for the city's AIDS cases in its monthly or quarterly surveillance reports.[27]

Moreover, my review of an internal SFDPH biannual State Department of Health report on duplicate AIDS cases raises the possibility that there are geographical biases in surveillance practices or policies that aggrandize the risk for transmitting the disease via gay sex in different California jurisdictions. Let me first explain something about the source of this information. This biannual report is a computer list of duplicate AIDS cases throughout the state, identifying AIDS patients who have been simultaneously reported as official cases in San Francisco and in a second jurisdiction in California. Ostensibly, the list is used to resolve duplicate records and establish which jurisdiction has priority for updating the health status and vital statistics of an individual case and for counting the case in a city's official surveillance reports.

Instead, however, I used the state's list of duplicate AIDS cases to compare and contrast how San Francisco and other jurisdictions differentially attributed HIV/AIDS risk to the same individual. For instance, on August 17, 1994, the state Department of Health reported 46 duplicate AIDS cases in San Francisco with discordant transmission risk categories; this means that San Francisco disease control investigators reported the patient with one risk and another jurisdiction in California reported the same person with a different risk for acquiring HIV/AIDS. Although I had no means of knowing which jurisdiction had reported the patient's risk most accurately, the available data did demonstrate a systematic tendency on the part of San Francisco's surveillance department to attribute HIV transmission to "homosexuality/bisexuality." Almost half (46 percent of the discordant cases) were reported with a transmission risk of "gay/bisexual" in San Francisco, versus only 28 percent of these same patients in other counties. Meanwhile, other jurisdictions were almost twice as likely to identify cases as "gay intravenous drug users" (39 percent of discordant cases outside of San Francisco County versus 24 percent within the county).[28] These highly disparate results are disturbing, not only for the homosexual bias they illustrate, but also for the distortions they produce in the very data that are used to understand the risk factors, modes of transmission, and prevention of AIDS. If this report is representative in its characterization of jurisdictional biases in attributing HIV/AIDS risk, then statistics produced from these surveillance activities are imbued with fundamental flaws.

Perhaps one might argue that an AIDS patient would be more willing to admit to homosexual/bisexual behavior in San Francisco, thereby accounting for the greater percentage of discordant cases reported in that transmission category in the city versus other jurisdictions. But the same argument cannot account for the disparity in the figures for gay IVDUs. It seems unlikely to rationalize the greater incidence of GIVDU case reports in outlying jurisdictions by arguing that AIDS patients are more closeted about this behavior only while residing in San Francisco. Instead, these results can be explained only by acknowledging that San Francisco surveillance practice is systematically less rigorous in ferreting out IV drug abuse among homosexual/bisexual AIDS cases, having already documented the "primary" risk factor for the disease in these men.

Certainly my own review of case files for the first 24 AIDS cases reported in San Francisco in 1981 would support such a bias, as I found that approximately a half-dozen gay injection-drug users had been erroneously reported as "homosexual/bisexual men with no history of intravenous drug use" in the first six months of AIDS surveillance in the city. And the results of a random telephone survey of gay and bisexual men in San Francisco conducted by the San Francisco AIDS Foundation and Communications Technologies in 1989 seem to support a similar conclusion. That report found that 26 percent of all participants in the survey who had tested positive for the HIV antibody said they were either current or former intravenous drug users.[29] This figure is more than double the number published by the city Department of Public Health: approximately 10 percent of the cumulative total of homosexual/bisexual men with AIDS are listed as GIVDUs,[30] and more than triple the number of intravenous drug users that Dr. Winkelstein et al. reported in their population-based San Francisco Men's Health Study (8 percent of the HIV-positive men in this cohort were identified as GIVDUs in 1984).[31] I am not arguing for the veracity of the number produced by the San Francisco AIDS Foundation survey, nor am I positing that one of every four gay AIDS patients in San Francisco acquired the disease by injecting drugs. However, all three sources of information cited above suggest that official AIDS surveillance statistics for the city underreport the prevalence of injection-drug use among gay AIDS cases in the city. Every example that I have cited tends to move the data in one direction only; in no instance is there any indication of a countervailing tendency toward overreporting gay injection-drug users.

Patient "X"—Diagnosis Cryptosporidiosis

A conversation I had with several disease control investigators at San Francisco's AIDS Seroepidemiology and Surveillance Branch in 1994 provides further anecdotal confirmation of the point above. While I was engaged in entering the results from a recent CD4 T-cell count into a patient's chart as part of a health status update, a conversation ensued with three DCIs who made it abundantly clear that they were collectively reluctant to further stigmatize an AIDS patient by amending an AIDS case file to include information about the patient's history of injection-drug use.

The patient, 36 years old and a native of France, had recently received a lab test confirming a CD4 T-cell count of 20. I asked a disease control investigator working nearby whether there was any way to know if Patient X had been reported as an AIDS case in France. "No, we don't check that" was the reply. Continuing to review his AIDS case file, I noted that Patient X had 728 CD4 T-cells on his first lab test in 1991. It seemed logical to conclude that he had been tested for the HIV antibody at that time as well (or presumed to be at risk for AIDS); otherwise a CD4 test would never have been ordered. The next lab result available for this patient was from the fall of 1993; he reportedly had a CD4 T-cell count of 127 (11 percent), indicating a depletion that automatically confers an AIDS diagnosis.

This patient's progression to AIDS was anomalous, as according to orthodox theories of progression, an HIV-positive person will lose on average 100 CD4 T-cells per year; this patient had lost 600 CD4 T-cells in two years, a progression three times the rate of an average HIV-positive person. So my question was "What's going on with this guy? He progresses from relatively healthy (728 CD4 T-cells in 1991) to an AIDS diagnosis (127 CD4 T-cells in 1993) in two years and now, just one year later (in the fall of 1994), has only 20 CD4 T-cells left?"

I perused his chart for any major opportunistic infections that might account for this sudden decline, but Patient X had only one diagnosis—cryptosporidiosis (an opportunistic infection of the intestinal tract that causes diarrhea), which the patient reportedly contracted six months after he was diagnosed with AIDS in 1993. Other than the bout with "crypto," Patient X had been symptom-free. But I was in for a greater shock when I noticed that a disease control investigator had initialed the entry for the patient's date of death four days previously.

My attention was riveted by this exceptional case: a 36-year-old gay man, relatively healthy in 1991, was dead less than three years later. He represented such a stark contrast to a previous AIDS case that I had recently updated, an "average" bisexual male, of similar age, with 180 CD4 T-cells in 1991 and no opportunistic infections as of 1994. This second AIDS case was still living, but Patient X from France had already been buried.

Because it was too soon to have an official death certificate, the immediate cause of this patient's demise remained a mystery. One DCI speculated that Patient X "could have died of pancreatitis or something like that we don't count." I argued that this deserves some attention, however: if 20 percent of AIDS cases are dying of something that isn't counted, then doesn't this argue for an expanded AIDS definition with 31 opportunistic infections instead of 29? I then asked, "How many men have died like this patient, with their only AIDS-defining condition a low CD4 count and no opportunistic infections— they just drop dead?"[32]

One disease control investigator then informed me that he knew that Patient X had cryptosporidiosis "for sure," because he was a friend of the French man. Forging ahead I inquired, "But doesn't he have to have several positive lab slips in order to establish a crypto diagnosis?" The AIDS case report specifies that a patient must have cryptosporidiosis continuously present for one month in order for it to constitute an AIDS-defining condition. This question catalyzed a roundtable discussion about the vagaries of diagnosing cryptosporidisis, factors contributing to Patient X's rapid decline, and the way in which different people subjectively interpret risks for acquiring AIDS. I transcribed the conversation between myself and the three disease control investigators I spoke with—they are identified as DCI A, B, and C for convenience. Explanatory comments have been provided in brackets.

DCI A: Crypto is really hard to culture, you can test several times without finding it, so they probably just put down crypto when he continued to have watery diarrhea that wouldn't resolve with treatment.

DCI B: I know crypto killed him, because he lost like 50 pounds in the previous two months before he died . . . although everyone was really surprised at how rapidly he progressed. After he got back from Mexico with crypto he really declined.

Author: So he went to Mexico, and then he got sick?

DCI B: Well, actually he wasn't all that healthy before he went to Mexico.

Author: So what kind of health problems did he have before then?

DCI B: Well, he was the sort of guy who really liked to party a lot. He had injected drugs, and well . . . even after he got sick he never really took care of himself, and he sort of gave up. For instance, even after he got crypto he never took care of himself, and he went to the Gay Games [June 1994 in New York City] because he wanted to be there—and then he came back and was hospitalized.

Author: So that's when we [SFDPH] picked him up [in the summer of 1994], getting his CD4 count done here in San Francisco after he returned from the Gay Games. And he shot drugs?

DCI B: Yeah, well, I just know that as a friend . . . and he sort of just gave up and refused all help [health care] et cetera.

Author: But his file [the ACR] says his risk is sex with men.

DCI B: Yeah, well, I just know that because I was a friend; I knew that he had shot drugs.

Author: But you haven't changed the file to reflect that risk?

DCI B: Well . . . I don't like to change charts.

DCI A: [Comments directed to the author] You've got to realize that for us . . . when I see my friends in there I don't even want to open their charts. I mean it's different for everyone . . . some people just don't want to change charts of their friends. You've got to understand that people get emotionally burned out after years of doing this . . . and IVDU is the one thing that most people are the most reluctant to talk about.

Author: I can understand how one can get burned out from doing this work after one month, but in this case the chart is already open, it's of interest because he declined so quickly, and if we're trying to get accurate information on disease progression and co-factors of disease progression it's important that information in the chart reflect his risk. If he was unhealthy before he went to Mexico then it shortens the progression even more. I mean, he went from totally healthy [728 T-cells] to AIDS in two years, and now he's dead at age 36. That's terribly quick.

DCI C: Well, you've been here long enough to see that this data [documentation of CD4 counts and opportunistic infections] isn't very good.

Author: [Comments directed to DCI A]: But wait . . . if your friend was listed as a homosexual and he was actually a heterosexual, since you believe in "het cons" [heterosexual cases of AIDS], wouldn't you feel that it's important that he be correctly listed as a heterosexual so that money and research would be directed at the "Epidemic of Heterosexual AIDS" and the figures wouldn't say heterosexual transmission is 7 percent [when] it's actually 20 percent?

DCI A: Well, that's you. I don't change friends' charts ever.

DCI B: Well, I changed one once . . . but I don't remember which one or why. I don't know, I just don't like to.

Author: But aren't you concerned that incorrect risk information misdirects research and interferes with an understanding of disease progression that could empower "Steve" in San Francisco to make an informed choice about how to live his life and what might keep him living longer—"If I do this, or I don't do that, I'll live longer," instead of thinking "if I just don't share needles, it's OK if I inject this heroin."

DCI A: But you don't even know how long he shot drugs, or when he shot up.

DCI B: Well, I was in this support group with [Patient X], and he was open about everything, about IV drugs. And he was very clear . . . he had been depressed and in a very hard time in his life and that's when— he knew that he got it from unsafe sex.

Author: So had he always been "unsafe," let's say . . . for eight years before becoming positive?

DCI B: No, once or twice, he said. . . . He was depressed and he knew that he got it from unsafe sex.

At the conclusion of this conversation I reflected on the way in which surveillance "knowledge" such as this is negotiated, filtered through a sieve and distilled. Anecdotal information was sufficient to record the date of this patient's death, and implicit knowledge about the vagaries of culturing pathogens was sufficient to record a diagnosis of cryptosporidiosis despite the presence of only one lab result when, technically, two positive tests in sequential months are needed to confirm this particular opportunistic infection. But amending a chart with anecdotal information about intravenous drug use was strictly off-limits. Again, conceptually, from the very earliest weeks of the epidemic the predominant risk factor for acquiring and transmitting the disease was engaging in homosexual intercourse; not unhealthy behavior, preexisting medical complications, dismal health care, homelessness, or the complex synergy of various social ills.

Establishing Heterosexual HIV Risks and Resolving NIR Cases

The issue of the heterosexual transmission of HIV/AIDS, especially from women to men, is only slightly less sensitive than the subject of IV drug use. Surveillance practice regarding this mode of transmission is rife with political debate. According to San Francisco's AIDS surveillance supervisor Kevin McKinney, the city's policy is that "if someone is a member of the heterosexual community we classify them as NIRs [an AIDS case with 'no identified risk' for acquiring the disease] . . . and we continue to follow them, until we interview them, or until death" continuing to look for risk factors. However, in a discussion with several female DCIs in San Francisco regarding AIDS cases whose HIV risk factor was heterosexual contact, they categorically stated: "We believe in het cons." And they dissented with the city's practice of only reluctantly accepting female-to-male HIV transmission cases. In San Francisco, male AIDS patients are not officially reported as heterosexuals who acquired the disease from a woman unless they can identify a female partner who tests HIV-positive. Without this evidence, these men continue to be reported as AIDS cases with no identifiable risk for transmission.

Kevin McKinney differed slightly with the assessment of department policy by the female disease control investigators above however, and he added the following caveat about establishing a male heterosexual case of HIV/AIDS:

> If the health-care provider is comfortable with that I.D. ["heterosexual"], and if the man's sexual partner has an independent HIV risk factor that we can verify through a chart review or health-care provider, then we will accept that this man is a heterosexual case of AIDS. We don't ask that the female partner of an HIV-positive heterosexual male be tested for HIV. I only want additional information that will help me get a feel for whether there is a regular female partner with an independent risk for HIV; or whether this is a phantom "bad woman" invented to cover guilt about morally proscribed activities.[33]

As a result of the rigor with which San Francisco investigates these men, there is a cumulative total of 44 heterosexual male cases of AIDS reported in the city since the beginning of the epidemic (0.2 percent of all male cases as of 1994). On the other hand, surveillance protocol is infinitely more lenient when reporting a female heterosexual with the disease, as a woman can merely claim she acquired HIV/AIDS via heterosexual intercourse, regardless of whether a sexual partner at risk for infection is identified. Again adding a caveat about

San Francisco surveillance policy, McKinney confirmed that "the San Francisco Department of Public Health tries to verify the source of HIV transmission/risk, but in the absence of an HIV-positive contact being identified, the case is accepted as a heterosexually transmitted AIDS case from male to female."[34] Correspondingly, the number of females in San Francisco who have reportedly acquired the disease via heterosexual intercourse is nearly four times the number for heterosexual men (the cumulative total is 185 female heterosexuals, which is approximately 29 percent of all females reported with AIDS in the city since the beginning of the epidemic). However, in toto, these 229 heterosexual AIDS cases constitute a mere 1 percent of all AIDS cases reported in San Francisco as of 1995. Furthermore, well over half of these heterosexual cases (59 percent) were reported subsequent to profound changes in surveillance practice that accompanied the CDC's expanded definition of AIDS in 1993—an elaboration of the clinical parameters of the disease to include tuberculosis, cervical cancer, and a low CD4 count as qualifying AIDS diagnoses in persons who test positive for HIV antibodies. In point of fact, however, even in the face of this elaborated definition, the majority of heterosexual AIDS cases reported in San Francisco acquired the disease through intravenous drug use, and their children account for the majority of the city's pediatric AIDS cases as well.

Because San Francisco's ASSB relentlessly investigates risk for non-IVDU, nonhomosexual AIDS cases, a mere 0.6 percent of all patients in the city's AIDS registry have been reported as "no-identified-risk cases. This is a local phenomenon, however, and solely the consequence of the exceptional personal integrity and professionalism of San Francisco's surveillance staff, which adheres to the letter of the law set forth in the CDC's policies for investigating heterosexual AIDS cases. As McKinney explained: "Risk [for acquiring HIV] is the most useful information gathered by surveillance . . . and if you can't get risk [information] out of your cases you're not doing that good of a job. So I take NIR reporting very seriously."

Fieldwork in New York City

I learned that surveillance practices and policies vis-à-vis NIR and heterosexual AIDS case reporting are different in other cities and states, however. While doing fieldwork at the AIDS Surveillance offices of New York City's Department of Public Health in December 1994, I received a tip from an anonymous informant that there had been a profound shift in the way the department reported heterosexual cases of AIDS. Until 1986, a cumulative total of 12 men had been reported as acquiring the disease through heterosexual intercourse; this figure increased at the rate of one man per year through 1992, at which time 20 heterosexual male AIDS cases had been reported in New York City out of a cumulative total of 45,276 cases (0.04 percent of all cases).[35]

However, sometime in 1993 this number began to increase exponentially, reaching a total of 372 male heterosexual cases by October 1, 1994. Obviously, something profound had taken place in 1993 in New York City to account for a 19-fold increase in heterosexual transmission to men. And buried within the surveillance report was another intriguing statistic: as of October 1, 1994, the New York City AIDS Surveillance Department had reported more than 7 percent of all of its AIDS cases with "no identified risk" for acquiring the disease— a figure more than 14 times greater than San Francisco's NIR rate. When I spoke with an AIDS surveillance coordinator (ASC) at the NYC Office of AIDS Surveillance, it became abundantly clear that these two extraordinary statistics were integrally related.[36]

I eased into my interview with the surveillance coordinator by asking how many AIDS cases in New York City had been captured by a review of death certificates. This is a reliable proxy measure of how timely AIDS surveillance is in the city and an indication of the integrity of information regarding risk in AIDS case reports. Obviously, if a disease control investigator does not uncover an AIDS case until death, then there is no opportunity to thoroughly investigate the individual's risk factors for the disease vis-à-vis an interview; identifying a primary health-care provider (if there was one) and conducting a thorough review of the patient's medical chart is also less likely. This surveillance coordinator responded that in New York City "at least 15 percent, and [possibly] 20 percent are picked up this way." Once again, this figure is in stark contrast with San Francisco, where less than 2 percent of all cases in the city have been captured from active surveillance at the Bureau of Vital Statistics. Hoping that the ice was now broken, I forged ahead with the primary reason for my visit to the department:

Author: In reviewing [NYC's] surveillance reports for the last several years, I've noticed that the number of male heterosexuals reported with AIDS has increased dramatically. I was wondering if you could explain the reason for this increase. Did you have a change in surveillance staff, or was it related to the 1993 change in the definition of AIDS perhaps? Something must have changed.

ASC: No, there was no change in surveillance staff. . . . [The number of] 250 heterosexual males as of 1994 reflects a change in policy. I think it was in mid-1993, we stopped investigating all claims of AIDS in heterosexual cases. Women are automatically classified as such, but based on our experience with men, [prior to 1993] we investigated all cases through a pretty extensive review, and additional chart reviews and interviews and so on, and most of the men did have another risk. This became problematic in that we have over 4,000 NIRs, so we got backed up.[37] A good number of [these cases] had claims of heterosexual transmission; so we thought, "Why don't we just treat them like the women?" Other places like Florida were classifying [similar cases] as heterosexual men; why was New York City using a different classification? So we caved in to outside pressure . . . and we decided to lighten up.

Author: Caved in to pressure? What type of pressure, from whom? The CDC?

ASC: Well, CDC pressure, and pressures from outside.

Author: What kind of pressure were you getting from the CDC?

ASC: Well, [it wasn't like] the CDC saying you have to add more, but, you know, the questions that came from the CDC; and mainly the Bureau of Disease Intervention, New York City.

Author: I'm not sure I understand about this pressure—was it related to the change in the definition of AIDS in 1993?

ASC: [It] had nothing to do with the change in the case definition, because we had been asked by the Bureau of Disease Intervention to treat male and female heterosexual cases the same before [in previous years]. We just decided not to resist anymore, and frankly, we don't get that many claims [of female-to-male transmission of AIDS], it's still less than 1 percent. Before, when the numbers were lower [in the years before 1993], it didn't reflect the real numbers of claims because our policy was to reflect them as NIRs until we investigated them further.

Author: And you said most of those men had other risks?

ASC: Based on our experience—most had another risk.

Author: So how do you establish a male heterosexual case of AIDS now?

ASC: Basically, if a client makes a claim.[38]

When I returned to the San Francisco AIDS Office in January 1995, I asked Kevin McKinney what could possibly motivate New York City's surveillance department to willfully manufacture such a factoid, thereby deliberately aggrandizing the risk for the heterosexual transmission of HIV/AIDS from women to their male sexual partners. He replied:

> According to CDC policy . . . in verifying NIRs, if you're backlogged, you're supposed to investigate your highest priority NIRs. If NYC is just checking a box, "heterosexual contact with female," they're fiddling the statistics. As a surveillance organization, funded by the CDC, you jeopardize your funding if you're awash in cases with no identified risk for AIDS. And if your NIR rate is higher than the national average, you'll look for other ways to dump the data.[39]

So in New York City, which accounts for one out of every five AIDS cases reported in the United States, the Office of AIDS Surveillance garners up to 20 percent of its cases from death certificates, consistently reports 10 percent of its cases without an identified risk factor for acquiring the disease,[40] and "dumps data" into artificially constructed categories of transmission, thereby potentially misdirecting AIDS prevention, planning, and treatment efforts. And if uncorrected, these local distortions in AIDS surveillance data are necessarily reproduced at the national level in the CDC's surveillance statistics.

Before moving on to a discussion of how raw surveillance data is integrated into public health policy and epidemiological research, I would like to address an additional interpretive dance that is unique to the process of establishing a "heterosexually transmitted" case of AIDS. The issue arose by accident one day in July 1994 at the hospital when I picked up a negative culture for *Pneumocystis carinii* pneumonia (PCP) in a 43-year-old white female with a previous diagnosis of Kaposi's sarcoma noted on her PCP lab report. I duly returned to the ASSB and checked the ACR and OOJ case files to see if we had previously reported her as an AIDS case with Kaposi's sarcoma. Admittedly, however, I also intended to do a thorough medical chart review and analysis of the information in her ACR file, as this particular woman piqued my interest on several counts: 1) I rarely encountered female AIDS cases during my surveillance activities; 2) I had never seen, and rarely heard reference to, a case of Kaposi's sarcoma in a female; and 3) I was curious about the patient's risk for acquiring KS, as the use of amyl/butyl nitrites (poppers) has frequently been epidemiologically associated with those who develop this rare form of skin cancer, which is characterized by disseminated violaceous spots or lesions—"purple stigmata," if you will.[41] For all of these reasons, a female AIDS case with KS justified several hours of my time rummaging through files.

The ACR file for this female patient was cross-referenced to a second ACR file (she had obviously used an alias at some time), a fact that in itself is not unusual: there were 28,000 names for the 20,000 cumulative AIDS cases reported in the city as of 1995. The patient's primary risk factor for the disease was reported as "heterosexual intercourse with a male at risk for HIV/AIDS"; it was noted that she had engaged in "sex with an IVDU." The diagnosis of Kaposi's sarcoma was definitive. After digging through handwritten notes appended to the patient's file, and returning to SFGH to review her chart—my curiosity was rewarded, and an exceptional AIDS case became exceptional in a rather different way. This "female heterosexual" AIDS case was a post-op transsexual—a male who had undergone sex reassignment surgery to become a female. A conversation ensued with supervisor Kevin McKinney about how such cases are classified in practice and in theory.

McKinney: This is a source of consternation here at SFDPH, this issue you've just brought up. Some people are not happy about the way that it is handled. The deal about transsexual people, the way the CDC wants us to classify these cases, is that your gender[42] is what you are biologically born with. And it avoids a burning question of how to classify men who are born male, then get new plumbing.

In the past, we experimented with the idea of "het cons," classifying them as heterosexual contacts, but the CDC clarified the situation, and I believe that it more meaningfully classifies their risk factor to classify them as men who have sex with men.

Author: But what about their [sexual] partners? Aren't their partners heterosexual men?

McKinney: There is also a definitional battle on this. I don't think that they [the partners] should be classified as "heterosexual" partners. I think the majority of their regular partners would be called "bisexual"; before their surgery they were men having sex with men, the great majority . . . and most of their regular sex partners understand their sexual history, I believe.

Author: And are there any studies on the level of HIV seroprevalence among bisexuals?

McKinney: No, there are no studies that I know of.

Author: OK, so San Francisco is very strict about this [classifying transsexuals as "men who have sex with men"] but are other states classifying transsexuals in "heterosexual contact" categories?

McKinney: Well, it's CDC policy . . . but there may be cases, perhaps a few cases in New York City, where you have a male-to-female transsexual that they're classifying as heterosexual contact. But pre-op transsexuals are always classed as male-to-male transmission.[43]

San Francisco's surveillance statistics were subsequently adjusted to reflect that this AIDS patient acquired the disease via male-to-male sex.

From Surveillance Data to Epidemiological Fact and Public Policy

My experience as a participant in an epidemiological research project at San Francisco's ASSB in July 1994 frames my concluding remarks about surveillance practices while illustrating how raw surveillance data become codified as medical knowledge. As an ASSB intern, I agreed to assist disease control investigators in gathering data for a study examining prophylaxis (preventative drug therapies) and the incidence of PCP.

Because I had joined the study at midpoint, a summary of the research proposal and a progress update was offered for my benefit. Staff involved with the study met in the department's main conference room with the principal investigator for this research, epidemiologist Dr. Sandy Schwarcz. Using the San Francisco AIDS database, Dr. Schwarcz had identified a study population of 420 Persons With AIDS (PWAs) who had been reported in San Francisco with *Pneumocystis carinii* pneumonia as their initial AIDS diagnosis between January and December 1993. Schwarcz gave a brief summary of the research, titled "Utilization of PCP Prophylaxis and Anti-Viral Agents," and its objectives.

Half of these patients are on prophylaxis for *Pneumocystis carinii* pneumonia and half of the patients are not.[44] Despite the fact that both groups developed PCP in 1993 as an initial A1 AIDS-defining condition, this does not indicate [that there is] no significant difference between patients receiving pneumonia prophylaxis and those not, because this is not a controlled study. Clinical trials have proven already that PCP prophylaxis is of significant benefit [in preventing PCP].[45]

The hypothesis for this study is that the occurrence of PCP depends on T-cell counts [i.e., it is expected that those patients who are not on PCP prophylaxis are developing PCP at higher CD4 counts or earlier in the disease process than those who are receiving prophylactic therapy]. I'm interested in prophylaxis and why people are not on it. Maybe it is because they're not in care; indicating a need to work on that. Maybe it is because they don't know their HIV status; if so, then we should emphasize testing.

At this point, Dr. Schwarcz opened the meeting to comments by the DCIs regarding the progress of their work and any problems they had encountered while reviewing the charts for patients in the study. In response, the DCIs raised several issues related to data input and missing or ineligible charts that potentially affected the integrity of the study. The first issue raised, was that the computer software designed expressly for the data collected in this study only had space for a three-digit CD4 count; thus 999 was the highest CD4 count that could be entered for a patient. The problem was that several patients (three men thus far) had CD4 counts that exceeded this number and therefore could not be accurately entered into the database.[46] Schwarcz responded that the correct CD4 information for these patients would be entered at a later date after the database software was amended to accept a four-digit entry.

Next, a member of the surveillance staff said that some charts were missing or inaccurate. Specifically with respect to patients reported from one hospital in San Francisco, "there are numerous ineligibles due to incorrect coding of initial PCP diagnoses in 1993." In other words, after reviewing the medical charts for hospital patients who were included in this study on the basis of a diagnosis of PCP in 1993, it was discovered that some patients were ineligible because (1) they never had this form of pneumonia, (2) they had other opportunistic infections prior to their PCP diagnosis in 1993, which disqualified them from the study, or (3) they had a previous diagnosis of PCP prior to 1993. As a consequence of this discovery of "numerous ineligibles," there would be considerably fewer individuals in this study than the original estimate of 420.

With respect to a third problem, several disease control investigators reported that many of the remaining charts yet to be reviewed were proving difficult to find. They had been requested from hospital storage, but the retrieval rate was slow. After we were reminded of the end date for the study, the meeting was adjourned and the surveillance staff, myself included, returned to the field to gather what data we could from what charts were available.

Once fieldwork was completed for the study, some surveillance staff privately voiced criticisms regarding its purpose and methods. A pilot study preceding this research had set out to prove that persons who presented with *Pneumocystis carinii* pneumonia had never received PCP prophylaxis before their diagnosis. That study (of 100 patients, nearly one-third as large as the subsequent study) did not confirm that hypothesis, however. Nonetheless, the researchers forged ahead with their proposed research, intending to use their data to answer a different set of questions. In the opinion of one DCI who spoke to me, this blind commitment to mine the data and salvage something relevant from the research effort meant that "the entire effort was a waste of time." The investigator elaborated on additional methodological problems with this study:

> The PI [principal investigator] requested information on CD4 counts before, during, and after the diagnosis of PCP. And CD4 counts . . . if they are written in the chart by a doctor . . . well, we know that what the Doctor writes is what the patient says. And as we know, there are a lot of patients who transpose numbers. Just from follow-up we know that it is not reliable when the patient says, for example, "They're in the 200 range."
>
> Furthermore, there is the whole thing with prophylaxis—halfway into the study this just came up, and the definition of what constituted "being prophylaxed" changed. People [the DCIs who were collecting data] thought if patients had been on Septra, AZT, or DDI at any time prior to the diagnosis of PCP then they should record this as prophylaxis. And then, in the late stages of the study, the PI decided to make it more definitive. What she meant to say was that a patient needed to be on it [AZT, DDI, or PCP prophylaxis] the month prior to presenting with PCP. So the whole definition of prophylaxis changed midstudy. That's why everyone got real discouraged with it . . . half of the data was not changed, and could not or would not be consistent with what came later. So what's the point?[47]

Naturally, AIDS surveillance staff have legitimate differences of opinion regarding various surveillance practices and policies. To be fair, a second disease control investigator admitted to some glitches in the study but felt that these had been adequately resolved in the latter stages of the research.

The final number of ineligibles and patients lost to follow-up totaled 86 when the research that commenced in July 1994 concluded several months later. Thus, from a study designed to evaluate 420 PWAs diagnosed with PCP in 1993, approximately 20 percent were subsequently dropped from analysis because of surveillance errors or loss to follow-up; in other words, there was a significant problem related to the quality or integrity of the surveillance information available about their diagnosis, or a medical chart could not be found to corroborate the AIDS case report for one out of every five AIDS cases in this "representative sample" of San Francisco's surveillance database. Though this might be seen as a sobering comment on the quality and accuracy of San Francisco AIDS surveillance data and its value in epidemiological research, Kevin

McKinney felt that there were extenuating circumstances unique to such a high error rate in this study, as "1993 is not typical of surveillance data in general [as it] was gathered while the staff was reporting two and a half times [the number of AIDS cases] that they [reported] in 1992."

The elision of data did not become part of the official record of this project as summarized by the principal investigator, however. When the first rough draft summarizing the PCP prophylaxis study was circulated in-house, the original population of PWAs selected for analysis had shrunk from 420 to "386 patients who were diagnosed with PCP as their AIDS-defining diagnosis in 1993." The very existence of a cohort of ineligible patients uncovered during the study was elided; and the reduction in the number of patients in the study (to 386) allowed the principal investigator to argue for the integrity of the project data as "medical charts were available for 88% of these patients."[48] As I've shown in numerous examples from daily surveillance practice, when AIDS research produces messy, contradictory, or inconvenient results, the data are deemed irrelevant or aberrant, subsumed in hypothetical speculation, or are simply tossed overboard.

VI

AIDS Surveillance Statistics
Changing the Subjects and Object of Study

As Nancy Krieger (1992), Sylvia Noble Tesh (1988), and others have argued, public health data are not apolitical, and biomedical assertions about the causes of illness and the characterization of symptoms denoting distinct disease entities are not, and have never been, value-free.[1]

> A first step in understanding the making of public health data is recognizing that the familiar word—"data"—is in fact a deceptive term. . . . [T]he singular noun "datum" in Latin, literally means "that which is given" . . . something known or assumed as a fact, and made the basis of reasoning or calculations. As many critics have noted, however, data of any type—including public health data—are not and never have been simply a "given." No data bases have ever magically arrived. . . . [I]nstead, their form and content reflect decisions made by individuals and institutions, and in the case of public health data, embody underlying beliefs and values about what it is we need to know in order to understand population patterns of health and disease. In other words, data are a social product, and are neither a gift passively received from an invisible donor nor a neutral collection of allegedly inevitable empirical facts.[2]

Public health data on HIV and AIDS are no exception: they are anything but a "neutral collection of facts." With this in mind, the public and scholarly perception of an exponential explosion in AIDS cases is to a significant degree the consequence of multiple and extensive changes in the methods by which the Centers for Disease Control (and thus local health departments) have captured and recorded patients during the past two decades. The frequent elaboration of the clinical criteria for diagnosing AIDS patients is largely responsible for the general impression that the epidemic's growth is unabated, and that the demography of risk for the disease is evolving and shifting to encompass nontraditional populations.[3] However, the danger of any historical analysis of the epidemiology of AIDS in the United States and other industrialized countries that fails to account for changes in the way AIDS cases are diagnosed and reported at different temporal periods or phases of the epidemic is that it risks compromising a critical assessment of how clinical therapies are affecting the course of the disease and whether HIV/AIDS prevention and education programs are effective—and if so, for which "high-risk" populations.

At the present time, most orthodox AIDS researchers would not challenge the statement that fewer new AIDS cases are reported now than during the late 1980s and early; however, it is not widely acknowledged that AIDS caseloads in San Francisco (and throughout the United States) began to decline much earlier than predicted (the epidemic peaked in the early 1990s) and that public health officials sought various means to obscure this welcome news for a number of years.

Cumulative AIDS Cases in San Francisco

As of the spring of 2002, San Francisco had reported 27,982 cumulative cases and 18,957 AIDS-related deaths since the disease was discovered in the summer of 1981.[4] A statistical summary of various attributes for all AIDS cases are disseminated in the city Public Health Department's monthly (now quarterly) *AIDS Surveillance Report.* Patients reported in the previous month and year-to-date are disaggregated in numerous tables by sex, age, race, transmission category, and so on. The report also summarizes cumulative mortality data, initial AIDS diagnoses (denoted "A1" in surveillance reports), and the number of patients who have qualified under each of the four successive definitions of the disease (in 1982, 1985, 1987, 1993). To remain consistent throughout this text and because the city's surveillance reports are now adumbrated vis-à-vis reports from previous years, I will reference the October 31, 1995, monthly *AIDS Surveillance Report* as the source for the data used in this chapter and as a touchstone for future quantitative analysis. As of the time of that report, San Francisco's AIDS Office had reported 22,185 cumulative AIDS cases and 14,892 cumulative deaths in the city, a mortality rate of 67 percent (see Figure 9).

Public health officials use surveillance statistics such as these to derive per capita AIDS incidence and mortality rates, evaluate the efficacy of prevention and education programs, and determine the fiscal toll of AIDS care and support services on city budgets. But these data embody particular political decisions and subjective criteria that have significant implications for understanding the past and future trajectory of the AIDS epidemic in this country. Moreover, surveillance statistics for AIDS are unique among those for diseases reported on by public health agencies. First, "AIDS is the first (and only) disease reported and recorded cumulatively."[5] Second, how the ASSB establishes San Francisco residency for AIDS patients "is contrary to the usual morbidity reports for other diseases which are based on residence."[6]

With respect to AIDS, and only AIDS, there is one overriding concept that guides San Francisco surveillance reporting practice: "if we capture a case it is ours," regardless of the patient's actual city, state, or country of residence.[7] To wit, if San Francisco is the first city to capture and report an individual's diagnosis with AIDS, then the city retains that patient as a reported AIDS case in official surveillance reports regardless of where the patient actually lives. This means that the October 31, 1995, reported figure of 22,185 cumulative AIDS

AIDS REPORTED CASES
(From 7/81 to 10/31/95)*

Total San Francisco Reported Cases:	22,185
Total San Francisco Reported Deaths:	14,892
Total S.F. cases reported month to date:	165
Total S.F. deaths reported month to date:	143
Total California reported cases: (as of 9/30/95)	86,853 cases; 55,421 deaths
Total U.S. reported cases: (as of 06/30/95)	476,899 cases; 295,473 deaths

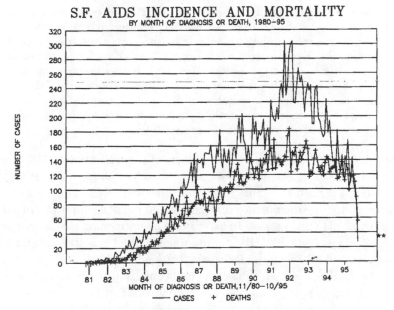

S.F. AIDS INCIDENCE AND MORTALITY
BY MONTH OF DIAGNOSIS OR DEATH, 1980-95

* Includes all persons diagnosed in SF and SF residents diagnosed in other jurisdictions.
** Reporting for recent months is incomplete.

San Francisco Department of Public Health AIDS Office

FIGURE 9   AIDS Reported Cases (from 7/31 to 10/31/95)
Source: San Francisco Department of Health Aids Office, Seroepidemiology and Surveillance
Branch, "AIDS Cases Reported through October 1995," *AIDS Surveillance Report* (October 31,
1995): 1.

cases includes patients from other jurisdictions who were reported as residents when they sought health care in San Francisco. As other cities and states do not follow a similar practice, the cumulative total of 22,185 AIDS cases also includes San Francisco residents who were diagnosed in other jurisdictions but then referred back to the ASSB. Surveillance practices such as these inflate the per capita incidence of AIDS in San Francisco, thereby complicating analyses of past or present projections of HIV transmission among risk populations in the city. Kevin McKinney, AIDS surveillance field unit coordinator at San Francisco's AIDS Seroepidemiology and Surveillance Branch, explains:

> We like to keep in our database, residents of San Francisco or those first diagnosed here. San Francisco is a bit different in reporting this information. We follow cases first diagnosed in San Francisco as if they were a San Francisco resident, even though they live in Santa Rosa or Oakland, et cetera. But when we report to the state, we only report San Francisco residents to the state. Then we send hard copies to other jurisdictions for them to report (so that that particular jurisdiction receives adequate funding for care). But we don't furnish them with a name for a case report . . . so sometimes this befuddles them, and the case doesn't show up in the registry. And also we notify them of death of their residents. This is contrary to the usual morbidity reports for other diseases which are based on residence. Approximately 8 percent of our cases we diagnose in San Francisco first, but they are not San Francisco residents.

Though 8 percent may be a credible estimate of the proportion of AIDS cases in San Francisco that are redundant patients from other jurisdictions within California, I pressed McKinney to give me some sense about how many AIDS cases reported by San Francisco surveillance staff might be duplicates of AIDS cases reported in other states.[8] In the example of one medical chart I reviewed, the patient was reportedly HIV-positive when he lived in South Carolina and was prescribed AZT while under care in that state. After moving to San Francisco he was diagnosed with an opportunistic infection and reported as a resident AIDS case shortly thereafter. Is it possible that San Francisco and South Carolina are both reporting the same patient as a resident AIDS case?

McKinney: In the evaluation of the 1993 definition [a future research project recently funded by the CDC], we'll attempt to assess that . . . how many HIV positives are from out of state but move to San Francisco when they are declining. There is no information on that now. . . . Definition of residence is so tricky, it's hard to specify. Do you mean their weekend home, their weekday residence, their second home?

Author: Well, in a specific case I just looked at, the patient was from South Carolina and HIV-positive since 1986 by self-report. He had been on AZT for three years. He became symptomatic in October 1992 after moving to San Francisco, and in February 1993 he had PCP.

The chart says "He wants to return home." Isn't it logical to assume that this guy has already been reported in South Carolina?

McKinney: Usually we wouldn't check this issue unless it is clear that he had opportunistic infections that met the definition before coming here. We want our statistics to be accurate, but we don't want to shoot ourselves in the foot.

Author: But isn't it likely that he had already been reported, given the fact that he knew he was positive in 1986 and was on AZT?

McKinney: Not necessarily, because perhaps the patient had no previous opportunistic infections and had 400 or 500 T-cells. . . . It is still standard therapy that AZT is given if a patient's T-cells drop below 500 or 400, and it is at the doctor's discretion to make this call. . . .

On average an HIV-positive person will drop 50 CD4 T-cells per six months, and on average, it is 10 years until AIDS, give or take. So easily one could take AZT for three years, if beginning at 500 T-cells, before becoming an AIDS patient at a CD4 count of 200. . . . Thus, he is a San Francisco case because we picked him up with the first opportunistic infection.

The logic behind McKinney's argument is based on the assumption that this patient never developed an opportunistic infection before moving to this city, despite being HIV-positive, despite being in care for AIDS, and despite being on chemotherapy (AZT) for the disease. Since San Francisco was the first jurisdiction to report his diagnosis, the patient is "our case."

Author: But with respect to duplicate reporting, is it possible that two cities could report the same AIDS case with the same name? Is there any mechanism to cross-check for that?

McKinney: In fact, CDC soundex only allows one soundex for a given date of birth, so subsequent, even legitimate, dates of birth for a different person with the same soundex code will not get reported.[9]

In the first six months of this year [1994] we deleted 8 percent of San Francisco's reported cases as duplicates from another jurisdiction within California. This was precipitated by a process of constant reviewing, plus cross-checking a computerized list from the state which prints out duplicate case reports attributed on a per-county basis.

Individual states are padding their numbers, but the CDC takes account of that and only counts a soundex and date of birth once. In 1986–1987, San Francisco reviewed its early cases [all reported AIDS cases] and eliminated within-state duplicate reports. But it would be years of bullshit, a pain in the ass, to clean up your records a little by, for instance, comparing early cases in New York and California for duplicate reports. It would be easier to pad cases if the state wasn't following up to eliminate this type of duplicate reporting between counties and jurisdictions. At least in California the state is stringent, but other states may vary.[10]

In the conversation below, the aggressive nature of the city's surveillance practices is evident in a DCI's explanation of a struggle s/he is embroiled in with public health officials in Alaska over a former resident of that state who was recently claimed as an AIDS case in San Francisco.

DCI: This case is ours in San Francisco because we reported it first. The logic behind this is that he receives his care for HIV disease here, thus the city needs the money from the government [for his care]. The same logic is used with Oakland—despite his residence in the East Bay, if he gets his care here and got reported with his first opportunistic infection or low CD4 count here—then he is a San Francisco case regardless of residence. The Alaskan Health Department doesn't get CD4 counts at the Department of Public Health as there are no CD4 labs in the state; all counts are done elsewhere and then mailed back to the doctor. If the doctor received the low CD4 count then he/she should have reported this case to the health department. Sometimes that doesn't happen, passive surveillance breaks down, or there is a delay with paperwork.

So I just called on this guy with 50 T-cells and discovered that they had no record on him. He arrived here in San Francisco one month ago, but probably was receiving care in Alaska before that, you'd think [given his low cell count]. Everybody wants the case, but this is our case.

Author: Why does everyone want the case?
DCI: Well, funding is allocated on the basis of AIDS caseloads. So there are fights between departments over duplicate reports; it gets battled out. (San Francisco) fights for it, or I get a phone call saying, "OK, this is so-and-so at the state," telling me to give her a case.

Well, everybody in the state of California, except San Francisco, goes by where the patient had the first opportunistic infection. Only the San Francisco AIDS Surveillance Department goes by who reports it first, and where they reported it first. If it was first reported in San Francisco, then it's our case.[11]

A month later, I resumed this conversation with McKinney because I had just begun a special project reviewing all AIDS cases reported in San Francisco between 1980 and 1982. Again, I was curious about the possibility of double-reporting early AIDS cases. In one instance, a man who lived all his life in

Washington, D.C., moved to San Francisco; within three months he had been reported as an AIDS case with Kaposi's sarcoma. After this diagnosis, the patient moved to New Jersey and subsequently to New York City, where he died.

Author: What is the guarantee that New York City and San Francisco haven't both claimed this guy as a case?

McKinney: There is no guarantee. The CDC only allows one soundex per one date of birth. Thus he can't get reported in duplicate there, at the CDC. However, there is no such cross-check mechanism between states' case reports. You would need to call each state individually and ask them . . .

Author: And what's your best guess about the extent of state-to-state duplicate reporting?

McKinney: In 1989, at the National AIDS Surveillance Conference, there was a report by the Centers for Disease Control that, in their database, there was a figure of 2 [percent] to 4 percent of duplicate soundex date-of-birth incidents.

Author: So the real figure of padding by states, versus the CDC's figures, might lie between 2 percent [the CDC's figure for duplicate Soundex incidents] and 8 percent [the number of in-state duplicate reports deleted from the San Francisco registry in early 1994]?

McKinney: Yeah.[12]

So the raw figures for AIDS incidence per capita and the cumulative number of cases that the ASSB publishes are inflated both in absolute terms, and relative to surveillance data from other cities that do not follow San Francisco's policies vis-à-vis residents.[13] First, with respect to the number of cases reported in the monthly *AIDS Surveillance Report* at any given point in time, an unknown number of these cases may be duplicates of AIDS cases reported in other jurisdictions or states. Second, San Francisco has the unique policy of reporting nonresidents if they were initially diagnosed with an AIDS-related opportunistic infection while visiting the city, whereas other cities must refer AIDS case information back here if San Francisco residents are diagnosed elsewhere. At a minimum, 8 percent of the 22,185 patients reported in the city are not San Francisco residents at all, in fact, but instead are patients who visited the city briefly and were captured as AIDS cases during their visits to area hospitals and clinics. Almost certainly, these AIDS cases are previously reported patients currently being followed by other public health departments. Another unknown percentage of this cumulative AIDS caseload is accounted for by those San Francisco residents who were diagnosed with the disease in another city, state, or country. These people may still reside elsewhere, in fact, or they may have returned to San Francisco. AIDS surveillance reports also necessarily include data for patients in regional prisons or other government

institutions, as well as data for an unknown percentage of homeless and/or transient PWAs.[14]

Cumulative AIDS-Related Mortality in San Francisco

When I reviewed the mechanics of capturing and reporting AIDS cases in a previous chapter, I noted that approximately 2 percent of San Francisco's recent AIDS caseload has been captured by reviewing death certificates. Obviously, for these individuals, the date of the patient's death is reported when the city first captures him/her as an AIDS case. For the remaining 98 percent of the city's caseload, however, death may be documented months, years, or even decades after an AIDS diagnosis. While disease control investigators sometimes glean mortality data from a patient's health-care provider, from medical charts, or anecdotally from friends or published obituaries, it is still necessary to obtain an official copy of a patient's death certificate before legitimately reporting AIDS case mortality. This means that disease control investigators in San Francisco must cross-reference their AIDS case reports against the databanks of two vital statistics registries: the California State Death Registry and the National Death Index. Kevin McKinney explained the process:

> On a weekly basis, San Francisco Disease Surveillance Staff checks with the Department of Vital statistics for deaths from AIDS for cases previously captured by the AIDS Seroepidemiology and Surveillance Branch (ASSB) and for unreported cases. This information is treated as a "health status update" and the disease surveillance officer returns to the ASSB with a photocopy of the death certificate and adds this to the patient's case file, or creates an AIDS case report for a new patient. Also on a weekly basis in San Francisco we download these data into the California AIDS registry updating them with new cases and with mortality.
>
> On a quarterly basis, AIDS-related ICD9 codes from San Francisco are matched to the California AIDS registry. The state death registry is matched by name, soundex, and date of birth to the ICD9 code [diagnostic code] for AIDS. This process initiates getting one, a death certificate on a previously reported case for our case files at SFDPH, or two, a death date for a San Francisco resident with AIDS that the ASSB has not previously reported. Once the name, soundex, and date of birth is matched, then a printout of the death certificate number is sent to San Francisco Department of Public Health with the location of death. Thereafter, SFDPH contacts the vital statistics out of state, and using the death certificate number, is able to get a hard copy of the death certificate to update the AIDS Case Report and file the death certificate for the case.
>
> Finally, there is an ongoing project at the ASSB regarding the health status of older cases. Each year the San Francisco AIDS Registry is matched to the National Death Index on the basis of soundex, date of birth, Social Security number, race, and sex. In this process, we may discover that a San Francisco resident diagnosed with AIDS has already died; we get a match and a death date. Then

surveillance officers write off for the death certificate to put in a health status up-date and into the patient's case file. In this latter project the ASSB never captures additional cases of HIV/AIDS but only updates mortality data for previously re-ported cases.[15]

Once a year, a disease control investigator travels to Research Triangle, North Carolina, to consult the National Death Index, carrying with him or her a tape (magnetic list) of names for people reported as still living with the disease in San Francisco. When the DCI compares this tape to the National Death Index and a match is found, death certificate numbers with the location of death are referred back to San Francisco's Department of Public Health. Subsequently, surveillance staff request a copy of the death certificate from out of state to as-certain the date and cause of death for the city's AIDS cases. One major draw-back of the National Death Index data, however, is that it is generally two years out of date. When I was conducting fieldwork at the AIDS Seroepidemiology and Surveillance Branch in 1994–1995, the latest death certificate information available from the NDI pertained to San Francisco AIDS cases that died some-time in 1992–1993. In light of this significant reporting delay, the cumulative mortality published in the October 31, 1995, *AIDS Surveillance Report* (14,892 deaths) appears to underestimate the number of AIDS patients in the city who have died from the disease.

The significance of this finding is offset, however, by countervailing tenden-cies embedded in surveillance practices and policy that overestimate AIDS-related mortality. Premier among these is the irrevocability of an AIDS diagnosis. By definition, an AIDS diagnosis once rendered is never rescinded; unlike cancer, for instance, a patient can never be "cured" or "recover" from the disease. Therefore, *all deaths that occur among persons diagnosed and reported with AIDS are deaths attributable to acquired immune deficiency syndrome.*

Consequently, the total of 14,892 cumulative AIDS deaths in San Francisco represents all deaths reported among patients from all causes as of the monthly surveillance report of October 31, 1995. Even if the AIDS patient died from cirrhosis, homicide, suicide, a drug overdose, a broken neck, or treat-ment side effects[16] the death is recorded as AIDS-related mortality. Again, this is an exception to the way in which case fatality rates are derived for other dis-eases. Moreover, public health officials do not routinely sift through mortality data to eliminate those patients who died from something other than AIDS-related opportunistic infections before publishing articles or reports assessing survival time following an AIDS diagnosis, or evaluating the efficacy of pre-vention programs or chemotherapy.

While I don't wish to appear glib, this peculiar practice is equivalent to claiming that "My father was shot in a bank robbery in 1994, but because he had been diagnosed with prostate cancer in 1987 he really died of cancer." I asked McKinney to explain the SFDPH policy of attributing non–AIDS-related mortality to the disease:

McKinney: If a PWA dies, then it's AIDS mortality.

Author: And what's your ballpark figure for the number of reported "AIDS deaths" in San Francisco that might actually be due to other causes of death?

McKinney: Of the people that we have cause-of-death information for . . . for 1990 deaths and before, we found 40 of 6,000 were suicides. Now, if you take a look at that for other accident-related mortality thrown in there, it would be a slightly higher number than that. And even if a person with AIDS dies in a car wreck, what's to say their vision or perception wasn't influenced by their AIDS diagnosis? But the National Vital Statistics report, which lists AIDS as the leading cause of death for people 25–44 years of age—now, they're just looking at cause of death from death certificates. And if the proximate cause of death is a car accident, then the cause of death is an accident; so those numbers are accurate.

I can't rule out that there aren't some non-AIDS related deaths in our mortality statistics, and that there are some PWAs who died with low CD4 counts and really died because of hepatitis B liver cancer, or really died because of lung cancer, or a drug overdose. So on survival data it would have some impact—but it would be minimal. We've never taken non-AIDS related mortality out of the survival analyses we've done; we've never, to my knowledge, looked at ICD codes for San Francisco Department of Public Health survival analysis publications.

Because it is a key tenet of orthodox AIDS discourse that AIDS struck down "previously healthy men" with no other risks for premature death, it is important to know that some epidemiological studies of AIDS cohorts similarly overestimate AIDS-related mortality and/or benignly neglect deaths within the cohort from unrelated causes. Moreover, after reviewing epidemiological studies of gay men in the early 1980s, one concludes that orthodox epidemiologists may have overstated their case about the general health and well-being of urban male homosexuals in the years immediately preceding and coincident with the emergence of the AIDS epidemic.

In 1985, for example, the CDC's Harold Jaffe published a study of AIDS and mortality among homosexual men after six years of follow-up study. Jaffe and his colleagues analyzed serum samples and patient data from the San Francisco City Clinic Cohort, made up of homosexual and bisexual men who were treated for sexually transmitted diseases at the clinic and members of the infamous hepatitis B vaccine studies. Of the 6,875 men in the cohort 166 (2.4 percent) had been reported with AIDS by December 31, 1984, and more than half had died. Although Jaffe et al. concluded that "mortality attributable to the syndrome in 1984 was 600 per 100,000"[17] we are not provided any further information on the specific cause of death for these 86 men.

You may wonder why I am problematizing the cause of death for these men, but ambiguity is actually introduced by the authors themselves, as they provide less than conclusive proof of a 100 percent correlation between HTLV-III/LAV (HIV) infection and AIDS in these patients. Jaffe et al. noted that serum samples, which were available for 111 of the 166 patients diagnosed with AIDS, showed only 24 of them, 22 percent, to be HIV-positive.[18] Hypothetically, it is possible that the remaining 78 percent of this cohort became HIV-infected sometime after they gave a serum sample (presumably between 1978 and 1981), but that would imply that the majority of these men were "rapid progressors" who developed AIDS within three years of becoming infected with HIV. And on this point, I demonstrated when I extensively reviewed findings of epidemiological studies conducted during the early 1980s (including this cohort) that there was no definitive evidence that significant numbers of cohort members progressed rapidly from HIV infection to AIDS in a matter of months or a couple of years. Neither can one argue that concurrent infections with hepatitis B, or receipt of the hepatitis B vaccine, or drug abuse were contributing factors for the swift decline of these "high-risk" men, because there are no co-factors for progression to AIDS, according to the tenets of orthodox AIDS discourse.[19]

Jaffe and colleagues then selected a "representative sample" from the remaining men in the hepatitis B cohort for follow-up study. These were high-risk homosexual men who had *not* been diagnosed with AIDS as of 1984. In the analysis of a subset of these men, "22 men were known to have died."[20] Only half of their deaths were related to opportunistic infections associated with AIDS, however; the other half (10 of 22) resulted from causes unrelated to the syndrome (e.g., chronic hepatitis and suicide). Clearly, in this subset of men from the San Francisco hepatitis B cohort, non-AIDS-related mortality (10 deaths) was nearly equivalent to AIDS-related mortality (12 deaths). Nevertheless, Jaffe et al. concluded that "AIDS is now the major health problem for gay men in San Francisco, particularly those who are members of the City Clinic cohort."[21]

I am not trying to diminish the significant toll exacted by AIDS in this cohort, caused principally by *Pneumocystis carinii* pneumonia and Kaposi's sarcoma. Rather, what I am highlighting is that other causes of premature death were exacting a significant toll among these high-risk gay men. And I am also suggesting that after acquired immune deficiency syndrome was discovered in 1981, some of these deaths were subsumed in AIDS mortality statistics.

A 1993 analysis of mortality among members of the San Francisco Men's Health Study (SFMHS) provides a final example, albeit less dramatic. In this cohort study, homosexual and bisexual men who were not infected with HIV died at four times the rate (7 of 367 men) of noninfected heterosexual men (1 of 214 men). Although AIDS was the overwhelming cause of death for members of the cohort, the excess mortality observed among HIV-negative gay men vis-à-vis their heterosexual peers is disturbing and seems to suggest that gay men at high risk of contracting AIDS may die in greater numbers and at younger ages than heterosexual men from causes not directly related to this epidemic.

Changing the Object (AIDS) and Subjects (Cases) of Surveillance

A study of the social construction of San Francisco AIDS surveillance data and national AIDS statistics demonstrates that frequent changes in the clinical criteria by which patients are diagnosed has contributed in large measure to the dramatic growth in the number of AIDS cases reported during the past two decades. A failure to grasp this central point of AIDS surveillance practices distorts analyses of the historical evolution of the epidemic, compromises a critical understanding of who is at risk for AIDS and why, and confounds evaluations of the efficacy of treatment and prevention initiatives.

Phase I: 1981–1986

When five homosexual men with severe immune deficiency were discovered in Los Angeles in the summer of 1981, the Task Force on Kaposi's Sarcoma and Opportunistic Infections was established at the Centers for Disease Control in Atlanta, Georgia.[22] Among the urgent priorities faced by the task force, one of the most immediate was to delineate a working case definition of the new disease syndrome that public health departments and physicians could use to standardize the way in which they diagnosed and reported patients with severe and inexplicable immune deficiency. The panel turned to the issue in September 1982:

> The CDC defines a case of AIDS as a disease, at least moderately predictive of a defect in cell-mediated immunity, occurring in a person with no known cause for diminished resistance to that disease. Such diseases include Kaposi's sarcoma (KS), *Pneumocystis carinii* pneumonia (PCP), and serious other "opportunistic" infections (OI). Diagnoses are considered to fit the case definition only if based on sufficiently reliable methods (generally histology or culture).
>
> However, this case definition may not include the full spectrum of AIDS manifestations, which may range from absence of symptoms (despite laboratory evidence of immune deficiency) to non-specific symptoms (e.g., fever, weight loss, generalized, persistent lymphadenopathy) to specific diseases that are insufficiently predictive of cellular immuno-deficiency to be included in incidence monitoring (e.g., tuberculosis, oral candidiasis, herpes zoster) to malignant neoplasms that cause, as well as result from, immunodeficiency.
>
> Conversely, some patients who are considered AIDS cases on the basis of diseases only moderately predictive of cellular immunodeficiency may not actually be immuno-deficient and may not be part of the current epidemic. Absence of a

reliable, inexpensive, widely available test for AIDS, however, may make the working case definition the best currently available for incidence monitoring.[23]

There had been 593 cumulative cases of AIDS reported in the United States when the CDC initially published this standardized AIDS case definition on September 24, 1982. The overwhelming majority of these patients (88 percent) were initially diagnosed with either PCP or KS or a combination of the two diseases. The remaining constellation of 10 "other opportunistic infections" accounted for only 12 percent of all AIDS cases.[24] The overwhelming predominance of just two clinical diagnoses was even more striking in San Francisco, as Kaposi's sarcoma and *Pneumocystis carinii* pneumonia constituted nearly 100 percent of the initial AIDS diagnoses among early cases. Of 118 cases reported in the city between June 1981 and December 1982, all were eventually reported as "homosexual/bisexual" men, and 117 had either KS or PCP. Only seven of these men suffered from an additional concurrent opportunistic infection when they were first reported to the San Francisco Department of Public Health.[25] As I will return to this point, it is important to note that the CDC Task Force specifically excluded diagnoses of tuberculosis, herpes zoster, and some malignant neoplasms from being reported under the AIDS case surveillance definition as these diagnoses were "insufficiently predictive of cellular immuno-deficiency."

The 1982 AIDS surveillance definition remained in effect until 1985, by which time "the probable cause of AIDS" had been discovered by Luc Montagnier, and the United States ELISA test kit had been licensed to detect antibodies to the LAV/HTLV-III (HIV). As the ELISA was originally designed to enable blood banks to screen donated blood products for the presence of viral antibodies, it had a considerable "false-positive" error rate. Nevertheless, its use as an instrument for diagnosis in patients at risk for AIDS was codified in 1985, when the CDC included the antibody test in its new revision of the surveillance criteria for the disease, and added histoplasmosis and isoporiasis to the list of opportunistic infections that constituted an AIDS diagnosis in a person who tested positive for LAV/HTLV-III/HIV antibodies.[26]

Phase II: 1987–1992

In August of 1987, the CDC profoundly revised the surveillance definition of AIDS, driven by the anticipation that the HIV antibody test would be increasingly used for patient diagnoses. Tautologically, the new definition fundamentally contributed to that very outcome by including a positive antibody result as a criterion for the diagnosis of several additional opportunistic infections. Prior to 1987, "fewer than 10% of all AIDS cases reported in (San Francisco had) included a laboratory result (for HIV infection)."[27] But when the CDC's new surveillance definition was instituted, the city's Department of Public Health aggressively encouraged health-care providers to test (and report) more patients.[28] By 1987, a positive HIV antibody test was reified as "prodro-mal" (a symptom of approaching disease) for AIDS in medical parlance and surveillance practice.

As the CDC specifically intended to capture more patients who suffered from a broader spectrum of AIDS-related conditions, the 1987 surveillance criterion necessarily increased the number and type of clinical symptoms that constituted an AIDS diagnosis. As expected, expanding the case definition caused significant growth in the epidemic, accounting for more than one of every three new AIDS patients reported after that date. The CDC reported that "in contrast to the 1985 revision, which increased the reported incidence of AIDS by no more than 3–4% . . . the impact of the 1987 revision on the num-ber of AIDS cases reported [has] been substantial,"[29] and was responsible for approximately 28 percent of all AIDS cases reported in the United States dur-ing the first 15 months of its use. Moreover, the CDC authors surmised that 28 percent was only a median estimate as the percentage of new cases attribut-able to the 1987 revision would continue to increase over time.[30]

Impact of 1987 Surveillance Definition

While a new geography of the American AIDS epidemic was also fashioned in 1987, quite literally, by incorporating new territories into the CDC's national surveillance reports (e.g., Guam, Puerto Rico, the Virgin Islands, etc.), most of the growth and shifting demography of the epidemic occurred because ad-ditional diseases were incorporated into the case definition and because physicians and disease surveillance officers changed the way in which they di-agnosed and documented opportunistic infections associated with AIDS.

Until July 1987, AIDS "diagnoses were considered to fit the case definition only if based on sufficiently reliable methods (generally histology or cul-ture)."[31] After August 1987 however, patients could be diagnosed with AIDS on the basis of a presumptive diagnosis of some opportunistic infections if they were also HIV-antibody-positive. This singular revision to diagnostic practices doubled the number of cases reported in the following year. More than half (56 percent) of the total number (8,044) of AIDS cases reported in the United States between August 1987 and December 31, 1988, were based on presump-tive diagnoses, primarily for *Pneumocystis carinii* pneumonia (34 percent) and esophageal candidiasis (12 percent of the total).

The impact of the change in the definition of the disease was not registered solely as a dramatic increase in the number of reported AIDS cases, however, as the 1987 revision also fundamentally altered the type, number, and range of infections that patients were diagnosed with, thus precipitating a concurrent shift in the demography of the disease. Recently captured cases meeting only the 1987 surveillance criteria were more likely to be "women, heterosexual IVDAs [intravenous drug abusers], blacks, Hispanics [or] cases from New Jer-sey or Puerto Rico."[32] And just two diagnoses accounted for nearly half (48 percent) of all newly reported AIDS cases: the ill-defined HIV encephalopathy ("dementia") and HIV wasting syndrome.

The changes introduced in 1987 also altered the attribution of the most likely mode of transmission for the disease and increased the number of persons reported with AIDS in two additional ways. First, AIDS had been uniquely defined as the susceptibility to opportunistic infections occurring in a person with no known cause for diminished resistance since the beginning of the epidemic in 1981. After 1987, however, patients with other causes of immune deficiency[33] could be counted as AIDS cases if they also tested positive for HIV antibodies. In other words, as of this date, patients who were *explicitly excluded* as AIDS cases in previous years given their preexisting predisposition to immune deficiency (congenital defects, chemotherapy, etc.) were now *explicitly included* in AIDS surveillance statistics and the cause of their immune deficiency attributed solely to the human immunodeficiency virus. Second, after August 1987, even a patient with laboratory test results *negative* for HIV infection could be counted as an AIDS case if s/he had no other cause for immune deficiency and presented with one of 12 (designated) opportunistic infections accompanied by a "CD4 lymphocyte count less than *400/mm³*."[34]

Geographic Differentials of Presumptive Diagnoses (by Race, Risk, and Sexual Orientation)

As previously noted, the greatest impact upon national statistics resulted from the inclusion of presumptive diagnoses, accounting for 56 percent of all AIDS cases captured via the new surveillance criteria. While this percentage was lower in San Francisco (44 percent),[35] the constellation of opportunistic infections that were most often presumptively diagnosed in this city differed from those similarly diagnosed elsewhere in the country. For example, the percentage of patients with presumptive PCP in San Francisco (42 percent) was higher than the national figure (34 percent), but that of patients reported with diagnoses of presumptive esophageal candidiasis was lower (8 percent vs. 13 percent).[36]

The significance of varying geographies of diagnosis, especially for patients in San Francisco vis-à-vis patients in other cities, is never made explicit in epidemiological literature. But homosexual/bisexual men constitute the bulk of reported AIDS cases in San Francisco, and they are overwhelmingly presumptively diagnosed with "gay pneumonia" (PCP), while heterosexual intravenous drug users, who account for a greater percentage of reported AIDS cases across the nation, are more frequently presumptively diagnosed with candidiasis. In a published study assessing the impact of the 1987 revised case definition on surveillance statistics in the city, even San Francisco Public Health Department researchers recognized that "the increase in presumptive diagnoses for PCP may represent less aggressive diagnostic practices for homosexual and bisexual men in a highly endemic city."[37]

The finding that patients are differentially diagnosed, depending on their race or ethnicity, risk, and sexual orientation holds true for national data as well, as the CDC acknowledged that Hispanics were more likely to be presumptively diagnosed with toxoplasmosis of the brain regardless of their risk factors for the disease, while an HIV-positive homosexual/bisexual of any race was more likely to be diagnosed with HIV dementia than was a heterosexual IVDU AIDS patient.[38]

Differentials of HIV Antibody Testing

Corresponding to the discovery of geographic differentials in the occurrence of presumptive diagnoses, the Centers for Disease Control also found that the patient's residence, sexual orientation, race, and transmission category (e.g., heterosexual, Gay IVDU, IVDU, hemophiliac, etc.) significantly influenced the likelihood that s/he would be tested for HIV antibodies. Moreover, geographical differentials for antibody testing demonstrated that "the proportion (HIV) tested was negatively correlated with the cumulative incidence of AIDS by area." Thus, while California and New York were responsible for almost one-third (29 percent) of all new AIDS cases reported between August 1987 and December 31, 1988, these two states were among those least likely to have tested their reported cases for the presence of HIV antibodies.[39]

Whether an individual AIDS patient was tested for HIV antibodies was not solely a function of geography, however; it was also a function of *identity,* as there were significant differences in the frequency with which the antibody test was administered to various risk groups. In both New York and California, a white heterosexual intravenous drug user was much more likely to have been tested for HIV antibodies than was a white non-IVDU homosexual. And when "area and exposure category were controlled," there were racial differences in the use of the test within risk populations.[40] Although minority homosexuals in California were more likely to have been tested for HIV antibodies than white gay men, the converse was true for heterosexual IVDUs in New York: minorities were less likely to have been tested than their white counterparts.

Results published by Selik et al. (for national statistics through the late 1980s) and Payne et al. (for San Francisco statistics) corroborate my empirical research of the differential ways in which homosexuals have been diagnosed and reported with AIDS in San Francisco. Because they constitute a population perceived as inherently high-risk, when homosexual/bisexual men become clinically ill with AIDS, they are less likely to be definitively diagnosed; rather, they are presumed to have gay-associated opportunistic infections. At least throughout the first decade of the epidemic (until the surveillance case definition changed in 1987 and more dramatically in 1993), it was easier to be reported as an AIDS case if you were a gay man.[41] Men who have sex with men are also less likely to be investigated for multiple risks for acquiring HIV/AIDS (e.g., IV drug use or transfusions); they are instead presumed to have been infected through sexual intercourse. Although "heterosexuals who have sex with injecting drug user(s)" account for nearly half of the cumulative total of heterosexuals who acquired AIDS via sexual intercourse in the United States, there isn't even an official surveillance risk category that would allow disease control investigators to report gay men whose sexual partners inject drugs.[42]

Sociopolitical Context of 1987 Revision

The 1987 expansion of the clinical parameters of AIDS did not occur in a social or political vacuum. In April 1987, four months before the revision, the French and U.S. governments agreed to share credit for the discovery of HIV and to split the patent rights to the antibody test.[43] There was now a considerable financial incentive for HIV test kits to be aggressively marketed and used diagnostically; it would be used not only to "confirm" AIDS diagnoses at clinics and in epidemiological studies, but also to test army recruits, women at prenatal screening clinics, and organ and blood donors. In the United States alone, royalties from the use of the HIV antibody test were $100 million annually. AIDS had become a big business. A second impetus for HIV testing and increased AIDS case reporting arose from pharmaceutical hype surrounding the benefits of early-intervention chemotherapy which accompanied the approval of the first antiviral therapy for persons diagnosed with AIDS or AIDS-related conditions. In February 1987, the FDA approved AZT (azidothymidine, aka zidovudine, marketed as Retrovir), the "most expensive drug of its kind" ever (at "$10,000 per person per year forever"),[44] specifically for HIV-positive persons and AIDS patients. "More than 10,000 persons received zidovudine from the manufacturer under a limited drug distribution system during March-September 1987";[45] within several years, the number of persons on AZT would increase tenfold.

Support for the 1987 revision was also bolstered by municipal departments of public health who were attempting to increase AIDS surveillance budgets and bureaucracies. An ever larger epidemic also enhanced the credibility and lobbying efforts of AIDS activists, educators, and researchers seeking increases in federal funding for research, treatment, and prevention efforts. The conflation of interests on the part of these institutions and community advocates, compounded by the evolution of clinical and biomedical knowledge on the "natural history" of the disease, amplified the magnitude of the AIDS epidemic in the United States and began to shift the perceived demography of risk for HIV infection. While these trends were abetted by incorporating AIDS caseloads from heretofore unreported geographical regions into U.S. surveillance totals and to ever expanding criteria for diagnosing patients, superficial analyses of rising local and national AIDS caseloads supported the claim that disease transmission was accelerating and diffusing into new populations of risk as the epidemic matured in the late 1980s.

The impact of the new 1987 surveillance definition was less dramatic in San Francisco than in the United States at large; nonetheless, its effect upon the cumulative AIDS caseload was substantial. After two years of follow-up, the city's AIDS Office estimated that the new case definition had increased case reporting in San Francisco by 23 percent, which was revised downward to 17 percent after accounting for those patients who subsequently developed opportunistic infections that qualified as AIDS diagnoses under previous definitions of the disease.[46] Only half of the city's 22,185 cumulative AIDS cases met the CDC's 1985 or earlier case definitions when they were first reported to the SFDPH; an additional 2,979 patients were reported under the 1987 AIDS case definition.[47] Thus, if there had been no changes to the roster of clinical syndromes and symptoms defining the disease after 1987, San Francisco would have reported a cumulative total of 14,216 AIDS cases—37 percent fewer patients than the ASSB claimed in 1995.[48]

The AIDS Epidemic Peaks and Declines
Phase III: 1993–Present

Despite the additional AIDS cases that were captured by virtue of the 1987 elaboration of surveillance criteria, the AIDS epidemic peaked in San Francisco by early 1990s and shortly thereafter nationally (1992). In fact, according to figures published in San Francisco's *Monthly AIDS Surveillance Report,* a salient harbinger of this welcome turn in the tide of the epidemic is embedded in surveillance data that tabulate the total number of AIDS cases reported in the city for each month of the epidemic from July 1981 through October 1995. And remarkably, one finds somewhat counterintuitively that the proportional increase in the total number of AIDS cases became smaller each year from the beginning of the epidemic until 1992.[49] Or to put it another way, the "doubling time" of the epidemic was becoming longer, which necessarily implied that rate of growth for the AIDS epidemic was slowing. This can be a confusing concept to grasp, but to illustrate my point, refer to the table of data below (Table 6) and compare the total number of number of AIDS cases reported in San Francisco in 1981 (23 patients) to the total caseload in 1982 (92 patients). Now divide the mathematical difference between the two years (69 patients) by the number of patients reported in the base year (23 patients in 1981) and convert your answer to a percentage (multiply by 100). This calculation tells you that the AIDS caseload in San Francisco increased by 300 percent during the first year of the epidemic. Following the same procedure for the following year demonstrates that the proportional increase in new AIDS cases was cut in half (147 percent) in 12 months; and declined further in 1984 (120 percent), and further still in 1985 (51 percent), and so on.[50]

So in spite of revised case definitions that cast a larger net to capture more AIDS patients, surveillance data from San Francisco reveal a consistently slower rate of growth in the epidemic in successive years. Moreover, these data

TABLE 6 AIDS Cases by Year and Month of Report to SFDPH, San Francisco, 1981–October 1995

Reported	Jan	Feb	Mar	Apr	May	Jun	Jul	Aug	Sep	Oct	Nov	Dec	Total
1981	0	0	0	0	0	0	8	4	3	3	0	5	**23**
1982	3	8	0	5	6	9	6	11	7	8	17	12	**92**
1983	15	12	25	11	20	11	16	27	20	24	21	25	**227**
1984	35	41	33	36	35	30	55	50	36	54	50	44	**499**
1985	59	61	67	65	64	54	63	66	59	62	70	62	**752**
1986	65	99	76	88	83	106	102	100	77	120	105	108	**1,129**
1987	91	107	122	103	117	92	140	116	126	167	154	131	**1,466**
1988	135	151	185	131	121	142	104	136	123	96	147	123	**1,594**
1989	138	115	180	204	163	158	147	161	145	138	144	121	**1,814**
1990	203	156	171	204	182	110	160	190	120	178	160	135	**1,969**
1991	151	180	167	184	140	171	159	224	144	163	145	136	**1,964**
1992	117	151	199	161	152	147	153	169	161	179	156	145	**1,890**
1993	701	673	599	502	411	426	321	264	292	238	221	234	**4,882**
1994	229	209	266	225	202	159	151	193	175	158	148	130	**2,245**
1995	166	163	180	165	185	134	140	206	135	165	—	—	**1,639**

Source: San Francisco Department of Public Health, "AIDS Cases Reported through October 1995," AIDS Surveillance Report (1995): 8.[[MR 1]]

trends have led some epidemiologists to infer a peak in HIV transmission between 1981 and early 1983, trailed by a parallel peak in annual AIDS caseloads approximately nine to ten years later (the median incubation period from HIV infection to AIDS for patients diagnosed in these years). Theoretically, a decline in annual caseloads should follow shortly thereafter (assuming, of course, that there is no explosion of new HIV infections in the intervening years). And indeed the annual AIDS caseload did decline as expected in San Francisco, leveling off at fewer than 2,000 cases per year in the early 1990s and then beginning to plummet.

By 1990/1991, San Francisco data clearly indicate that the epidemic had peaked at annual caseloads of 1969 and 1964 in each respective year. In the subsequent year (1992) the annual caseload declined by 4 percent (1,890 new cases). Any relief from a decade of bad news on the AIDS crisis would be short-lived, however, and the explosive growth of the epidemic seemingly rekindled, as the CDC contemporaneously engineered the most dramatic revision in the definition of the disease to date. Whatever successes had been achieved by promoting safe sex and needle exchanges among high-risk populations was soon obscured, yet again, by a profound revision of the constellation of clinical symptoms indicative of an AIDS diagnosis.

Sociopolitical Context of 1993 Revision

As in previous years, patient advocates, political lobbyists and those with financial and institutional interests at stake provided momentum in support of the proposed redefinition of AIDS. Public health researchers in San Francisco acknowledged as much, in an article evaluating the impact of the 1993 revised definition in San Francisco (a change initially proposed to begin in 1992):

> The 1987 revision . . . included presumptive diagnoses of certain indicator diseases, with the result of that revision being an increase in the number of persons, particularly intravenous drug users, women, and African Americans, identified as having AIDS. . . . The 1992 revision follows intense criticism that the 1987 revision is too restrictive and, in particular, that it does not include manifestations of HIV disease common among women and intravenous drug users. The 1992 definition, by using a marker of immune deficiency to define AIDS, avoids the problem of piecemeal addition of newly recognized manifestations of HIV infection. . . .
>
> Although the original purpose of the CDC AIDS definition was to monitor the epidemic, the case definition has taken on a broader social and economic significance. For some individuals, an AIDS diagnosis determines their eligibility for Social Security, Medicaid, and community-based services. For localities, in turn, the proportion of individuals covered by Social Security and Medicaid determines reimbursement for care. In addition, the number of AIDS cases, as classified by the CDC definition, governs funding allocations to HIV epicenters.[51]

According to Elinor Burkett, the April 1990 authorization of the Ryan White Comprehensive AIDS Resources Emergency Act (the Care Act) meant that federal dollars would be allocated to states and municipalities according to two tiers of eligibility.

> Title I funds which went to the original epicenters of the plague, were distributed according to the total number of AIDS cases since the beginning of the epidemic, although 60% of that number were dead. That meant that everyone could stop dying, even stop getting infected, in New York or San Francisco and those cities would still get the bulk of the Care Act funds.
>
> Title II money, which went to state governments, was distributed according to the number of people living with AIDS in each state.[52]

The financial windfall associated with the Care Act presented further incentives for local surveillance departments to increase the number of AIDS cases that they reported in their districts, a sentiment echoed by San Francisco health officials when they published a public health directive that "it is critical that reporting be as complete as possible since the distribution of Federal and State AIDS funds to cities and counties is determined by the number of reported cases."[53]

According to Burkett, the inequity in the distribution of these monies, "$6,000 per person with AIDS [in San Francisco, while] Pittsburgh and Cincinnati were lucky to see $1,100 per case," unleashed bitter municipal and state battles over each region's slice of the fiscal pie.[54]

> [San Francisco] has benefited from the Care Act windfall more than any other city in the country. For fiscal year 1994, San Francisco received $44.2 million in funds, based on a cumulative caseload of AIDS patients that gave the city the nation's highest per capita incidence of the disease.[55]

As long as Care Act funds and surveillance monies were forthcoming, most cities and states favored the expanded definition of AIDS. The San Francisco AIDS Office was already offering its endorsement as early as 1991, with the proviso that "additional resources [be] allocated for surveillance activities" and Ryan White Care funding be "commensurate" with the increasing caseload.[56] Public Health officials in the city also recommended that the CDC evaluate the impact of the revised case definition in "selected localities"; San Francisco, of course, would be an ideal candidate for such an impact assessment.[57]

Impact of 1993 Surveillance Definition: Changing Demographics

On January 1, 1993, the CDC rendered data from the first decade of the AIDS epidemic incommensurate with data after 1993 by officially expanding the case definition to include numerous clinical manifestations associated with HIV infection—irreversibly altering fundamental attributes of an AIDS diagnosis:

> [The CDC has] expanded the AIDS surveillance case definition to include all HIV-infected persons who have < 200 CD4 T-lymphocytes/uL, or a CD4+ T-lymphocyte percentage of total lymphocytes < 14(%). This expansion also includes the addition of three clinical conditions—pulmonary tuberculosis, recurrent pneumonia, and invasive cervical cancer—while retaining the 23 clinical conditions in the AIDS surveillance case definition published in 1987. It is to be used by all states for AIDS case reporting effective January 1, 1993.[58]

At the very moment that the epidemic appeared to be in decline, overnight, the CDC's elaboration of the constellation of symptoms signifying an AIDS diagnosis doubled the number of patients reported in the United States. A significant proportion of this skyrocketing caseload resulted from the inclusion of diseases (e.g. pulmonary tuberculosis) specifically excluded from the original definition of acquired immune deficiency syndrome in 1982. Certainly it is possible to argue that AIDS was underreported during the first decade of the epidemic, but one cannot use post-1993 surveillance data to prove that the epidemic was continuing to grow unabated or disseminating into new populations of risk. To the contrary, current AIDS prevalence and incidence data are skewed vis-à-vis surveillance data from years prior to 1993.

Shortly after the new surveillance definition was employed at local health departments, the number of reported AIDS increased nationally by 111 percent. Had the revision not taken place, AIDS cases would have declined in the United States by 2 percent in 1993 as is starkly evident in the following graph juxtaposing the nation's AIDS caseload before and after January 1, 1993 (Figure 10).

As this CDC graph illustrates, more than 90 percent of all new cases were asymptomatic and qualified for an AIDS diagnosis solely on the basis of "HIV-related immunosuppression" (CD4 T-cells fewer than 200 in number or less than 14 percent of total lymphocytes). Moreover, the epidemiology of risk for AIDS appears to be shifting even more dramatically toward "females, blacks,

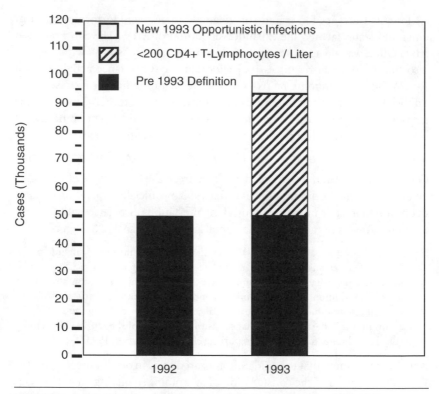

FIGURE 10   Number of Adolescents and Adults with AIDS—United States, 1992–1993
CDC, "Update: Impact of the Expanded AIDS Surveillance Case Definition for Adolescents and Adults on Case Reporting—U.S., 1993," *Morbidity and Mortality Weekly Report,* March 11, 1994: 161.

heterosexual injecting drug users (IDUs), and persons with hemophilia [who] were more likely than others to be reported with 1993-added conditions,"[59] while the proportion of new AIDS cases among homosexual and bisexual men correspondingly decreased.

For the most part, this artifactual amplification of the AIDS epidemic was disseminated uncritically in the news media, as exemplified by the following article in the *San Francisco Examiner:*

> In the United States, almost half of all AIDS cases in the 14-year history of the epidemic have been reported within the past three years. Of cumulative AIDS cases, 50,352 (10%) were reported from 1981 to 1987; 203,217 (41%) from 1988 to 1992; and 247,741 (49%) from 1993 to 1995, according to new data from the federal Centers For Disease Control and Prevention. Since the beginning of the U.S. epidemic . . . the proportion of cases among women increased to 18 percent from 8 percent at the beginning of the epidemic. The CDC data also indicate that the proportion of AIDS cases among [IVDUs] continues to climb, to 27 percent from 17 percent. The proportion of cases attributed to heterosexual trans-

mission increased to 10 percent from 3 percent . . . gay sex accounted for 64 percent of cases at the beginning of the epidemic but only 45 percent today.[60]

To one uninitiated in the arcane machinations of changing AIDS surveillance definitions, press reports such as this corroborated an infectious epidemic that was rapidly evolving and posing increasing risks for heterosexuals, especially women. What Krieger elided from this passage however, is that the CDC's elaborated surveillance criteria in 1993 had produced a one-time doubling of the nation's epidemic.[61] She also neglected to account for the increasing proportion of female AIDS patients reported, an anticipated result of the changes foreshadowed in 1987 and instituted in 1993, which explicitly incorporated opportunistic infections specific to women into the revised criteria for diagnosing AIDS.

As Elinor Burkett chronicles in *The Gravest Show on Earth* (1995), the CDC's 1993 revision was a conscious response to women's health-care advocacy:

> Throughout 1990, McGovern (a 34-year-old attorney . . . a certifiable AIDS heroine . . . waging a one-woman crusade to protect the nation's forgotten AIDS patients),[62] a small band of female activists and a group of physicians with large numbers of female AIDS patients inundated the CDC with data on women-specific manifestations of AIDS. . . . Finally CDC officials admitted that vaginitis, pelvic inflammatory disease [PID] and cervical cancer were showing up more frequently, or more severely, in HIV-infected women. But they asked, with perfect scientific composure, for proof of a cause-and-effect relationship.
>
> The women were dumbfounded. No one had proven a causal relationship between HIV infection and *Pneumocystis carinii* pneumonia, or Kaposi's sarcoma and HIV, when the first AIDS definition was published. If correlation was sufficient evidence in men, why was it insufficient for women? . . . Exasperated by the intransigence, McGovern filed suit against the U.S. government on October 1, 1990, alleging that the operative definition of AIDS discriminated against women. . . . [For] thousands of women dependent on the CDC's definition in order to qualify for presumptive disability, . . . it was the difference between sleeping on a park bench and renting an apartment.
>
> Just as McGovern was on the verge of concluding that government bureaucrats were impervious to reason, the Social Security Administration (SSA) announced a new set of criteria for AIDS-related disability. . . . The preface openly acknowledged that gynecological problems were more aggressive in women with HIV; the revised list of AIDS-related illnesses included pelvic inflammatory disease and vaginal candidiasis.[63]

Although incorporating opportunistic infections specific to women into the AIDS case definition had some effect on increasing national caseloads, a greater increase in the number and proportion of heterosexuals reported with AIDS after 1993 derived from recategorizing pulmonary tuberculosis as an AIDS-defining opportunistic infection; a disease explicitly excluded in the earliest definition of a emergent syndrome of immune deficiency in 1982. This

TABLE 7 AIDS Cases by Year and Month of Report to SFDPH, San Francisco, 1981–October 1995

Reported	Jan	Feb	Mar	Apr	May	Jun	Jul	Aug	Sep	Oct	Nov	Dec	Total
1981	0	0	0	0	0	0	8	4	3	3	0	5	**23**
1982	3	8	0	5	6	9	6	11	7	8	17	12	**92**
1983	15	12	25	11	20	11	16	27	20	24	21	25	**227**
1984	35	41	33	36	35	30	55	50	36	54	50	44	**499**
1985	59	61	67	65	64	54	63	66	59	62	70	62	**752**
1986	65	99	76	88	83	106	102	100	77	120	105	108	**1,129**
1987	91	107	122	103	117	92	140	116	126	167	154	131	**1,466**
1988	135	151	185	131	121	142	104	136	123	96	147	123	**1,594**
1989	138	115	180	204	163	158	147	161	145	138	144	121	**1,814**
1990	203	156	171	204	182	110	160	190	120	178	160	135	**1,969**
1991	151	180	167	184	140	171	159	224	144	163	145	136	**1,964**
1992	117	151	199	161	152	147	153	169	161	179	156	145	**1,890**
1993	701	673	599	502	411	426	321	264	292	238	221	234	**4,882**
1994	229	209	266	225	202	159	151	193	175	158	148	130	**2,245**
1995	166	163	180	165	185	134	140	206	135	165	—	—	**1,639**

(1) Cases reported through 10/31/95.

quantum shift in surveillance policy caused reported AIDS cases among minorities, the urban poor, and injecting drug users to rise correspondingly.[64]

I am not suggesting that the 1993 surveillance definition of AIDS is somehow more political or less accurate than the previous (1987 or 1985 or 1982) definitions of AIDS; what I am saying is that one cannot meaningfully compare AIDS surveillance data from prior years with data collected subsequent to January 1, 1993. Superficially juxtaposing the relative proportions of different populations reported with AIDS in the 1980s versus 1993, as Kreiger did in the passage above, and thereby concluding that the AIDS epidemic is increasingly spreading to women or IV drug users, is like comparing "apples and oranges," and thereby distorting our understanding of the evolution of the epidemic and the efficacy of interventions to contain it.[65]

Amplifying the Epidemic after the Fact

The impact of the 1993 AIDS case revision on annual caseloads in San Francisco is starkly evident from two tables of data published within the city's monthly *AIDS Surveillance Report* of October 31, 1995, and reproduced in this text (Tables 7 and 8).

When I argued that the AIDS epidemic began to decline in San Francisco in the early 1990s, I used unadjusted data from Table 7 ("AIDS Cases by Year and Month of Report") to show that the annual number of AIDS cases peaked in 1990/1991, and declined by 4 percent in 1992. But note the effect of the revised AIDS case definition in 1993; instead of continuing its downward trajectory, the annual caseload jumps 158 percent, and the lingering effect of the new definition trails on through 1994 and 1995. However, data in Table 8 tell a different story; here annual caseloads are higher in every year through 1992. And

TABLE 8 AIDS Cases by Year and Month of Primary Diagnosis, San Francisco, 1981–October 1995

Diagnosed	Jan	Feb	Mar	Apr	May	Jun	Jul	Aug	Sep	Oct	Nov	Dec	Total
1981	1	3	2	1	1	2	3	3	5	3	3	7	**34**
1982	6	5	0	6	6	15	12	10	10	14	19	13	**116**
1983	24	19	31	25	19	21	27	36	28	31	26	31	**318**
1984	46	32	39	43	39	48	67	59	70	54	61	56	**614**
1985	77	62	72	77	74	80	94	89	76	88	70	89	**948**
1986	104	94	115	100	103	110	121	137	112	149	99	142	**1,386**
1987	137	137	142	130	150	150	149	149	161	139	123	131	**1,698**
1988	157	145	182	141	130	156	139	137	155	117	134	157	**1,750**
1989	158	142	179	198	164	204	168	162	137	159	142	143	**1,956**
1990	201	176	193	161	180	174	179	196	154	179	184	155	**2,132**
1991	222	201	196	193	212	196	235	245	226	304	229	245	**2,704**
1992	287	300	304	219	218	246	267	247	256	240	206	230	**3,020**
1993	246	236	243	190	189	240	242	197	192	178	171	176	**2,500**
1994	224	178	194	160	138	141	122	181	135	125	147	116	**1,861**
1995	145	137	168	129	108	144	109	100	81	27	—	—	**1,148**

Source: San Francisco Department of Public Health, "AIDS Cases by Year and Month of Primary Diagnosis, San Francisco, 1981–1995," *AIDS Surveillance Report* 1995: 8.

because Table 8 contains adjusted data, these figures are constantly in flux, as new AIDS cases are thrown backward in time, increasing and decreasing annual caseloads as patients are enumerated as of the first date at which they met 1993 diagnostic criteria, a surveillance practice known as "backdating."

In order to fully appreciate the dramatic effect of the 1993 revision on the cumulative AIDS caseload in San Francisco and why the new case definition skews an interpretation of how the epidemic has evolved through time, one needs to understand how new AIDS cases are backdated and tabulated as cases for previous years. Once a patient has been captured by surveillance staff and qualifies as an AIDS case according to the CDC's most recent criteria for the disease (e.g., by virtue of a low CD4 count and/or a diagnosis of tuberculosis or cervical cancer, etc.), this "new" case is subsequently backdated and reported as of the earliest date by which s/he first met the current AIDS case definition. For example, let us suppose that the SFDPH captures a 29-year-old male AIDS case in July 1994 because the patient is diagnosed with *Pneumocystis carinii* pneumonia. During a medical chart review, the disease control investigator discovers that the man's physician stated that the patient tested HIV-positive in 1987, and had only 132 CD4 T-cells in December 1991. Given this knowledge, the patient, although captured and initially reported by the SFDPH in July 1994, is backdated to the earlier date and entered into Table 8 as an AIDS case with a primary diagnosis (HIV-positive, less than 200 CD4 T-cells) as of December 1991. Because of the sweeping changes introduced on January 1, 1993, this patient is officially reported as an AIDS case *two years before* he was clinically diagnosed with PCP, and two years before he came to the attention of AIDS surveillance staff in San Francisco.[66]

By throwing AIDS cases backward in time (and into Table 8), the city's annual caseload for the 1980s and early 1990s was amplified after the fact (e.g., the 24 AIDS cases actually reported in the first six months of surveillance in 1981 had grown to 34 cases as of the monthly surveillance report of October 1995). Simultaneously, because the 1993 case definition necessarily captured AIDS patients earlier in the course of their disease, San Francisco's annual AIDS caseloads for the immediate year (1993) and for the near future (1994 and 1995) were also amplified, as primarily asymptomatic (albeit HIV-positive) patients were captured several years in advance of when they would have been diagnosed with AIDS according to pre-1993 criteria. These patients were thus pulled forward in time and reported both in Table 7 (the year they were initially captured by the SFDPH) and Table 8 (on the date they first qualified for an AIDS diagnosis on the basis of the 1993 case surveillance definition; e.g., TB, low CD4 T-cell counts, cervical cancer, etc.).

The practice of backdating, coupled with the profound clinical and diagnostic changes introduced by the 1993 AIDS case definition, complicates efforts to track epidemiological trends in AIDS caseloads, mortality, and opportunistic infections by comparing aggregate data from the 1980s to data from the 1990s. First, the number of AIDS cases currently being reported is inflated in comparison to caseloads from previous years, as today more patients qualify for an official AIDS diagnosis with a broader range of symptoms than in past years, and current patients are captured by surveillance departments much earlier in the course of their illness. Second, the "peak" of the AIDS epidemic was delayed in time (seemingly occurring in 1993/1994 versus 1991/1992) and significantly amplified when it did occur, because newly captured patients were backdated and reported as cases during earlier years, and because patients who would have been diagnosed in future years were pulled forward in time and reported approximately 1.6 years earlier than they otherwise would have been under previous case definitions.[67] Bringing forward AIDS cases that would have trickled in throughout 1993, 1994, 1995, and so on, more than doubled the number of AIDS cases actually reported in San Francisco in 1993 (4,882 vs. about 1,850 under the old definition) and, because of backdating, also increased the number of AIDS cases "diagnosed" in 1990 (by 8 percent), 1991 (by 38 percent), and 1992 (by 60 percent) as shown in the table below (Table 9).

Clearly, the 1993 definition enabled San Francisco and other major cities in the nation to forestall the acknowledgment that the AIDS epidemic as defined historically was beginning to decline. Instead, overnight, the annual number of reported AIDS cases in San Francisco more than doubled, and Public Health officials predicted that the number of PWAs living in the city would triple (from 3,785 PWAs to more than 9,500 projected under the new case definition).[68] Both of these developments, in turn, increased San Francisco's allocation of Title I funds (cumulative AIDS caseload), and California's allocation of Ryan White

TABLE 9 AIDS Cases Reported in 1990, 1991, and 1992 before and after Adjusting for the 1993 Case Definition

Year	Cases Reported	Cases after Adjusting*	Difference
1990	1,969	2,132	+ 163 cases (8%)
1991	1,964	2,704	+ 740 cases (38%)
1992	1,890	3,020	+ 1,130 (60%)

*Data are adjusted not only because of backdating but because of reporting delays, although in San Francisco 90 percent of all cases are reported within six months of their capture, according to Kevin McKinney of the ASSB.

money under Title II (living PWAs per state). And with the Care Act coming up for reauthorization in 1994, a larger national AIDS epidemic also provided additional leverage for lobbyists.

As it turned out, not all of the figures that were projected by San Francisco's AIDS Office materialized. But in this city and nationally, as a result of the changes introduced by the 1993 AIDS case definition, contemporary AIDS surveillance practice and its product (statistical information) make fundamentally different claims about the disease vis-à-vis past representations. In a mechanical sense, the revision altered the very character of surveillance practice as it authorized disease control officers to track and monitor HIV-positive persons with fewer than 200 CD4 T-cells (or CD4 T-cells totaling less than 14 percent of total lymphocytes), regardless of whether the patient had developed any opportunistic infections or other clinical abnormalities associated with the disease.[69] In an epidemiological sense, the 1993 revision also continued to shift the characterization of populations at risk from AIDS, causing more cases to be reported from populations allegedly undercounted in previous AIDS statistics (specifically female patients and heterosexual IVDUs). In San Francisco however, this latter epidemiological shift was muted, Kevin McKinney said in an interview for this book:

> The 1993 definition was meant to bring in women and IVDUs, but now the cases have returned to gay men.[70] [Heterosexual] IVDUs [were] 5 percent of the cumulative total before 1993, and now are 9 percent of the total [cases in] 1993. . . . Cumulatively, females were 2.6 percent of the total before 1993, and now are 4 percent of the cases in 1993. So there is some excess, but obviously [the 1993 definition] hasn't opened the floodgates. . . . Basically, it didn't pan out in San Francisco as the activists were saying, that there are massive numbers of women and drug users out there that are not being counted the same as gays and bisexuals due to their unique symptoms.[71]

While McKinney's observations hold true for San Francisco, as men who have sex with men and gay IVDU comprise the overwhelming majority of reported AIDS cases in the city since 1981 (more than 94 percent of all cases), the Centers for Disease Control reported that the 1993 case definition caused AIDS cases among heterosexuals to skyrocket in the United States, especially in black and Hispanic communities.

> From 1985 through 1993, the proportion of persons with AIDS who reported heterosexual contact with a partner at risk for or with documented HIV infection increased from 1.9% to 9.0%, respectively. In 1993, AIDS cases attributed to heterosexual contact increased 130% over 1992. . . .
>
> Editorial Note: . . . Persons at highest risk for heterosexually transmitted HIV infection include adolescents and adults with multiple sex partners, those with sexually transmitted diseases (STDs), and heterosexually active persons residing in areas with a high prevalence of HIV infection among IDUs [intravenous drug users]. In addition, a disproportionate number of persons with AIDS who acquired HIV infection through heterosexual contact are black or Hispanic.[72]

Despite the CDC's conclusion that "the number of persons infected through heterosexual transmission is increasing rapidly," McKinney opined that an unintended consequence of picking patients up sooner in the disease process is that both patients and primary health providers may be less accurate when reporting risk factors for the disease:

McKinney: When a person finds out earlier in the course of the disease, or when a health-care provider sees them earlier in the disease, people tend not to say, and providers don't always ask, about risks. . . .

Author: So the 1993 definition, and cases diagnosed subsequent to it, may have a little less honest transmission data in it . . . and therefore the reported increase in the percentage of cases attributed to heterosexual transmission might be simply an artifact of changing HIV/AIDS surveillance practices?

McKinney: It's just that when people have a major illness [an opportunistic infection] they tend to be more forthcoming with information. That, and another thing is that drug users [IVDUs] clean their needles but aren't very good about using condoms.[73]

Although the demography of risk for the disease did not shift dramatically in San Francisco, the impact of the revised case definition was immediately registered by a 158 percent increase in the annual AIDS caseload in 1993, and monthly caseloads that were 30 percent higher in the first six months of 1994 than during previous years.[74]

Burgeoning caseloads put increasing pressure on San Francisco's surveillance staff, who were now capturing and reporting nearly double the number of AIDS cases that they had reported in previous years; most likely, the increased workload had a overall deleterious effect on the quality of surveillance data.

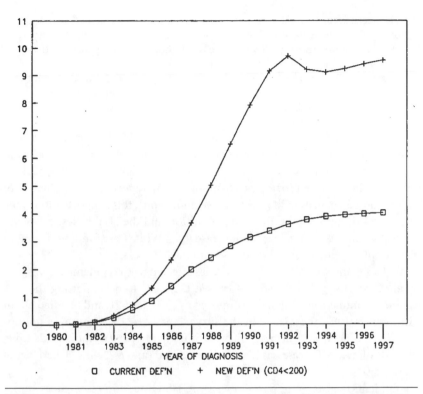

FIGURE 11 Projected Living Persons with AIDS—Current vs. Proposed New Case Definition, San Francisco
Source: A. M. Hirozawa, "Projections of the AIDS Epidemic in San Francisco through 1997: Impact of the New Case Definition." Presentation at the Seventh International Conference on AIDS. Amsterdam, The Netherlands, July 19–24, 1992.

"Sitting On News that the Epidemic Is in Decline"

Indisputably, the greatest impact of the 1993 revision was upon the projected number of persons with AIDS (PWAs) living in San Francisco; ASSB officials projected the number of PWAs needing services in the city would triple once the new definition was put into effect (Figure 11).[75]

Concern over this issue had been raised early on by SFDPH officials, prompting them to offer only provisional support for the 1993 case definition. Their approval of the revision was necessarily contingent upon an increase in funding for surveillance staff and for patient care and services. The San Francisco AIDS Office was also worried that the Social Security Administration (SSA) would back away from its position that "Californians with an AIDS diagnosis have presumptive eligibility for Medi-Cal and (disability) if they meet financial criteria."[76]

> The Social Security Administration has decided not to accept the 1992 definition of AIDS [implementation of the new definition was delayed until January 1, 1993] as presumptive eligibility for benefits. Without federal support to individuals and localities, the new definition will result in more cases but the same level of services. Rather than benefiting from the change, service providers will be placed in the difficult situation of choosing which of the people with AIDS are in the most need of care.[77]

As early as December 1991, George Lemp of the SFDPH AIDS Office expressed similar sentiments about the necessity of tying care, prevention, and health services money to the CDC's case definition. "Although the majority [of clinicians and health-care providers in San Francisco] appear to be supportive [of the proposed changes in the surveillance definition], this support could wane if the SSA decouples from the CDC definition and the Health Resources and Services Administration does not increase Ryan White Care funding commensurate with the increase in the number of new AIDS cases."[78]

In San Francisco and other major cities affected by the epidemic, it was precisely concerns such as these that caused the CDC to delay putting the new definition into effect. Originally proposed as early as 1991, and bandied about throughout 1992, the change in the surveillance case definition was not approved as official surveillance policy until January 1, 1993. And all this time, the tide of new AIDS cases, as historically defined (and re-defined), had begun to recede.

Epidemiologists in the San Francisco AIDS Office and researchers studying cohort data in the city had foreseen the decline in new AIDS cases for years. As early as 1989, UCSF epidemiologists studying cohorts of gay men at risk for AIDS in the city had projected that the epidemic would begin to level off as early as 1989, but no later than 1991.[79] In an unpublished report by the AIDS Office commissioned in July 1992, public health officials predicted that "based on the current [1987] AIDS case definition . . . the epidemic curve will peak at 2,173 cases during 1992."[80] The authors of this report repeatedly emphasized the dramatic effect that the 1993 case definition would have on the number of PWAs living in the city. But even with the amplification of the epidemic following the January 1993 revision, San Francisco surveillance data still registered a peak in new AIDS diagnoses in 1992 (see Table 8).

In the 1992 report, the authors provided six tables projecting the annual number of AIDS cases and PWAs that the city could expect under the 1987 definition. They used these projected data to illustrate their conclusion that the "epidemic curve" for AIDS would peak in San Francisco in 1992. However, the authors included only one table to illustrate the impact of the proposed 1993 revision, and it was this table, of course, that contained the dramatic data that projected a trebling in the number of PWAs in the city if the proposed revisions were adopted.[81] In the seven figures that accompany this report, nowhere is there any information on the projected impact of the 1993 revisions on the city's annual caseload. One week after this 1992 report, SFDPH officials presented a 15-page summary of their conclusions to the Eighth International Conference on AIDS. This presentation included just one graph and one concluding remark addressing the decline of the AIDS epidemic in San Francisco. The SFDPH researchers clearly acknowledged that the "epidemic curve will peak at 2,173 cases during 1992 [under the 1987 definition, or] . . . if the definition of AIDS were expanded in September 1992 [it was delayed until January 1993], the number of AIDS patients diagnosed each year would peak at 3,649 in 1991."[82]

Therefore, regardless of which definition of AIDS is used, the SFDPH is on record in 1992 with its assessment that the city's AIDS epidemic was already in decline. Any effect from the proposed revision in the case definition would only move the decline backward in time, to 1991. But at the time of this presentation (July 1992), San Francisco officials were working from projected data; their conclusions were provisional. Any confirmation of their estimates would have to await the official use of the 1993 case definition in surveillance practice.

It was almost two years, however, before any such confirmation arrived from the SFDPH. And this is remarkable, given that news of the decline of the AIDS epidemic in its very epicenter was the best news about the disease in the past decade. Seemingly, public health officials and politicians in San Francisco delayed the release of this information as long as they possibly could. And subsequent to a press conference in 1994 announcing the decline of annual caseloads in the city, they attempted to mitigate the significance of this profound shift in the trend of the AIDS epidemic by speculating about a "second wave" of HIV infection on the horizon, or by suggesting that vast numbers of AIDS patients had gone unreported in the city.

According to press coverage at the time, some politicians and activists in San Francisco even resented a limited and tardy acknowledgment that the peak years of the epidemic had passed. They suggested that surveillance data corroborating a decline in the epidemic should never have been released by the health department in the first place as it served only to exacerbate problems in finding legislative dollars for AIDS prevention and services in the city. When the announcement was finally made by SFDPH officials, albeit belatedly, it unleashed vehement criticism from some members of the gay community and threats of sanctions by at least one member of the city's board of supervisors.

The following excerpts are from the official press release, embargoed until 1 P.M. on February 15, 1994, wherein the San Francisco AIDS Office announced the release of a new report projecting trends in the epidemic:

The report . . . shows that the annual number of new AIDS cases has peaked at 3,326 in 1992 and is expected to decline to 1,204 annually by 1997. The number of persons living with AIDS has also peaked according to these projections, and is expected to decline gradually from a high of 9,109 persons living with AIDS in 1992 to 6,460 living with AIDS by the end of 1997.

These trends reflect the dramatic reductions in new HIV infections which occurred a decade ago and which were achieved as a result of successful prevention campaigns waged in San Francisco during the past 10 years. The number of new AIDS cases are only now reflecting this change, because of the average 10-year incubation period between infection with HIV and development of AIDS.

The trends are also affected by the recent expansion of the definition of AIDS, which resulted in AIDS being defined earlier in the course of HIV infection for many people. . . . This has caused the epidemic curve to shift, resulting in an earlier and sharper peak than what would have been expected under the old case definition.

It is estimated that 28,000 men, women, and children are currently living with HIV infection in San Francisco, representing almost 4% of the City's population. San Francisco has the highest number of HIV-infected persons per capita of any major city within the United States.

"This study is important because it identifies the number of people who will be needing AIDS-related care over the next four years," said Dr. Sandra Hernandez, Director of the Department of Public Health. "Since the number of persons living with AIDS is projected to decline only slightly over the next four years, we should take care not to become complacent or withdraw support for programs for persons with AIDS. The fact that more of these new cases will be among injection drug users suggests that increased resources may be required."[83]

Characteristic of the media's treatment of established AIDS science and discourse, the SFDPH press release was uncritically disseminated on the front pages of local newspapers and in the *New York Times* and *The Wall Street Journal.* Included below are graphs that accompanied the text of two of these articles: the *San Francisco Chronicle* article (Figure 12) and the *New York Times* article (Figure 13).

The press release begins with the announcement that the AIDS epidemic peaked in San Francisco in 1992 with 3,326 cases. Given the vastly different visual representations of the SFDPH data in the *Times* and the *Chronicle* however, it is hard to believe that the newspapers were depicting the same epidemic. The way in which the graphs are annotated in each newspaper also differs significantly. In the graph accompanying the *Chronicle* article (Figure 12), the peak of the AIDS epidemic in 1992 is clearly marked with 3,326 AIDS cases. It is only in the small print beneath the graph that the reader is advised that the illustration was constructed from projected data, and that "the number of observed cases may vary from projections." In contrast, the *Times* article specifically informs the reader that only data for the years 1994 through 1997 are "projected." In fact, every number in the SFDPH press release is projected data.

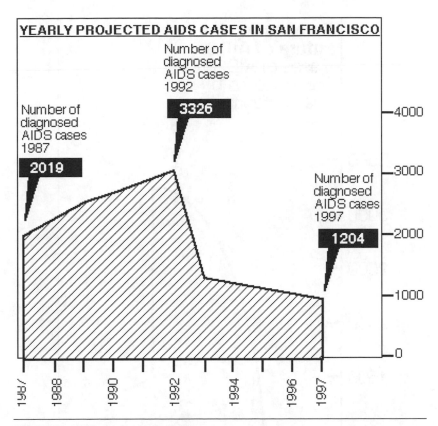

FIGURE 12 AIDS Prevention Methods Work
"AIDS Cases Decline in San Francisco," *San Francisco Chronicle,* February 16, 1994.

One has to wonder why the SFDPH used a projection of the number of AIDS cases in 1992 for the content of a press statement issued in February 1994. Surely, after two years, officials at the SFDPH were confident about the actual observed number of AIDS cases in the city in previous years. In the *AIDS Surveillance Report* for the most recent month (January 1994) available to officials at the time of their announcement, 3,049 AIDS cases were reportedly diagnosed in 1992, nearly 8 percent lower than the figure announced.[84] Referencing the 39-page report upon which the press release was based, one finds that the larger caseload was generated by adding a fudge factor to the observed number of AIDS cases to "adjust for reporting delay."[85] After a reporting delay of two years, however, the additional 277 AIDS cases projected by the SFDPH never materialized; to the contrary, some cases reported in 1992 had disappeared by October 1995, when an adjusted total of 3,020 cases were reported in the monthly surveillance report.[86]

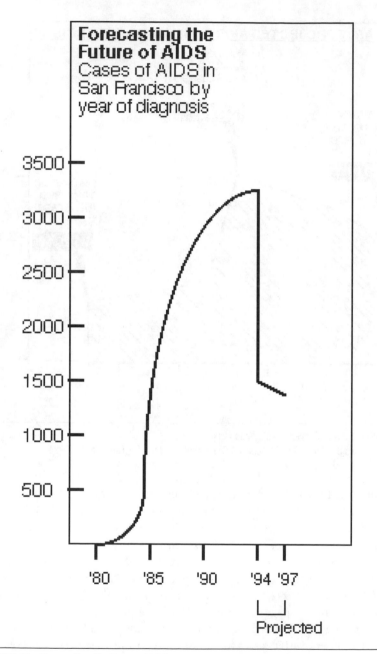

FIGURE 13   Forecasting the Future of AIDS
Source: "Forecasting the Future of AIDS," *New York Times,* February 16, 1994.

While all of the surveillance data cited in the SFDPH press release can be deconstructed, I have already reviewed in considerable detail the way in which demographic projections of populations at risk for AIDS (e.g., gay men in San Francisco) are estimated in previous chapters. My primary focus here is the representation by the San Francisco AIDS Office that the 1993 revision prematurely caused the observed decline in the AIDS epidemic. This claim is patently false; as reviewed, internal SFDPH documents and SFDPH presentations at the Eighth International Conference on AIDS stated explicitly that the AIDS epidemic would peak no later than 1992, regardless of which surveillance case definition was used. To reiterate, research by epidemiologists in the city also predicted a decline in the epidemic as early as 1989, while monthly AIDS surveillance reports in San Francisco record a peak in the epidemic in 1990/1991 under the 1987 case definition. Therefore, it is somewhat disingenuous for a SFDPH press release in 1994 to assert that the changes introduced in 1993 "caused the epidemic curve to shift, resulting in an earlier and sharper peak than what would have been expected under the old case definition."[87] The implication is that the decline of the AIDS epidemic in San Francisco is an artifact of recent surveillance practice, and had the definition not caused future cases to be reported "prematurely," the increase of the AIDS epidemic (as historically defined) would have continued throughout the decade. To the contrary, each subsequent revision of the case surveillance definition of AIDS has *delayed* a decline in the epidemic by increasing the number of patients who qualify as AIDS cases.

It appears that the SFDPH's measured comments were designed to mollify angry politicians and key stakeholders who felt increasingly financially vulnerable as a consequence of the SFDPH's acknowledgment of a waning epidemic. Dr. Hernandez, the director of the San Francisco Department of Public Health, attempted to thwart any criticism attendant to the press release by adding the caveat that "since the number of [PWAs] is projected to decline only slightly over the next four years, we should take care . . . not to withdraw support for programs. . . . The fact that more of these new cases will be among injection drug users suggests that increased resources may be required."[88]

Dr. Hernandez demonstrates the negotiated political stance of the SFDPH as she deemphasizes the future decline of PWAs in the city and stresses the growing number of AIDS cases among IVDUs. But according to the department's own projected data, the number of PWAs in San Francisco was expected to decline by 2,649 persons (a decrease of 29 percent) between 1992 and 1997,[89] which Dr. Hernandez concluded was only a "slight" decrease. Meanwhile, she suggested that "additional resources" may be needed in San Francisco because "more of these cases" will be among IVDUs. Presumably, Hernandez is referring to the 16 percent increase between 1992 (571 IVDUs) and 1997 (660 IVDUs) in the number of intravenous drug users who will be living with an AIDS diagnosis in San Francisco.[90] So she is arguing that the financial impact from a decline of more than 2,600 PWAs overall will be "slight" while an increase of 89 PWAs who may require additional evaluation for substance abuse supports an increase in funding.[91]

Although a community forum had been held to discuss the SFDPH's report several weeks before the press release, the contents of the report proved to be so controversial that a "special joint hearing between the San Francisco Board of Supervisors Health and Budget Committees" was convened to discuss its conclusions. As reported by the *San Francisco Sentinel*, during this meeting a member of San Francisco's Board of Supervisors vehemently critiqued the release of the SFDPH press release and called for future censorship of similar reports that would potentially jeopardize funds to combat the epidemic:

> Supervisor Angela Alioto was concerned that the report would be used by politicians to justify a decrease in AIDS funds for the city . . . Alioto chastised the AIDS Office for releasing the report to the public and the media, insisting that the data never should have been compiled and released. . . . "If you want to sit around and do surveys that make you feel good about the AIDS epidemic, fine, but . . . I go back to Washington [D.C.] and these people throw your survey in my face and question why they should give me more money. Stop doing surveys; keep it among yourselves." (Alioto was so incensed, she introduced a resolution the following week that urged the Department of Public Health to create a community review process to screen all future reports on the AIDS epidemic.)[92]

Other members of the Board of Supervisors, and representatives from the AIDS Office, defended the report and its conclusions by arguing that the SFDPH data supported a continuation, not a retrenchment, in the level of funding for San Francisco's successful prevention and education programs. They also argued passionately that the report did not signal an end to the AIDS epidemic, because "28,000 men, women, and children are currently living with HIV infection in San Francisco, representing almost 4% of the City's population." Nor did the report imply a reduction in Care Act funding, argued the director of the AIDS Office, because the SFDPH estimated that 1,000 new HIV infections still occurred annually in the city, a level of infection that could potentially signal a second wave of HIV infections among "17–22 year-olds who are ignoring safer sex guidelines and by older gay men who have relapsed into unsafe behavior."[93]

Setting aside the hyperbole associated with AIDS statistics becomes problematic, if not impossible, as a result of the constant metamorphosis of the object under study (the disease itself).[94] At first glance, the clinical manifestations and absolute number of AIDS cases reported in the United States during the past two decades implies a biological explosion in the disease and a shift in the demographics of risk factors for HIV transmission as the AIDS epidemic has matured. This case study of the social construction of surveillance data in San Francisco, however, demonstrates that observed trends in these data are significantly influenced by successive elaborations of the criteria by which patients are diagnosed with AIDS and multiple shifts in surveillance practices and policies that have altered the manner in which cases are reported. These changes in the methods by which AIDS cases are diagnosed and reported are, in turn, mediated by social and political interests and by the force and influence of evolving biomedical knowledge on the disease. For example, of the 22,185 cumulative AIDS cases reported in San Francisco as of October 31, 1995, only 50 percent of these patients met the CDC's 1985 and earlier case definitions when they were first reported to the SFDPH; the remainder were captured as a result of the changes instituted in 1987 and 1993.[95]

By disaggregating AIDS surveillance data in San Francisco and elsewhere, I am not arguing that the 1982/1985 definitions of AIDS were written in stone and inviolate for all time. Obviously, there is a learning curve associated with the study of any newly emergent disease, and it is rational to assume that additional clinical phenomena associated with profound immune suppression would be uncovered by physicians over time and added to the CDC's surveillance definition. But the profound changes in the definition of this disease, beginning in 1987 and elaborated upon in 1993,[96] have fundamentally altered basic attributes of AIDS surveillance statistics, thereby distorting historical research on trends in the diffusion and epidemiology of the disease.[97] More important, failing to critically interrogate AIDS surveillance statistics and epidemiological data potentially confounds survival analyses and evaluations of the efficacy of antiviral therapies and prevention efforts.[98] And given that "the cure" for AIDS seems as elusive now as it was when the epidemic began, understanding when, why, and for whom treatments and prevention interventions have or have not worked is surely the most important thing we need to understand as we enter the third decade of the epidemic.

VII
Conclusion
Alternative Theories of AIDS

Diseases are not natural immutable categories waiting to be discovered. They must be examined as contingent and historically specific struggles over who, and for what purpose, provides the definition and makes the diagnosis.

—K. Jones and G. Moon,
Health, Disease and Society: A Critical Medical Geography

The Price of a Premature Commitment to a Single-Virus Cause

Prying open the black box of AIDS surveillance practices and policies and exploring in rich detail how AIDS diagnoses were constructed for individual patients at San Francisco's Department of Public Health AIDS Office in the early years of the epidemic reveals that much of received knowledge on HIV/AIDS epidemiology is a social construction of reality by those actors with sufficient institutional power and cultural capital to gain credibility for their own representations and research on the disease and to marginalize or elide alternative HIV/AIDS facts and knowledge(s).

Constructivist views of science, such as this ethnography of AIDS surveillance and epidemiology in San Francisco, "regards scientific knowledge primarily as a human product, made with locally situated cultural and material resources, rather than as simply the revelation of a pre-given order of nature."[1] Revisiting early epidemiological research and patient archives, and observing scientific facts in the making at San Francisco's hospital clinics, diagnostic laboratories, and at the AIDS Seroepidemiology and Surveillance Branch offices of the city's Department of Public Health destabilizes some orthodox knowledge claims by providing greater context for patients' diagnoses while demonstrating the process by which clinical and epidemiological observations constructed a local and global consensus of "facts" about the disease and how official HIV/AIDS surveillance policies and practices evolved.

Other historians of science have "identif[ied] and examin[ed] episodes of controversy" to uncover the "social forces that protect and sustain" historically triumphant scientific paradigms and knowledge claims.[2] In this methodological vein, exploring "episodes of controversy" regarding AIDS can lead to more complex and holistic theoretical models that suggest alternative ways to understand the genesis of the epidemic, the pathogenesis of the disease, and different research and prevention programs to ameliorate its social impact and reduce the incidence of new HIV/AIDS cases. One controversial episode in AIDS historiography concerns orthodox versus alternative theories of the cause(s) of AIDS. How this debate was historically resolved necessarily provided both the impetus and direction for current scientific research into understanding the pathogenesis of the disease (how exposure to a virus leads to disability and death), and strategically directed local and global AIDS treatment, prevention, and education priorities. Reviewing AIDS etiological debates (theories of the cause of the disease) sketches a broad outline of the theoretical significance and practical consequences that derive from alternative constructions of the cause and pathogenesis of AIDS.

This topic has been the subject of exhaustive review by Steven Epstein and by Joan Fujimura and Danny Chou in several articles and books on the sociology of scientific knowledge on HIV/AIDS and provided fodder for several controversial debates among scientists, community activists and lay experts, and the "AIDS establishment."[3] Epstein and Fujimura and Chou generally agree that scientific consensus in support of a new infectious agent (a virus) as the cause of AIDS was legitimized and deemed credible by national public health authorities and scientific research institutions far in advance of conclusive empirical evidence to support this single-germ theory. For Epstein, the "endorsement of a viral etiology hardened 'ahead of' the accumulation of the putatively requisite evidence" when "HIV became what Bruno Latour has called an 'obligatory passage point,' a necessary way station between a wide variety of actors and the places they wanted to go."[4] Similarly, for Fujimura and Chou, "the very construction of AIDS as a single problem was a collectively produced phenomenon . . . established relatively quickly." The viral etiology of the AIDS epidemic was not (and is still infrequently) asserted on the basis on any one observation or piece of experimental evidence. Rather, the thesis that HIV is the single viral cause of AIDS was initially justified, and continues to be defended, by employing what Fujimura and Chou call a "mosaic or patchwork quilt"[5] style of reasoning whereby epidemiologists revised their historical understanding of disease etiology to incorporate new technologies and new knowledges from the allied disciplines of virology, microbiology, evolutionary biology and genetics, immunology, biostatistics, clinical medicine and pharmacology, and the social sciences.[6] Meshing observations and data generated by different ways of knowing and by scientific disciplines that frequently employ incommensurable methods of adjudicating "facts" produced a consensus opinion that there was overwhelming evidence that the human immunodeficiency virus was the single necessary and sufficient infectious agent causing the emergent syndrome of immune deficiency.

The theory that HIV causes AIDS has remained the preeminent AIDS paradigm throughout the course of the epidemic, despite the fact that orthodox researchers readily admit to the existence of multiple lacunae or paradigmatic anomalies that this theory of specific etiology does not resolve. Examples in this regard include the following: there is still no effective treatment to cure the disease; there is still no vaccine against HIV that can evoke protective immunity for populations at risk for the disease; and orthodox AIDS science and research communities have failed to construct an adequate theoretical model that can describe or model the "pathogenesis of HIV infection" (e.g., the exact mechanism or means by which the human immunodeficiency virus induces immune suppression in a host infected with the retrovirus).[7]

With respect to the episodes of controversy evoked by these theoretical anomalies and etiological debates, Epstein and Fujimura and Chou have differing methodologies for analyzing issues of power, knowledge, legitimation, and tracing the means by which scientific credibility is established and maintained by various social actors engaged in AIDS etiological debates. Epstein reconstructs how given scientists historically forged and sustained their professional credibility by leveraging the "dual supports of power and trust" to legitimate knowledge claims and bolster their authorial voice.[8] In contrast, Fujimura and Chou focus on the critical significance of different "styles of scientific practice" which temporally coexist and lead to the "co-production of facts and the rules for verifying facts over time."[9] The latter authors' epistemological calculus of how different scientific disciplines establish causality or "proof" thus differs from Epstein's conclusion that social actors' differential access to power and professional legitimacy plays the critical role in explaining how and why a majority of scientists reached the consensus that HIV caused AIDS and were able to fend off paradigmatic challenges from dissenting scientists and lay actors.

Although I obviously borrowed more from Steven Epstein in my study of the social construction of AIDS epidemiological and surveillance data and discourse, all of these authors make valuable contributions to the theory and methodological practice of the sociology of scientific knowledge by directing attention to moments of disciplinary debate and paradigmatic controversy that "forced HIV/AIDS researchers to respond by making their arguments and assumptions explicit."[10] Moreover, these texts and other critical histories of the AIDS epidemic are crucial for corroborating my own empirical investigations of literature from the early 1980s by temporally locating the moment at which consensus around a viral etiology hardened (mid-1982 to early 1983),[11] thereby concentrating my initial fieldwork at the ASSB to intense review of primary source materials from 1980 through 1982,[12] the years of the epidemic immediately preceding the discovery of HIV and therefore the period most likely to yield empirical evidence in support of alternative constructions of the disease.

Still, vehement debates about the cause of AIDS have never wholly subsided, and lay experts and loose consortia of AIDS dissenters continue to produce and disseminate data and research challenging orthodox constructions of

AIDS and positing a number of alternative theories for the genesis of the epidemic. And the roots of theoretical dissent for those who challenge official AIDS science and discourse can be traced to the first year of the epidemic, when three hypotheses were championed to explain the discovery of a growing number of patients suffering from severe and often fatal immune deficiency. In 1981, hypotheses for the AIDS epidemic included:[13]

1) **Germ Theory or a Disease of Specific Etiology:** A new and previously unknown infectious agent (most likely a virus) had recently been introduced into the United States;

2) **Multifactorial Theory:** Repeated and frequent exposure to a number of common and preexisting infectious agents leads overtime to chronic antigenic "overload" (in other words, chronic stimulation or immune activation among patients), which eventually causes a host's immune system to collapse and lose the ability to fight off common pathogens and cancers. Multifactorialists believed that AIDS patients shared an epidemiological profile that included prolonged and repeated exposure to an historically unprecedented number of infectious disease agents which they acquired through promiscuous sexual behavior, by directly injecting foreign body fluids, or by receiving blood products pooled from multiple donors;

3) **Lifestyle/Toxic Exposure:** Proponents of this view hypothesized that some qualitatively or quantitative difference associated with the "lifestyle" of some gay men and intravenous drug users in major urban centers was responsible for the emergence of uncommon opportunistic infections and cancers among these populations. These lifestyle attributes included substance abuse and the chronic consumption of recreational drugs, especially inhalants such as amyl/butyl nitrites, as well as designer drugs (GHB, Special K, and MDA) and drugs injected intravenously or smoked (cocaine, crack, and heroin).

Although this is not an exhaustive list of all alternative constructions of AIDS, I've sought a better understanding of some of the social forces that protect and sustain orthodox constructions of the epidemic by examining the dissident views of one scientist articulating a multifactorial theory of AIDS. In turn, imagining an alternative construction of AIDS necessarily leads to its paradigmatic implications for research on the etiology and pathogenesis of AIDS and for designing effective public health prevention and education.

I acknowledge that my own case study of AIDS knowledge and surveillance in San Francisco is also a socially constructed "story" of "science in the making," and as such does not represent the entire truth of this epidemic. Nonetheless, taking a "reflexive" view of scientific knowledge does not mean that I believe all knowledge claims about AIDS are equally valid, or that I cannot support a thesis that alternative stories of the AIDS epidemic offer theories and facts that contribute to a greater understanding of the pathogenesis and epidemiology of this disease and more effective public health interventions.[14] As Jan Golinski argues in *Making Natural Knowledge,* "I do not identify the constuctivist outlook with a generalized relativism, if by that is meant a determination that all claims to knowledge are to be judged equally valid. . . . [C]onstructivism [is instead] based on a degree of methodological relativism, which stipulates that all forms of knowledge should be *understood in the same manner*—which is not the same thing."[15]

The Multifactorial Model: A Profile of Dr. Joseph Sonnabend

Trained as a physician in South Africa during the 1950s, Joseph A. Sonnabend, MD, spent the following decade as an infectious disease specialist with qualifications from the Royal College of Physicians of Edinburgh, Scotland. He subsequently worked as a laboratory virologist in London's National Institute for Medical Research, researching the properties of interferon under the mentorship of Alick Isaacs, who discovered interferon in 1957.[16] Although Isaacs was already investigating this naturally occurring glycoprotein as a possible antiviral treatment, Sonnabend's work made a significant contribution to our understanding of interferon's antiviral action, knowledge that would factor into his own multifactorial theory of AIDS 20 years later.[17]

Moving to New York City in the 1970s, Sonnabend continued laboratory research at the Mt. Sinai School of Medicine and subsequently at the State University of New York until his research grants expired. Concurrently he moonlighted at NYC's Department of Health, Bureau of Venereal Disease city disease clinics. Sonnabend ended these affiliations shortly before AIDS emerged and established a private practice in Greenwich Village where he primarily treated gay men, many of whom he had already met at the city clinic or through volunteer work at the Gay Men's Health Project. Sonnabend was, in his own words, uniquely and "ideally" suited to formulate a hypothesis for the disease as he was one of the nation's first physicians to recognize the epidemic of cancer and opportunistic infections emerging among his gay male patients in the early 1980s.

> When this disease first started, I was in the situation, as a physician to many of the men who actually developed the disease, to observe the guys in their setting, the conditions in which—I'm speaking now about a particular lifestyle which involved having sex with many, many different partners in settings where the prevalence . . . of many diseases had become very high. . . . I well knew, as every other doctor and every socially active person involved in this particular lifestyle would know, that there was a constant barrage of infections. Men were getting gonorrhea, hepatitis, syphilis, let alone non-specific viral infections, strep throat, parasitic infections, several times a year. It was a completely unhealthy lifestyle.[18]

And when Kaposi's sarcoma, *Pneumocystis carinii* pneumonia, and other diseases associated with depressed immunity did emerge in his patients,

Sonnabend concluded that the specific correlates of disease in the "fast-track" urban gay lifestyle were the historically unprecedented number of sexual contacts among his patients and thus their frequent and repeated exposure to, and chronic infection with, a multitude of infectious diseases (syphilis, gonorrhea, giardia, shigella, herpes, cytomegalovirus, hepatitis A, hepatitis B, Epstein-Barr virus etc.). For Sonnabend, the critical factor was one of "quantitative" changes in gay male sexual behavior that caused epidemic levels of bacterial and viral pathogens in many metropolitan areas in the United States and Europe, meaning that even a single sexual encounter carried with it a high risk of an infection of some sort.[19]

Empirically grounded by his patients' medical histories and his own clinical observations, Sonnabend and several colleagues "tried to use only things that were known" by immunologists and virologists to create a theoretical model that could explain the AIDS epidemic.[20] As formally articulated in subsequent publications, the multifactorial theory of AIDS proposed that the immune deficiency associated with AIDS, at least among gay men, was not caused by exposure to any *single* pathogenic agent or *single* sexual encounter, but represented instead the cumulative damage to the immune system of repeated "exposures to multiple environmental factors."

> Among homosexual men, it appears that the disease has been occurring in a rather small subset characterized by having had sexual contact with large numbers of different partners in settings where the prevalence of carriage of cytomegalovirus [CMV] is high. Such conditions were met in New York City, San Francisco and Los Angeles in the 1970s as a result of changes in lifestyle that became apparent in the late 1960s.
>
> The specific factors we propose that interact to produce the disease in homosexual men are: (1) immune responses to semen; (2) repeated infections with cytomegalovirus; (3) episodes of reactivation of Epstein-Barr virus; and (4) infection with sexually transmitted pathogens, particularly those associated with immune complex formation such as Hepatitis B and syphilis. The new element is the extremely high prevalence of CMV carriage particularly in the semen of sexually active homosexual men in large cities in the United States during the past decade.[21]

Sonnabend emphasized the role of CMV in his multifactorial model because it was already widely known that this particular herpes virus caused immune suppression and altered the ratio of T4 helper cells to T8 suppressor cells in infected individuals. By virtue of early research with his own AIDS patients, Sonnabend was also able to demonstrate that monogamous homosexual men did not manifest the symptoms of immune dysregulation characteristic of the disease, while healthy nonmonogamous homosexuals did.[22] In future work, he produced evidence that patients at risk for AIDS had high levels of circulating immune complexes and reduced specific immunity,[23] which implied that patients were producing tons of antibodies in response to infections but had few cells that could effectively identify, target, and kill infected cells.[24]

Sonnabend summarized the complicated balancing act of the immune system in an interview in 2003: "The immune system responds to the introduction into the body of foreign material in an extraordinary specific manner. While tolerating 'self' components, it recognizes and attacks foreign material in two general ways. Antibodies are made that specifically recognize a foreign protein, which may be part of a virus or bacterium. This is the humoral component of the immune system. The second component is the cell mediated immune response, where specialized cells that recognize other cells infected with a specific microorganism are generated. These immune system cells are able to destroy the infected cells. These two types of response can work together and both are regulated in a complex manner, to preserve specificity and to ensure that the magnitude of the response is appropriate to the degree of threat."

Other studies of gay men at risk for AIDS corroborated Sonnabend's research by demonstrating that AIDS patients often had some hyperactive components of their immune systems (i.e., evidence of a plethora of antibodies to foreign tissues and antigens such as sperm), while other host immune system responses were functionally impaired, rendering patients unable to rid their bodies of existing intracellular infections. Recalling his earlier research with Alick Isaacs in London, Sonnabend followed an intuitive hunch and demonstrated that the majority of his AIDS patients also had high levels of interferon circulating in their blood, a clinical discovery that correlated to more rapid progression to severe AIDS-related complications and patients' poor prognosis for surviving the disease.

In toto, Sonnabend's multifactorial model of AIDS pathogenesis described a positive-feedback mechanism that explained the progressive deterioration of patients' host immunity. But intriguingly, the theory also raised the hypothetical possibility that there could be several stages in the development of the disease and that gay male patients might even potentially slow or reverse progression to full-blown AIDS by dramatically reducing or avoiding additional exposures to foreign body fluids, semen, antigens, and infectious agents that continually reactivated latent viruses within their bodies (CMV, EBV, herpes, etc.) and kept their immune systems in a state of perpetual stimulation and hyperactivity. Sonnabend also incorporated elements of autoimmunity into his theoretical model, as his patients demonstrated multiple and varied circulating antibody complexes in their blood, implying that some aspects of AIDS pathogenesis bore striking resemblance to other diseases of autoimmunity, such as lupus.[25]

But as early as 1983, when Sonnabend published his multifactorial model, he was already lamenting the fact that more research was not being pursued on this hypothesis; rather, "a single etiologic hypothesis—that of a specific AIDS agent—has almost entirely dominated the field." He was never opposed to further extensive research on HIV "the killer virus," but cautioned colleagues that focusing on one disease agent to the exclusion of "alternative approaches could only be justified if evidence in its favor were overwhelming. This is clearly not the case."[26]

There have been few modifications to Sonnabend's original multifactorial thesis in the ensuing decades, other than factoring in a better understanding of the mechanisms by which HIV transmission can be precipitated and/or enhanced by the synergistic interactions between the virus, other pathogens, and the socioeconomic environment of the host.[27] His analysis of the pathogenesis of the disease over the course of 20 years of the epidemic is still predicated on an intimate knowledge of the medical histories of his own patients with HIV and AIDS, and his conviction that the multifactorial thesis is superior to the HIV theory of specific etiology in explaining the unique demography of AIDS risk groups and the distinct epidemiological pattern of the disease in the United States. For Sonnabend, almost without exception, all infectious diseases are best understood as multifactorial in origin and pathogenesis, which led to his belief that "the early debate on the causation of AIDS was taking place in an historical vacuum regarding the history of thought on disease causation (back to the time of Hippocrates). My multifactorial theory was more in keeping with what had become orthodox thinking on disease (in line with Rene Dubos and others). The notion of a single cause of disease—particularly a killer virus acting alone to obliterate everyone it infected (a hypothetical attack rate of 100 percent) was actually pretty radical. (Yet vis-à-vis AIDS in the early 1980s) all of a sudden orthodoxy had been transformed into radical dissent, and what was really primitive thinking—already discredited, became the new orthodoxy." As evidenced by my own epidemiological study of San Francisco and belated admissions by the CDC and public health officials, the fact that the "risk groups" for AIDS have not changed significantly since 1983 when the multifactorial theory was first proposed also bolsters the credibility of this thesis.

A Critique of Orthodox AIDS Science

Orthodox AIDS researchers claim that this retrovirus is the singular cause of the disease because HIV and a clinical syndrome associated with acquired immune deficiency were discovered in tandem "in time, place and population group,"[28] and eliminating HIV from the nation's blood supply subsequently reduced the incidence of new AIDS cases among transfusion recipients and hemophiliacs. While Sonnabend agrees that orthodox AIDS researchers have "shown beyond a doubt" that HIV and AIDS are correlated in populations, that association alone does not necessarily constitute proof that the virus is the single cause of the disease.[29] Alternatively, it is possible that there are members of the general population who harbor latent HIV infections with no apparent clinical effect—in other words, that there are people who carry HIV within their bodies but fail to test positive for HIV antibodies.

In the absence of evidence such as this, Sonnabend suggests that the observed association between HIV infection and an AIDS diagnosis could just as reasonably support the hypothesis that the "ability of human immunodeficiency virus to cause disease might be dependent on its activation by other infections, as well as the modest immunosuppression associated with many common infections, nutritional deficiencies and so on." Perhaps latent HIV infections (no expression of HIV antibodies) are relatively common in populations, while the expression of HIV antibodies (seroconversion to HIV-positive status) occurs only in those persons repeatedly exposed to pathogens that reactivate HIV from latency—just as the Epstein-Barr virus and cytomegalovirus are reactivated from latency during the course of this disease.[30]

As a virologist, Sonnabend also criticizes the lack of correspondence between orthodox representations of the natural history or biology of the (HIV) virus and the epidemiology of the disease (AIDS). A brief list of these criticisms include the following observations:

- as there are no models for retroviral infections in humans, it is impossible to know if infection with a retrovirus is always followed by seroconversion, or when that may occur;
- it is hard to understand how HIV could survive in nature when there is little epidemiological evidence that females can transmit the infection to males (in industrialized countries) with any efficiency;[31]
- orthodox AIDS researchers initially argued that HIV was the cause of AIDS based on two circumstantial observations: 1) that HIV was widespread in populations at increased risk for developing AIDS; and 2) HIV demonstrated an affinity for infecting CD4 cells—the very cells of the immune system that were notably lacking in the blood of AIDS patients. As originally conceived by Robert Gallo, the single-virus theory claimed that HIV was killing these cells (i.e., that the virus was "cytotoxic" to T4-lymphocytes). But research has shown that HIV "didn't destroy T-cells the way they claimed,"[32] and subsequent speculations regarding "indirect mechanisms" by which HIV might induce immune deficiency have yet to be demonstrated.

In Sonnabend's opinion, the surveillance practice of lumping together all cases of immune deficiency without a known underlying cause necessitated a "unifying hypothesis—a single cause," based on the "similarities of disease manifestations" of patients.[33] However, he was one of the first to argue that with the exception of homosexuals and transplant recipients, the "clinical presentation" of AIDS patients differs according to risk group (for instance, gay men and blood recipients constitute the bulk of Kaposi sarcoma and PCP diagnoses).[34]

Sonnabend also calls into question the other assumptions upon which the viral hypothesis is built; namely that 1) AIDS "is the same disease in 'disparate groups'"; 2) that AIDS is "spread by contagion between" those groups; and 3) that "the disease is new in all groups." While he thinks that the latter assumption is true for homosexual men, once again Sonnabend argues that given the multiple pathways to immune deficiency it is conceivable that different risk groups for AIDS (namely blood recipients and IV drug users) have different risks for developing disease. For instance, prior to AIDS, it was known that blood transfusions induced immune suppression because patients were exposed to foreign antigens and blood contaminants such as CMV. Persons injecting drugs are also at risk for developing immune deficiency because of the "known immunological consequences to the use of opiates"[35] and their repeated exposure to numerous infectious pathogens; these well-known health risks are further exacerbated by their marginalized socioeconomic status and the social context that structurally produces and perpetuates their drug-using behavior.

Meanwhile Sonnabend's theories have marginalized him. His "fundamental belief that the root of AIDS is essentially social, rather than medical . . . has kept him at odds with mainstream thinking about AIDS."[36] The failure on the part of established AIDS researchers to look at the "totality" of the disease and "the overall environment of the patient" led epidemiologists to construct homogenous categories of homosexuals (and Haitians), whom were presumed to share nothing in common other than sexual intercourse.[37] Referring to the CDC's infamous Los Angeles Cluster Study in June 1982 that provided the revolutionary paradigmatic moment in support of the single-virus hypothesis, Sonnabend argues that such a conclusion is "only possible if the population of homosexual men in Los Angeles county are assumed to be homogenous with respect to the frequency of their sexual contacts. An alternative explanation is that the cases occurred in a relatively small subset of homosexual men who shared a similar lifestyle."[38]

Believing that the rapid scientific consensus in support of the single-virus theory of the AIDS epidemic was premature and overdetermined because of a conflation of interests among biomedical researchers, leaders in the gay community, and the conservative sociopolitical context of the early 1980s, Sonnabend surmised that the cultural politics of the early 1980s and the theoretical and ideological preeminence accorded the germ theory of specific etiology all served to divorce AIDS from the social conditions that gave rise to the epidemic:

> People who wanted to promote family values liked it, because it was nice to say extramarital sex could be lethal. Others like it because they could promote celibacy before marriage. Gay men liked the idea, because they could avoid thinking about the behavioral part. For them, a killer virus that would not discriminate

became a way of saying that promiscuity was less important. Even in Africa, with a killer virus theory, it was easy for politicians to say our economic policies and the fact that many people live in squalor have nothing to do with this disease. And for scientists and health workers, there were going to be a lot more funds for fighting a virus that was a threat to everyone than for a condition affecting special groups.[39]

Moreover, one hypothesis was able to dominate discourse on the disease within such a short period of time because prominent government officials and researchers affiliated with large academic institutions had savvy public relations departments able to exploit their relationships with the media and connections at prestigious journals that enabled them to get their research published. In an interview in 1992, Sonnabend reluctantly acknowledged that theories "have to be sold" and marketed. "This information in turn is what the world believes."[40]

In a history of experimental science, Steven Shapin and Simon Schaffer construct a model of "polity of science" comprising interdependent relations among the "polity" of an intellectual scientific community and the "wider polities" of both state and society to study the problem of generating and legitimating scientific knowledge. In their conclusion, when historical controversies bring to light credibility struggles between proponents for alternative constructions of scientific reality, the outcome of this contest "depends upon the political success of the various candidates in insinuating themselves into the activities of other institutions and other interest groups. He who has the most, and the most powerful, allies wins."[41] Throughout this text I have demonstrated how the "polity" of an orthodox scientific community invested in research on HIV and the political economy and bureaucracy of the nation's public health surveillance infrastructure wields power over media, over scientific research and publication, and over funding priorities and provides the means to contain challenges to its exclusive control over the production of credible and authoritative knowledge on HIV/AIDS. Whether through public censure or sanctions, peer-review panels, or its appropriation of scientific funds and legitimate research agendas, the orthodox research community ensures theoretical consensus within the biomedical community by restricting access to the material and "intellectual space(s)"[42] where experimental research on AIDS can be produced and accredited.

Nonetheless, alternative constructions of the reality, as exemplified by Joseph Sonnabend's promotion of a multifactorial AIDS theory and his success at implementing research and treatment interventions premised on this alternative thesis, suggest the possibility for creating and sustaining spaces for alternative AIDS knowledge, discourse, and treatment and prevention practices. Although lacking tenure, institutional affiliation, or access to public research capital, Sonnabend and other community-based research activists have managed to generate a body of clinical research and treatment knowledge about HIV/AIDS and to successfully lobby government officials for changes in AIDS treatment and care.

Opportunity Costs and Implications of Premature Consensus

> In 1982, there were several directions of AIDS research that were articulated and not pursued . . . they're still stalling. That translates into the most unspeakable suffering.
>
> —Joseph Sonnabend, quoted in *Out*

In the epigraph above from 1992, Sonnabend cites the collective failure of the nation's AIDS research establishment to pursue research on the role of CMV, interferon, autoimmunity, and "allo-immunization" in the pathogenesis of AIDS as the direct cause of increased morbidity and mortality. While clinical and epidemiological studies repeatedly confirm the presence of CMV and interferon as predictive of a rapid progression of AIDS,[43] more than a decade has elapsed without significant headway against these opportunistic infections and developing new therapeutic agents. Despite a few preliminary studies that showed "encouraging results" in some patients,[44] the AIDS establishment also neglected to support further research on promising experimental therapies such as plasmapheresis (in which the plasma is removed from whole blood and the cellular components of blood are returned to the patient's circulatory system) which might have eased the debilitation that AIDS patients suffered as a result of high blood levels of interferon and circulating immune complexes.

The failure of the nation's AIDS, scientific, and research establishment to develop comprehensive "patient management strategies" is perhaps even more distressing given recent studies that conclude the duration of an AIDS patient's survival following diagnosis is directly attributable to the quality of care that he/she receives. While acknowledging that the "timely receipt of medical care can reduce morbidity associated with [HIV] infection [and] slow disease progression," SFDPH officials were chastened to find that two-thirds of all of the patients in this San Francisco clinic survey had no medical insurance, and that "receipt of general preventive care for HIV-infected and at-risk persons was low."[45]

> There has been an unbelievable neglect in developing patient management strategies, although things may be a little better in this respect now. Patients with AIDS die—for the most part—from opportunistic infections [OIs] which, while not generally curable, may be preventable, and manageable, with . . . a structured program of care that includes prophylaxis, early diagnosis of OIs, aggressive treatment and provision of support—whether nutritional or psychological. Why did it take so long to study PCP prophylaxis? In fact, why was it not offered since Bactrim was known to work in leukemic children. . . . Although AIDS pa-

tients do show a high frequency of adverse responses to Bactrim, did we really think that Bactrim would not work in an AIDS patient even though it was effective in a transplant patient?[46]

As a laboratory virologist, physician, and infectious disease specialist, Sonnabend articulated some of the earliest criticisms of AIDS orthodoxy and has remained an outspoken critic of established AIDS science and discourse for two decades, taking great personal and professional risks to pose "awkward questions about 'what everybody knows.'"[47] To this day, he continues to treat scores of AIDS patients suffering from acute immune suppression, many of whom survive for remarkable periods of time because of innovative patient management strategies that prioritize early diagnosis and aggressive treatment for opportunistic infections.[48]

As government institutions committed to the theory that HIV causes AIDS neglected this research in the mistaken belief that the development of a vaccine against HIV, or effective antiretroviral therapies, would make the treatment of OIs redundant, it fell upon community research organizations to prioritize the study of prophylaxis and conduct the clinical trials necessary to approve pentamidine for the prevention of PCP.[49] And in this specific example, during the two years that Sonnabend and PWAs fought for FDA approval of the treatment, 16,929 PWAs died of *Pneumocystis carinii* pneumonia[50] that could have been prevented if the FDA had only approved the use of prophylaxis (e.g., Bactrim, or aerosolized pentamidine, etc.) and mandated its use as standard and recommended care.

Sonnabend has also been the driving force behind a number of community initiatives in New York City:

- He was the force behind the initial articulation of "safe sex" guidelines, which led to a self-published pamphlet, coauthored by Richard Berkowitz and Michael Callen (1982);[51]
- He initiated the nation's first AIDS antidiscrimination suit (1983);
- He was responsible for implementing what is arguably the single most important clinical treatment for AIDS patients, as he was among the first physicians in the country (1982) to advocate the use of PCP prophylaxis (at the time, PCP was the number one cause of death for PWAs) and was instrumental in getting the FDA to approve the use of pentamidine as standard care for AIDS patients. Although Sonnabend made a strong argument that prophylaxis could head off recurrence of PCP, approval of its use was inexplicably delayed by the federal government until 1989;[52]
- He founded the first independent medical research organization on AIDS in the United States (*AIDS Medical Foundation*, 1983);[53]
- He was the founding editor for the first medical journal exclusively devoted to the disease (*AIDS Research*, 1983–1986);[54]

- He founded, and acted as associate medical director for, one of the country's first independent, nonprofit, community-based AIDS research organizations (CRI-NY, 1987),[55] and was subsequently appointed as medical director for CRIA;[56]
- He worked with Michael Callen to organize the Persons With AIDS Coalition (1986), a consortium of AIDS activists and patients who lobbied for better treatments for the disease and protection from discrimination;[57]
- He founded, with Michael Callen and Tom Hannon, the PWA Health Group in 1986, the first buyer's club for AIDS drugs in the United States. No longer in operation today, the PWA Health Group was instrumental in searching for pharmaceutical distributors and importing drugs such as fluconazole (for thrush), Biaxin (for mycobacterium avium), and pentamidine (for pneumonia);
- He was one of the first vocal opponents of the "promiscuous" use of long-term treatment with AZT, a form of chemotherapy that he concluded was "incompatible with life." Sonnabend said initial approval of the drug was based on "inept research."[58] He is, however, enthusiastic about the judicious use of combination retroviral regimens in appropriate patient populations.

The multifactorial theory suggests an alternative way to understand AIDS epidemiology and the pathogenesis of the disease, and clearly articulates a specific research agenda and alternative priorities for HIV/AIDS prevention, education, and treatment interventions. The theory offers a plausible hypothesis for why the disease began, and remains entrenched, in narrowly circumscribed risk groups within the United States and other industrialized countries, and is prescient in predicting that HIV infections and the AIDS epidemic would never diffuse widely throughout the heterosexual population in industrialized nations.

In addition to offering guidelines for progressive patient management strategies, perhaps the seminal palpable benefit of the multifactorial theory is that it enables persons with AIDS to have some measure of hope in confronting their illness and offers both a means of preventing the disease and of surviving a diagnosis that is otherwise said to be irreversible and terminal. Michael Callen, one of Sonnabend's former patients, explains how this alternative construction of his illness fostered in him a cautious skepticism toward scientific and medical experts and empowered him to envision a means of safe sexual expression that jeopardized neither him nor his partners:

> I have never believed that HIV, or any other "new" virus, is the cause of AIDS. By the age of 27, when I was diagnosed, I'd had thousands of sexual contacts and as a consequence, developed dozens of sexually transmitted diseases—viral, bacterial, parasitic, and fungal. When I got AIDS, the question was not why, but rather

how I had been able to remain standing for so long! Whether I'm right or wrong in my belief that AIDS is really the result of repeated assaults on the immune system by common infections, the important thing is that I always believed that if I stopped doing what I thought was making me sick, I could get better.

Believing that I could survive is probably the precondition necessary for my survival. Unlike many other people with AIDS who considered themselves "ticking time bombs," my world view admitted from the first at least the possibility of recovery. My doctor's shared skepticism about the etiological party line led him to discourage me from jumping on many a bandwagon of experimental treatments. This also probably saved my life.

The uncritical repetition of the myth that everyone with AIDS dies, denies the reality of—but perhaps more important, the possibility of—our survival.[59] If I have this disease because an unknown virus [is] ticking away in my body, there's no hope. . . . The concept of multifactorality—think of it like dominos— my history of syphilis, gonorrhea, venereal warts: You could really direct therapy at several of them. In other words, Joe's [Joseph Sonnabend's] model offered to me the first ray of hope that I might not die of this disease. . . .

The other implication . . . was that safer sex could be invented. . . . We didn't think that a single unlucky contact could give you this disease; it built up over time. Which meant if you followed the safer-sex guidelines that we proposed and you made a mistake . . . it wouldn't be the end of the world.[60]

While humbly admitting that he cannot explain every AIDS case, Sonnabend adds that it "should be sufficient" that he offers a plausible explanation for the majority of those cases among homosexual/bisexual men, and a plausible model for the generalized HIV/AIDS epidemic in sub-Sahara African countries where ubiquitous exposure to infectious agents is likely to similarly enhance Africans' increased vulnerability to acquiring and transmitting HIV/AIDS during heterosexual intercourse.[61]

Competing Ideologies of Public Health

In a larger sense, the contentious debate between those in support of the theory that HIV causes AIDS and those who favor alternative constructions of AIDS (and other illnesses) is simply a contemporaneous example of the theoretical divide that has traditionally polarized the history of medicine and undergirded competing ideologies of public health, setting germ theorists and attendant practices of biomedical reductionism against social epidemiologists and proponents of socioeconomic change who argue that both chronic and epidemic infectious diseases are socially produced and socially mediated. As Rene Dubos, Nancy Krieger, Sylvia Tesh, and others representing this position have argued, "social conditions give rise to behavior"—"lifestyle" choices, and biological agents in and of themselves are insufficient to explain who gets sick and why. While socioeconomic class, race, gender, or discretionary income are significant factors in health and influence access to treatment, care, and prevention services, these aggregate categories inadequately capture the social relations that condition a given individual's differential power to access information, secure public entitlements, or negotiate sexual risks to protect their own health.[62] Nancy Kreiger's analyses of high rates of infant mortality within families headed by college-educated African Americans and increased relative risks for losing a child vis-à-vis white families exemplifies this point by demonstrating that there is another element (or other elements) conferring vulnerability for disability and death inherent to membership in socially marginalized or subaltern populations.

Retheorizing AIDS as a chronic, and infectious disease, Nancy Kreiger and Elizabeth Fee argue that better HIV/AIDS prevention policies and practices "require a greater appreciation of the historical and social contexts in which AIDS occurs."[63] By neglecting the study of these other elements that structurally frame the lives and reproduce the risks of AIDS patients (whether race, sex, class, sexual orientation, discrimination, social isolation, or internalized homophobia), the single-germ theory as promulgated by national research agendas, the CDC, and AIDS prevention campaigns depoliticizes the disease and makes the epidemic more difficult to contain.[64] The single-germ theory's "ideological commitment to individualism [pays] no attention to social power, voice, conflict or non-rational behavioral choices mediated by social structures, class, 'race,' (or) how behaviors are related to social conditions and constraints on how communities [e.g., social relations] shape individual's lives. These attitudes [of biomedical individualism] implicitly accept inequalities in health and fail to challenge the social production of disease."[65]

Sylvia Tesh argues in *Hidden Arguments* that "a public health policy that consists mainly of exhorting individuals to change their behavior appears at best to be shortsighted. At worst it seems less a policy directed at attaining health for the public than one bent on protecting the institutions threatening that health."[66] Because it protects the status quo and reifies dominant social norms, such a policy perpetuates disease. It limits government prevention and education efforts to changing individual behaviors to reduce exposure to HIV, irrespective of the social context in which these behaviors occur. While Virchow and Engels developed a theory of "the social production of disease" which advocated radical social changes in the national political economy, the social relations of production, and capitalistic forms of production, more radical descendants of Virchow argue for the theoretical primacy of an "unjust social system" and the critical need to identify and locate the "social roots of disease" if one hopes to create effective and sustainable prevention policies.[67] In light of these critiques, we need a new theoretical and structural framework for understanding the uneven geography and unequal demographic distribution of HIV infections and AIDS.

Identifying the social determinants and correlates of this disease would have been more straightforward if the disease had not first appeared—or rather, had not been represented—as an epidemic of affluent and previously healthy white gay men. Empirical evidence contradicting this representation was clearly evident in medical journals from the late 1970s, which published studies claiming that the health of a subset of gay men in major cities of the United States resembled "the tropics in the Third World," with epidemic levels of sexually transmitted diseases, hepatitis B, CMV, gay bowel disease, and other infectious diseases (even cholera and typhoid).[68]

When AIDS Began details many instances of striking dissonance between the (private) record of AIDS and the (public) representations promulgated by those with sufficient institutional authority and cultural capital to author an "official" history of the epidemic. While research focused on a specific (retro)viral agent, and public health officials and AIDS educational organizations beat the drumbeat of a threat of this disease rapidly disseminating to members of the 'general' population, the epidemiology of this disease clearly indicated otherwise until April 1984 when the human immunodeficiency virus was discovered. Those patients who developed the clinical symptoms of AIDS during the first four years of the epidemic were widely recognized to have markedly increased risk factors/vulnerability for infectious disease. Almost universally, AIDS patients in the early years of the epidemic used large quantities of recreational drugs, and/or belonged to socioeconomically marginalized populations, and/or had frequent and extensive exposure to a variety of infectious diseases that cumulatively degraded their host immunity and lowered their resistance to epidemic diseases.

In numerous instances, official public health data and discourse, epidemiological research, and HIV/AIDS surveillance practices and policies collectively elided the multiplicity of social and behavioral risk factors that characterized those populations most likely to acquire the disease, instead favoring an explanation based on the random chance of being exposed just one time to a single highly infectious and fatal virus. Throughout the course of the epidemic, the general tendency inherent in surveillance activities and epidemiological research was to magnify the role of gay male or (hetero)sexual intercourse in driving the HIV/AIDS epidemic and minimize the contribution of chronic urban poverty, poor public health care and services, and injection-drug use and substance abuse in producing and sustaining this epidemic.

As Ian Hacking argues, "These representations do cultural work. . . . [W]e represent in order to intervene, and we intervene in the light of our representations."[69] By reducing the representation of AIDS to that of a simple and singular sexually transmitted infection, public health interventions focused on curtailing gay male sexual expression and prohibiting "high-risk" populations from donating blood or sharing needles. This hygienic campaign was fully consonant with the conservative political climate of the Reagan years. Had representations of AIDS included the more complex and multiple social, political, and economic correlates of the disease, public health interventions would have necessarily required an expansion of government services to the homeless, to substance abusers, and a program of national health care. Instead, during the Reagan decade, Americans witnessed a massive deinstitutionalization

192 • When AIDS Began

of the mentally ill, a rise in drug abuse (especially cocaine and heroin), a rise in tuberculosis, and an amplification of the AIDS epidemic. Public health officials and the AIDS research establishment abrogated their responsibilities to educate the public about the social and economic risk profile of early AIDS patients by claiming that "AIDS is an equal-opportunity disease"; one broken condom can kill you; heroin is blessedly nontoxic;[70] there are no co-factors for the disease other than age;[71] and nutrition, recreational drug use, socioeconomic status, and social marginalization play no role in increasing one's vulnerability for acquiring the disease or its progressing to full-blown AIDS.[72]

Listen carefully to the words of one 34-year-old office worker who was diagnosed with *Pneumocystis carinii* pneumonia in San Francisco in the spring of 1982. After answering 19 pages of questions regarding his income, his prior medical history, his recreation drug use habits and his sexual behavior, the San Francisco surveillance officer asked this AIDS patient if he would like to comment on "any other aspect of [your] sexual experiences that we should talk about?" The young man replied:

Unemployment, lack of a warm relationship, socially isolated . . .[73]

Notes

Preface

1. Author's notes, author's case "John Doe;" medical chart review. The 261,000 figure is an approximation based on CDC data for cumulative AIDS deaths as of July 1994.
2. DNCB is chemically known as 1-chloro-2,4-dinitrobenzene. Those who support and promote the use of DNCB claim that it primes the cell-mediated arm of the immune system and causes an increase in CD8 and natural killer T-cells, thereby controlling the intracellular pathogens that cause opportunistic infections in persons with AIDS. See literature from ACT-UP San Francisco regarding DNCB, at the DNCB Study Group, 2261 Market Street #436, San Francisco, CA 94114.
3. Author's notes, author's case "John Doe," July 1994.
4. The figure is a very rough estimate based on San Francisco AIDS mortality statistics from July 31, 1994. The details of Doe's case are peculiar, though not unusual. Because John Doe was initially reported as an AIDS case in another state, that state remains the sole repository for all information about him. Consequently, despite the fact that Doe lived in San Francisco for his last decade and died there, his death certificate was mailed out of state, and the metropolis that initially "captured" this case counted him among its AIDS mortality statistics.

Introduction

1. R. Shilts, *And the Band Played On: Politics, People, and the AIDS Epidemic,* New York: St. Martin's Press, 1987; W. A. Rushing, *The AIDS Epidemic: Social Dimensions of an Infectious Disease,* Boulder, Colo.: Westview Press, 1995; L. K. Clarke and M. Potts, eds., *The AIDS Reader: Documentary History of a Modern Epidemic,* Boston: Branden Publishing, 1988; and E. Fee and D. M. Fox, eds., *AIDS: The Burdens of History,* Berkeley: University of California Press, 1988, and E. Fee and D. M. Fox eds., *AIDS: The Making of a Chronic Disease,* Berkeley: University of California Press, 1992.
2. For examples, see B. D. Schoub, *AIDS and HIV in Perspective: A Guide to Understanding the Virus and Its Consequences,* Cambridge, UK: Cambridge University Press, 1994; A. S. Fauci, "The Human Immunodeficiency Virus: Infectivity and Mechanisms of Pathogenesis," in *The AIDS Reader: Social, Political and Ethical Issues,* ed. N. F. McKenzie, New York: Penguin Books, 1991.
3. See J. Mann, D. J. M. Tarantola, and T. W. Netter, eds., *A Global Report: AIDS in the World,* Cambridge, Mass.: Harvard University Press, 1992; and G. J. Stine, *AIDS Update 1994–1995,* Englewood Cliffs, N.J.: Prentice Hall, 1995.
4. See C. Patton, *Inventing AIDS,* London: Routledge, Chapman & Hall, 1990; C. Patton, *Last Served? Gendering the AIDS Epidemic,* London: Taylor & Francis, 1994; C. Patton, *Sex and Germs: The Politics of AIDS,* Boston: South End Press, 1985; P. A. Treichler, "AIDS, Homophobia, and Biomedical Discourse: An Epidemic of Signification," in *AIDS: Cultural Analysis, Cultural Activism,* ed. D. Crimp, Cambridge: MIT Press, 1988: 31–70; P. A. Treichler, "AIDS, HIV, and the Cultural Construction of Reality," in *The Time of AIDS: Social Analysis, Theory and Method,* ed. G. Herdt and S. Lindenbaum, London: Sage Publications, 1992: 65–100; P. A. Treichler, *How to Have Theory in an Epidemic: Cultural Chronicles of AIDS,* Durham, N.C.: Duke University Press, 1999; S. Watney, *Policing Desire: Pornography, AIDS and the Media,* Minneapolis: University of Minnesota Press, 1987; S. Gilman, *Disease and Representation: Images of Illness from Madness to AIDS,* Ithaca: Cornell University Press, 1988, and other references in the bibliography.
5. S. Epstein, *Impure Science: AIDS, Activism, and the Politics of Knowledge,* Berkeley: University of California Press, 1996.
6. Books include G. W. Shannon et al., *The Geography of AIDS: Origins and Course of An Epidemic,* New York: Guilford Press, 1991; P. Gould, *The Slow Plague: A Geography of the AIDS*

Epidemic, Cambridge, Mass.: Blackwell Publishers, 1993; articles include M. R. Smallman-Raynor and A. D. Cliff, "Acquired Immune Deficiency Syndrome (AIDS): Literature, Geographical Origins and Global Patterns," *Progress in Human Geography* 14(2), 1990: 157–213; M. Loytonen, "The Spatial Diffusion of Human Immunodeficiency Virus Type 1 in Finland, 1982–1997," *Annals of the Association of American Geographers* 81(1), March 1991: 127–151; and W. B. Wood, "AIDS North and South: Diffusion Patterns of a Global Epidemic and a Research Agenda for Geographers," *The Professional Geographer* 40, 1988: 266–279, among others.

7.   A reformulation of a geography of health, as exemplified by R. A. Kearns and W. M. Gesler, *Putting Health into Place: Landscape, Identity, and Well-Being,* New York: Syracuse University Press, 1998.

8.   Ibid., 5.

9.   D. Haraway, "The Biopolitics of Postmodern Bodies: Constitutions of Self in Immune System Discourse," *Simians, Cyborgs, and Women: The Reinvention of Nature,* New York: Routledge, Chapman & Hall, 1991: 203–230.

10. P. A. Treichler, "AIDS and HIV Infection in the Third World: A First World Chronicle," *Remaking History,* Seattle: Bay Press, 1989: 48.

11. Centers for Disease Control, "Pneumocystis Pneumonia—Los Angeles," *Morbidity and Mortality Report,* June 5, 1981: 4.

12. R. Gallo, *Virus Hunting. AIDS, Cancer, and the Human Retrovirus: A Story of Scientific Discovery,* New York: Basic Books, 1991: 193. This thesis was reiterated in other orthodox texts, including Shilts, *And the Band Played On;* Fauci, "The Human Immunodeficiency Virus"; Clarke and Potts, *The AIDS Reader.*

13. "AIDS Research, Keystone's Blunt Message: It's the Virus, Stupid," *Science* 260, April 16, 1993: 292–293.

14. As of 1996, the Group for the Scientific Re-appraisal of the HIV-AIDS Hypothesis comprised well over 300 scientists, academics, and political activists, and published a monthly newsletter in addition to managing an electronic listserve. See the newsletter, subsequently renamed "Reappraising AIDS," 7514 Girard Avenue, #1-331, La Jolla, CA 92037. philpott@wwnet.com publisher/editor.

15. For several reviews and critiques of HIV/AIDS dissidents, see "Debunking Doubts That HIV Causes AIDS," *New York Times,* March 11, 1993; ABC-TV's *Day One* news program, broadcast March 23, 1993; and a plethora of articles and letters to the editor in *Spin, Science, Nature.*

16. San Francisco Department of Public Health, HIV Seroepidemiology and Surveillance Section, AIDS Surveillance Unit, "AIDS Cases Reported Through March 2002," *Quarterly AIDS Surveillance Report,* March 31, 2002: 1.

17. AIDS histories include Shilts, *And the Band Played On;* M. D. Grmek, *History of AIDS: Emergence and Origin of a Pandemic,* Princeton: Princeton University Press, 1990; and E. W. Etheridge, *Sentinel for Health: A History of the Centers for Disease Control,* Berkeley: University of California Press, 1992. Studies of the natural history of the disease include those by W. Winkelstein Jr. et al., "Sexual Practices and Risk of Infection by the Human Immunodeficiency Virus: The San Francisco Men's Health Study," *Journal of the American Medical Association* 257(3), January 16, 1987, and many others by Winkelstein; and Schoub, *AIDS and HIV in Perspective.* For examples of San Francisco as the nation's bellwether for trends in the epidemic, see Centers for Disease Control, *Morbidity and Mortality Weekly Report,* September 27, 1985, and March 11, 1994; and "Forecasting the Future of AIDS," *New York Times,* February 16, 1994.

18. Current caseloads are reported in San Francisco Department of Public Health, *Quarterly AIDS Surveillance Report: AIDS Cases Reported through March 2002.* Until 1994, the per capita incidence of AIDS was greater in San Francisco than in any other urban center in the United States. The annual rate of AIDS cases per 100,000 population was 284.2 in 1993 and 158.0 in 1994. As of 1995 and 1996, the annual rate of AIDS cases per 100,000 in the city/county had dropped to 108.5 and 83.1 (1995 and 1996 midyear data respectively) and been surpassed by the rates in New York City (131.0 and 117.2), Jersey City (114.5 and 109.8), and Miami (115.1 and 86.6). (CDC, 1997: 6–7).

19. San Francisco's former AIDS Surveillance Unit (which had a staff of three in 1983) was rechristened the AIDS Seroepidemiology and Surveillance Branch (ASSB) in the early 1990s and employed approximately 37 people in 1995. The ASSB is funded by a CDC

grant which is subject to annual revisions; for fiscal year 1995, the department received a renewal of its annual surveillance grant for approximately $1.13 million along with $2.4 million for HIV seroprevalence research, and an additional $340,000 for a special research project evaluating the 1993 revised AIDS clinical definition (in fiscal year 1994, this grant totaled $1,128,486 for surveillance activities and $895,000 for seroprevalence research).

20. The strength of constructivism, according to D. Demeritt, "Social Theory and the Reconstruction of Science and Geography," *Transactions of the Institute of British Geographers* 21(3), 1996: 486.

Chapter 1

1. See D. Harvey, "Population, Resources, and the Ideology of Science," *Economic Geography* 50(3), July 1974: 256–277.

2. P. L. Berger and T. Luckmann, *The Social Construction of Reality: A Treatise in the Sociology of Knowledge*, New York: Anchor Books, 1966: 5–8. Cf. Howard Waitzkin, "A Critical Theory of Medical Discourse: Ideology, Social Control, and the Processing of Social Context in Medical Encounters," *Journal of Health and Social Behavior* 30, June 1989: 220–239.

3. Berger and Luckmann, *The Social Construction of Reality*, 6. When Berger and Luckmann argued for a radical reconfiguration of the discipline, however, they distinguished themselves from Mannheim, and others who followed in his wake (Merton, Parsons et al.), who held out the possibility of *transcending* the "social location" of knowledge through utopianism, "relationism," or the accumulation of multiple "socially grounded positions" (2–18).

4. P. Wright and A. Treacher, *The Problem of Medical Knowledge: Examining the Social Construction of Medicine*, Edinburgh: Edinburgh University Press, 1982; C. E. Rosenberg, and J. Golden, *Framing Disease: Studies in Cultural History*, New Brunswick, N.J.: Rutgers University Press, 1992; B. Turner, *The Body and Society, Explorations in Social Theory*, Oxford: Basil Blackwell, 1984, and *Medical Power and Social Knowledge*, London: Sage Publications, 1987; N. Black et al., *Health and Disease: A Reader*, Milton Keynes, England: Open University Press, 1984; K. Jones and G. Moon, *Health, Disease and Society: A Critical Medical Geography*, London: Routledge & Kegan Paul, 1987; Gilman, *Disease and Representation*; A. Mack, *In Time of Plague: The History and Social Consequences of Lethal Epidemic Disease*, New York: New York University Press, 1991.

5. S. N. Tesh, *Hidden Arguments: Political Ideology and Disease Prevention Policy*, New Brunswick, N.J.: Rutgers University Press, 1988.

6. H. Waitzkin, "A Critical Theory of Medical Discourse," 220–239.

7. Ibid., 222, 224–225.

8. J. B. Thompson, *Ideology and Modern Culture*, Stanford, Calif.: Stanford University Press, 1990: 56.

9. Waitzkin, "A Critical Theory of Medical Discourse," op. cit., 1989: 226.

10. P. Farmer, *AIDS and Accusation: Haiti and the Geography of Blame*, Berkeley: University of California Press, 1992; Fee and Fox, *AIDS: The Burdens of History* and *AIDS: The Making of A Chronic Disease*; C. Patton, *Sex and Germs*; T. Boffin and S. Gupta, *Ecstatic Antibodies: Resisting the AIDS Mythology*, London: Rivers Oram Press, 1990; Watney, *Policing Desire*; P. Aggleton, G. Hart, and P. Davis, *AIDS: Social Representations, Social Practices*, New York: Falmer Press, 1989; D. Crimp, *AIDS: Cultural Analysis, Cultural Activism*, Cambridge: MIT Press, 1988, 1989.

11. M. Foucault, *Birth of the Clinic: An Archaeology of Medical Perception*, New York: Random House, 1975; and *The History of Sexuality. Volume 1*, New York: Random House, 1978.

12. C. Patton, *Inventing AIDS*, 77.

13. Ibid., 80, 82.

14. Ibid., 84, 86–87.

15. Ibid., 87–88. Patton finds the term "compassionate use" particularly specious, as the term was originally developed to justify the expanded access to experimental treatments for "terminally ill" persons, not to legitimate the risks of exposure to an experimental vaccine on a healthy population.

16. Ibid., 88–89.
17. Ibid., 92.
18. For similar analyses of the ideological and metaphorical content of biomedical research in Africa, see M. Vaughan, "Syphilis in Colonial East and Central Africa: The Social Construction of an Epidemic," *Epidemics and Ideas: Essays on the Historical Perception of Pestilence,* ed. T. Ranger and P. Slack, Cambridge: Cambridge University Press, 1992; M. Vaughan, *Curing Their Ills: Colonial Power and African Illness,* Stanford, Calif.: Stanford University Press, 1991; and J. and J. Comaroff, "Medicine, Colonialism, and the Black Body," *Ethnography and the Historical Imagination,* San Francisco: Westview Press, 1992.
19. C. Patton, *Last Served?,* 6.
20. J. Weeks, "AIDS: The Intellectual Agenda. Moral Panic (1982–5)," *Against Nature: Essays on History, Sexuality, and Identity,* London: Rivers Oram Press, 1991: 118–120.
21. Ibid., 124.
22. Ibid., 130.
23. Watney, "Moral Panics," *Policing Desire,* 43, 53.
24. "and up to five per cent for women." See Watney, *Policing Desire,* 128.
25. Ibid., 134.
26. Quoting Dr. Allan Pred, professor of geography, University of California at Berkeley, 1997.
27. Bergman and Luckmann, *The Social Construction of Reality,* 5–8.
28. J. Golinski, "The Theory of Practice and the Practice of Theory: Sociological Approaches in the History of Science," *ISIS* 81, 1990: 492.
29. T. S. Kuhn, *The Structure of Scientific Revolutions,* Chicago: University of Chicago Press, 1970, 3–6.
30. Kuhn, *The Structure of Scientific Revolutions,* 35–51. Cf. also J. Rouse, *Knowledge and Power: Toward a Political Philosophy of Science,* Ithaca: Cornell University Press, 1987: 31, for the following quote: "Normal science involves shared practices, not shared beliefs These shared practices take place within a common field of operations, which Kuhn has more recently called a 'disciplinary matrix' . . . the 'field' within which the shared concepts, symbols, apparatus, and theories are applied. It opens up a domain of objects for comprehension, manipulation, and intervention. This domain constitutes a field of research possibilities and opportunities arising out of prior activities and achievements. . . . What is shared, however, is a sense of what is at issue, why it matters, and what must be done to resolve it."
31. L. Fleck, *Genesis and Development of a Scientific Fact,* ed. T. J. Trenn and R. K. Merton, trans. F. Bradley and T. J. Trenn, Chicago: University of Chicago Press, 1979.
32. Kuhn, *The Structure of Scientific Revolutions,* 10.
33. D. Bloor, *Knowledge and Social Imagery,* Chicago: University of Chicago Press, 1991.
34. D. Haraway, "Teddy Bear Patriarchy: Taxidermy in The Garden of Eden, New York City, 1908–1936," *Primate Visions: Gender, Race, and Nature in the World of Modern Science,* New York: Routledge, Chapman & Hall, 1989: 26–58; B. Latour, *Science in Action: How to Follow Scientists and Engineers through Society,* Cambridge, Mass.: Harvard University Press, 1987; B. Latour and S. Woolgar, *Laboratory Life: The Construction of Scientific Facts,* 2nd ed. Princeton, N.J.: Princeton University Press, 1986.
35. Latour, *Science in Action,* 4, 15. Italics in original.
36. S. Shapin and S. Schaffer, *Leviathan and the Air-Pump: Hobbes, Boyle, and the Experimental Life,* Princeton, N.J.: Princeton University Press, 1985: 7.
37. I. Lowy, "Ludwick Fleck on the Social Construction of Medical Knowledge," *Sociology of Health and Illness* 10(2), 1988: 150. This "conception of the sociology of science" is almost identical to that espoused by Barry Barnes in *Interests and the Growth of Knowledge,* London: Routledge & Kegan Paul, 1977: 2. "Knowledge is not produced by passively perceiving individuals, but by interacting social groups engaged in particular activities. And it is evaluated communally and not by isolated individual judgments. Its generation cannot be understood in terms of psychology, but must be accounted for by reference to the social and cultural context in which it arises. Its maintenance is not just a matter of how it relates to reality, but also of how it relates to the objectives and interests a society possesses by virtue of its historical development." As cited in S. G. Epstein, "Impure Science: AIDS, Activism, and the Politics of Knowledge," Ph.D. dissertation, Department of Sociology, University of California at Berkeley, 1993: 39.
38. Lowy, "Ludwick Fleck," 134.

39. Wright and Treacher, *The Problem of Medical Knowledge*. Other notable exceptions among feminist studies of medical sociology include such works as Emily Martin's deconstruction of premenstrual syndrome in *The Woman in the Body: A Cultural Analysis of Reproduction*, Boston: Beacon Press, 1987; and several studies of the evolution of paridigms within immunology. Cf. D. Haraway, "The Biopolitics of Postmodern Bodies: Constitutions of Self in Immune System Discourse," *Simians, Cyborgs, and Women: The Reinvention of Nature*, New York: Routledge, Chapman & Hall, 1991: 203–230; E. Martin, "Toward an Anthropology of Immunology: The Body as Nation-State," *Medical Anthropology Quarterly* 4(4), December 1990: 410–426; and B. Patton, "Cell Wars: Military Metaphors and the Crisis of Authority in the AIDS Epidemic," in *Fluid Exchanges: Artists and Critics in the AIDS Crisis*, ed. J. Miller. Toronto: University of Toronto Press, 1992: 272–286.

40. "The concept of cultural construction . . . takes for granted metaphor and other forms of linguistic representation; it presupposes that ideas are produced out of concrete contexts and have concrete effects; it takes for granted hermeneutic activity; it is a complex of ideas and operations sustained over time within a given community; hence it is institutionalized. . . . Although meaning is indeed arbitrary and fluid, this does not mean that it is arbitrary and fluid within a given signifying system. The predictability and stability provided by a given history, society, culture, and set of disciplinary conventions are anything but arbitrary. . . . No wonder then that we expend great effort to preserve belief in a given system where meaning appears stable, indeed, even universal. Recognition that reality is culturally constructed makes such belief impossible." Treichler, "AIDS, HIV, and the Cultural Construction of Reality," 89–90. Cf. also additional titles by Treichler: "AIDS and HIV Infection in the Third World"; "AIDS, Africa, and Cultural Theory," *Transition* 51, 1991: 86–103; "AIDS, Homophobia, and Biomedical Discourse"; "Seduced and Terrorized: AIDS and Network Television," *A Leap in the Dark: AIDS, Art and Contemporary Cultures*, ed. A. Klusacek and K. Morrison, Montreal, Quebec: Véhicule Press, 1992: 136–151; *How to Have Theory in an Epidemic*.

41. Treichler, "AIDS, HIV, and the Cultural Construction of Reality," 74, 84–85, citing the work of K. D. Knorr-Cetina, *The Manufacture of Knowledge: An Essay on the Constructivist and Contextual Nature of Science*, Oxford: Pergamon, 1981.

42. Treichler, "AIDS, HIV, and the Cultural Construction of Reality," 74, 88.

43. J. Feldman, "French and American Medical Perspectives on AIDS: Discourse and Practice," Ph.D. dissertation, University of Illinois at Urbana-Champaign, 1993; J. Feldman, "Gallo, Montagnier, and the Debate over HIV: A Narrative Analysis," *Camera Obscura* 28, January 1992: 101–132.

44. Feldman, "Gallo, Montagnier, and the Debate over HIV," 103. It has now been far more than 7 years, and accusations continue to be made and charges of misconduct pronounced and then retracted. As of 1994, Gallo was contemplating countersuing for libel, and Congressman Dingell vowed to continue his efforts to see Gallo charged with scientific misconduct (see *Science*, February 1994). As of 1996, Dingell's influence over the investigation had been undermined by the dissolution of the Office of Scientific Integrity and its reconstitution as the Office of Research Integrity; Gallo had left the National Institutes of Health to set up his own $12 million AIDS research program at an independent virology institute at the University of Maryland after admitting that Montagnier's team at Pasteur Institute deserved credit for the initial discovery of LAV/HIV; and the NIH, under new leadership, unilaterally acquiesced to French demands for "sole credit" for the isolation of the virus and thus a greater share of patent royalties from the sale of HIV-antibody test kits. See also D. R. Foster, "Back to the Future: Dr. Robert Gallo Seeks to Put His Controversial Past Behind Him with Plans for a Major New AIDS Research Initiative," *Advocate*, January 23, 1996: 56–58; J. Crewdson, "Inquiry Rejects Gallo's Claim to AIDS Test: Leaves Little Doubt French Scientists Discovered Virus," *San Francisco Examiner*, June 19, 1994; "Baltimore: AIDS Doctor Lured with $12 Million," *Sentinel*, March 25, 1995; "Dingell Pursues AIDS Patent 'Cover-Up,'" *Science* 261, July 30, 1993: 539; and L. M. Krieger, "Losses Exacted by AIDS Probe: With Leading Scientist Exonerated, Researchers Look Back at 4-Year Distraction," *San Francisco Examiner*, November 14, 1993.

45. The quote is from a press conference held by the U.S. Department of Health and Human Services in April 1984, wherein Margaret Heckler of the department, stated that "the probable cause of AIDS" had been discovered by Robert Gallo at the National Cancer Institute within the National Institutes of Health.

46. Feldman, "Gallo, Montagnier, and the Debate over HIV," 101–132.
47. Ibid., 116: "As part of this settlement, Gallo and Montagnier co-authored a chronological history of AIDS research up to March 1985, and agreed 'not to make nor publish any statement which would or could be construed as contradicting or compromising the integrity of said scientific history.'"
48. Ibid., 117.
49. Ibid., 114, 126. Other examples include the following quote by San Francisco AIDS clinician Dr. Paul Volberding in 1993: "I think the sense of science as an unethical, perhaps illegal enterprise to boost one's own career has been part of how people have seen this. It is clearly not how science generally operates, and maybe this [the end of the investigations of Gallo for misconduct] will help restore what's been lost of its image." Quoted in L. M. Krieger, "Losses Exacted by AIDS Probe."
50. Feldman would agree, however, that this instance of scientific "fact making" is exceptional by virtue of its longevity and visibility, and because the debate was opened up to a larger audience of lay persons and journalists.
51. Treichler, "AIDS and HIV Infection in the Third World," 48.
52. Italics in the original. See R. C. Bleys, *The Geography of Perversion: Male-to-Male Sexual Behavior outside the West and the Ethnographic Imagination, 1750–1918,* New York: New York University Press, 1995: 1, citing Kobena Mercer in B. D. Adam, *The Rise of a Gay and Lesbian Movement,* Boston, 1987. For just one of many empirical studies of the sexualization of colonial medicine, see M. Vaughan, "Syphilis and Sexuality: The Limits of Colonial Medical Power," *Curing Their Ills: Colonial Power and African Illness,* Stanford, Calif.: Stanford University Press, 1991: 129–154. "Whatever analytical status one would want to accord the preoccupation with sex in European writings on the 'black' and on the 'African,' its presence is inescapable and, as Gilman argues, pre-dates Freud. But representations of African sexuality in the nineteenth and twentieth centuries need also to be seen in the context of a more general history of ideas about sexuality in Britain. . . . Foucault's contention, after all, was the modern European history of sexuality is not one of repression so much as of the power of description and production" (131). For the parallel constructions of race and sex, see A. L. Stoler, "Making Empire Respectable: The Politics of Race and Sexual Morality in 20th-Century Colonial Cultures," *American Ethnologist* 16(4), November 1989: 634–660. "Probably no subject is discussed more than sex in colonial literature and no subject more frequently invoked to foster the racist stereotypes of European society. The tropics provided a site of European pornographic fantasies long before conquest was underway, but with a sustained European presence in colonized territories, sexual prescriptions by class, race and gender became increasingly central to the politics of rule and subject to new forms of scrutiny by colonial states" (635).
53. S. O. Murray and K. W. Payne, "The Social Classification of AIDS in American Epidemiology," *Medical Anthropology* 10, 1989: 115–128.
54. "Because early (AIDS) cases were urban gay men, the syndrome from the beginning was presumed to be a 'sexually transmitted disease,' an already trendy classification in the zeitgeist of 'sexual counter-revolution.' The CDC penchant for the emotion-charged category 'sexually transmitted disease' contributes more to stigmatizing victims than to identifying how diseases such as hepatitis-B and AIDS are transmitted." Murray and Payne, "The Social Classification of AIDS," 117–118.
55. Murray and Payne, "The Social Classification of AIDS," 116, citing P. Conrad and J. W. Schneider, *Deviance and Medicalization: From Badness to Sickness,* Philadelphia: Temple University Press, 1990.
56. Murray and Payne, "The Social Classification of AIDS," 199, citing J. Lauritsen, "CDC's Tables Obscure AIDS/Drug Connection," *Coming Up!* 6(7), 1985: 6–18.
57. Murray and Payne, "The Social Classification of AIDS," 122.
58. Ibid., 118.
59. "Asymptomatic HIV infection is itself debilitating given its relation to the medical emergency we have come to know as AIDS" (23). N. F. McKenzie, introduction to *The AIDS Reader: Social, Political, Ethical Issues,* New York: Penguin Books, 1991: 1–18. As a counterpoint, a few AIDS dissident patient organizations, including HEAL, argue that the AIDS diagnosis itself and the stigma it carries physiologically produce the disease in some cases.
60. Murray and Payne, "The Social Classification of AIDS," 123.
61. For a related argument see the comments of Dr. Selma Dritz, the former assistant director of San Francisco's Bureau of Disease Control, when she identified the decision by the state

of California to decriminalize sodomy in California as the catalyst for unleashing public health emergencies such as the AIDS epidemic. S. K. Dritz, "Medical Staff Conference: Venereal Aspects of Gastroenterology," *Western Journal of Medicine* 130, March 1979: 238.

62. J. A. Miller, "Jeremy Bentham's Panoptic Device," *October* 41, 1987: 3. "The Panopticon is not a prison. It is a general principle of construction, the polyvalent apparatus of surveillance, the universal optical machine of human groupings. And such was Bentham's intention: apart from various minor details, the panoptic configuration could be used for prisons as well as schools, for factories and asylums, for hospitals and workhouses. . . . Surveillance confiscates the gaze for its own profit, appropriates it, and submits the inmate to it."

63. S. Schecter, *The AIDS Notebooks*, Albany: State University of New York Press, 1990: 10.

64. Witness the support groups offered by just one Bay Area HIV/AIDS service provider: the UCSF AIDS Health Project offers eight groups "for HIV-positive clients" (both symptomatic and asymptomatic), three groups for "HIV-negative clients," and two groups for "HIV-affected clients" (including those who care for "someone with HIV disease" or "anyone with HIV concerns including HIV-negative individuals"). See the monthly bulletin "AHP: Events and Services," UCSF AIDS Health Project, July 1996.

65. Gilman, *Disease and Representation*, 7.

66. For many researchers the issue of sexual orientation (homosexuality) itself has moved from the realm of psychology and the medicalization of deviance into the realm of genetics. Since 1991, a continuous stream of NIH-funded studies have posited that homosexuality is neither a choice nor a socially constructed preference for partnering with the same sex, but rather is at least partially caused by a genetic or biological predisposition; in the former case, the "gay gene." Simon LeVay, a gay researcher at the Salk Institute, was the first to propose a biological basis for homosexuality in 1991; see S. LeVay, *The Sexual Brain*, Boston: MIT Press, 1993. LeVay's research (which claimed to find an anatomical difference between the brains of homosexual men and those of heterosexual men) has been critiqued methodologically, as he based his study comparing the size of the hypothalamus in men who had been autopsied, presuming that those men who died of AIDS were homosexual, and presuming that all other dead males autopsied were heterosexual. This was followed by a study by Dr. Gorski at UCLA Medical Center, who "reported that the anterior commissures of dead gay men were on average 34 percent larger than their heterosexual counterparts." Gay columnist Michael Botkin summarized the problems with much of this research in the following comments: "Autopsy studies are relatively easy to do, as the study participants are very compliant. The main problem with them is that the identified 'homosexuals' are always PWA's, which means they died from a disease which is known to affect the brain. This makes it impossible to say if the differences found are the result of queerness or of AIDS. But gay brain stories are playing well in the mainstream media, and these rather feeble data have launched a surprisingly popular theory." See Michael Botkin, "Queer Watch: Big Gay Brain," *Bay Area Reporter*, November 23, 1994: 22. Similar methodological critiques followed the publication of Dean Hamer's NCI-funded research in the pages of *Science*, July 16, 1993, and D. Hamer and P. Coperland's, *The Science of Desire*, New York: Simon & Schuster, 1994. Hamer's study concluded that there was a genetic region on the X chromosome (inherited from the female parent) that correlated significantly with sexual orientation among sets of gay brothers. In 1995, however, the *Chicago Tribune* reported that "nearly two years later, no other laboratory has confirmed Hamer's findings . . . [and] Hamer and his lawyers are defending his study before the Office of Research Integrity, which is investigating allegations by one of Hamer's collaborators that he selectively reported his data in ways that enhanced the study's conclusions" (" 'Gay Gene' Findings Come under Fire: Study's Author Faces Allegations on Data," *Chicago Tribune*, June 25, 1995: 1. For additional coverage of this research, which made headlines throughout the Western world, see S. Connor, "Homosexuality Linked to Genes: Ethical Dilemmas Loom as Genetic Study of Gays' Families Suggests Predisposition Is Inherited through Men's Mothers," *Independent*, July 16, 1993: 1; N. Angier, "The Science of Desire: The Search for the Gay Gene and the Biology of Behavior," *New York Times Book Review*, October 16, 1994: 9; "Is There a 'Gay Gene'? Why New Findings are Causing a Storm—Especially among Homosexuals," *U.S. News and World Report*, November 13, 1995: 93; and C. Burr, "Homosexuality and Biology," *Atlantic*, March 1993: 47–65. Criticisms against this type of research can be found in K. Davidson, "Psychiatrists Debate Biology's Role in Sexuality," *San Francisco Examiner*, May 28, 1993: A-5; and J. Horgan, "Hierarchy of Worthlessness," in "Trends in Behavioral Genetics: Eugenics Revisited," *Scientific American*, June 1993: 123–131.

67. Dritz, "Medical Staff Conference," 238.
68. C. Patton, *Inventing AIDS,* 89 and footnote 25.
69. See J. A. Wiley and S. J. Herschkorn (University of California, Berkeley), "Homosexual Role Separation and AIDS Epidemics: Insights from Elementary Models," *Journal of Sex Research* 26(4), November 1989: 434–449. In this NIAID-funded research the authors concluded that "as expected, role differentiation in anal intercourse and mixing preferences affect the course of an AIDS epidemic in crucial ways. As Trichopoulos and his colleagues (1988) have inferred, if HIV can be transmitted sexually only from an infected insertive partner to a receptive partner in unprotected anal intercourse, an epidemic will be of smaller size in a population with a correspondingly smaller segment which takes both roles. . . . Most interestingly, a worst-case epidemic occurs not with random mixing . . . but in a situation where dual-role individuals prefer to mix with themselves to a certain degree" (447–448).
70. See the Physiology Series: Immunology. Perma-Chart Quick Reference Guide, LLS-17F, Concord, Ontario: Papertech Marketing Group, Inc., 1993: Clinical Focus, Side 2. See also "How The Virus Attacks, and How to Attack the Virus," *Newsweek,* June 25, 1990: 22. The actual process by which HIV gains entrance to a lymphocyte is poorly understood, but is thought to occur when a receptor on the external coat of HIV "docks" to a complementary receptor or receptors on the external coat of the T-cell (for instance, the CD4 marker), perhaps with the assistance of enabling proteins; once fused, HIV then disgorges its genetic contents into the CD4 T-cell. But the transfer of genetic material from the virus to the host's cell does not take place via actual penetration of the body of the virus into the cell. "Although CD4 is the high-affinity receptor for HIV, studies have shown that expression of CD4 by a cell is not sufficient for HIV infection . . . some other membrane molecule must participate in the process of HIV entry" (J. Kuby, *Immunology,* New York: W. H. Freeman, 1994: 528.) As of 1994, the molecule hypothesized as an aid to HIV infection was CD26. However, as of the spring of 1996, several additional "helper" proteins were proposed: "fusin," and a "chemokine receptor . . . CC-CKR-5." Cf. Associated Press, "Key Protein in Attack of AIDS Virus Discovered," *Los Angeles Times,* May 10, 1996; and M. Ritter, "New Chemical Footholds Identified for HIV in Cells: Research on How Killer Virus Invades," *San Francisco Examiner,* June 19, 1996: "Scientists have long known that to get inside cells HIV needed another foothold as well. Last month, government researches reported that for some strains of HIV, this second foothold is a cell protein called fusin. But fusin does not appear to be used by HIV strains that are most commonly transmitted between people. . . . Now, scientists have identified a foothold for these strains. It's a protein found on blood cells, and it normally acts as a docking site for chemokines—chemical messages that summon blood cells to the sites of inflammation."
71. Broadcast on April 24, 1994 by KTEH/PBS as part of what the station called its "educational campaign against AIDS." The credibility of the broadcast's claim of educational value was enhanced by the participation of Dr. David D. Ho, a prominent AIDS researcher at the Aaron Diamond Foundation for the past several years. In a recent citation analysis of AIDS publications, Ho ranked second only to Robert Gallo (at the NIH) in the number of citations in the period of 1993 to 1995; Ho had 83 papers published during this time. In addition, "Ho and colleagues accounted for the most-cited paper published in 1995, a *Nature* report on viral and immune-system dynamics in HIV-1 infection . . . one of two 1995 AIDS reports that garnered more than 100 citations in their first year of publication." "RESEARCH: Citation Analysis Reveals Leading Institutions, Scientists Researching AIDS," *Scientist,* July 22, 1996: 12.
72. Professor Opendra Narayan of Johns Hopkins Medical School, quoted in Leo Bersani, 1998: 197. I have yet to see the epidemiological study that supports her contention that the average PWA had 3,000 anal-receptive sexual partners per year; some may have had 3,000 sexual contacts in a lifetime, but the disaggregation of these contacts (in other words, whether they engaged in anal sex, insertive or receptive, or oral sex) was infrequently done. The earliest epidemiological questionnaires administered by the CDC between 1981 and 1982 did ask AIDS patients to estimate the number of their lifetime sexual partners, and to estimate, by percentage, how frequently they engaged in various sexual acts, as did some of the early epidemiological work by Winkelstein et al. Although I did not have access to all of the CDC interviews, those questionnaires that I reviewed in San Francisco did not support anywhere near the figure of 3,000 anal-receptive partners per year or per lifetime for that matter. Cf. also a 1992 study wherein the mean number of "lifetime male sexual intercourse

partners" was 501 for HIV-positive men who progressed to AIDS within five years of infection, versus a mean of 322 partners for HIV-positive men who did not develop AIDS within five years after HIV infection. J. Phair et al., "Acquired Immune Deficiency Syndrome Occurring within Five Years of Infection with Human Immunodeficiency Virus Type-1: The Multicenter AIDS Cohort Study," *Journal of Acquired Immune Deficiency Syndromes* 5, 1992: 492 ("Table 1. Distribution of specific characteristics of cases and controls").

73. Fleck, *Genesis and Development of a Scientific Fact,* 93.
74. Lowy, "Ludwig Fleck," 151. For a lengthy discussion of how some observations and not others are transformed into facts, first, by a process of legitimation by authorities within the field, and second, through repeated citations in scientific texts, cf. Bruno Latour, *Science in Action,* 29. "By looking only at them [a fact or a machine] and at their internal properties, you cannot decide if they are true or false, efficient or wasteful, costly or cheap, strong or frail. These characteristics are only gained through *incorporation* into other statements, processes and pieces of machinery. . . . To sum up, the construction of facts and machines is a *collective* process." (Italics in the original.)
75. D. Gregory, *Geographical Imaginations,* Cambridge, Mass.: Blackwell Publishers, 1994: 6.
76. J. Abu-Lughod, "On the Re-Making of History: How to Re-invent the Past," in *Dia Art Foundation: Discussing Contemporary Culture, Remaking History,* ed. B. Druger and P. Mariani, Number 4, Seattle: Bay Press, 1989: 112–113.

Chapter 2

The epigraph is from comments by Dr. Selma Dritz, assistant director of the Bureau of Communicable Disease Control of the San Francisco Department of Public Health, to colleagues at the University of California at San Francisco in 1980. Cited in Shilts, *And the Band Played On,* 40.

1. Murray and Payne, "The Social Classification of AIDS," 115–128. Italics in the original.
2. Selma Dritz, "Medical Aspects of Homosexuality," *New England Journal of Medicine,* 302 (8), 1980: 463–464. For some of this quote, Dritz cited B. Goldman, "Profile of the Gay STD Patient," 105th Annual Meeting of the American Public Health Association, Washington, D.C., October 30–November 3, 1977.
3. Medical Staff Conference, "Venereal Aspects of Gastroenterology," 240.
4. Dritz, "Medical Aspects of Homosexuality," 464.
5. Medical Staff Conference, "Venereal Aspects of Gastroenterology," 242.
6. As there was no test for the hepatitis B antigen until 1974, consequently there could be relatively few confirmed cases before this time. Venereal transmission of hepatitis B was not even recognized until the late 1970s, as the invention of an antigen test was necessary before researchers were able to reliably study the incidence and prevalence of the virus. See Medical Staff Conference, "Venereal Aspects of Gastroenterology," 239, for the following quote: "Before 1974, when the hepatitis-associated antigen (HAA) test became generally available, hepatitis B diagnoses were based on a history of probable parenteral contamination. Diagnoses of hepatitis A were accepted on the physicians' clinical impression, if tests were negative for hepatitis B antigen."
7. Medical Staff Conference, "Venereal Aspects of Gastroenterology," 239.
8. *San Francisco Chronicle,* "Judge Blocks Health Fund Cuts For Poor, Seamen," June 5, 1981: 12; *San Francisco Chronicle,* " 'High Risk' Reported: U.S. Surveys Gays and Disease," September 1, 1981: 6. Although this report was officially published in September 1981 following the first announcement of AIDS, the survey itself took place in 1977, and the CDC's results had been presented at the 107th Annual Meeting of the American Public Health Association in New York in November 1979. See W. Darrow et al., "The Gay Report on Sexually Transmitted Diseases," *American Journal of Public Health,* September 1981, 71(9): 1004–1011.
9. Murray and Payne citing the research of John Lauritsen in their article, "The Social Classification of AIDS," 119. After 1985, homosexual/bisexual men with no history of IV drug use (GM) were classified separately from gay IV drug users (GIVDU), at least theoretically, if not in actual practice. Conversely, heterosexuals with a history of IV drug abuse (IVDU) have always been listed as a distinct risk category from heterosexuals who never injected drugs.
10. S. B. Thacker et al., "The Surveillance of Infectious Diseases," *Journal of the American Medical Association* 249(9), March 4, 1983: 1181.
11. Author's telephone interview with Dr. Selma Dritz, August 1995.

12. Shilts, *And the Band Played On*, 75–76.
13. Author's recorded lecture of Dr. Paul A. Volberding, September 15, 1994, at the Fairmont Hotel, San Francisco, California.
14. See also Centers for Disease Control, "Kaposi's Sarcoma and Pneumocystis Among Homosexual Men—New York City and California," *Morbidity and Mortality Weekly Report,* July 3, 1981.
15. And even this is a matter for some debate; as the patient's medical chart records his age as both 22 and 29—neither given more credence than the other.
16. Author's files; medical chart review, case number 1008.
17. A grant proposal from the files of Dr. W. Winkelstein Jr., principal investigator, "The Natural History of Acquired Immune Deficiency Syndrome (AIDS) in Homosexual Men," 1983.
18. Summarized in the CDC's "Update on AIDS—U.S.," *Morbidity and Mortality Weekly Report,* September 24, 1982: 508. By their own definition, therefore, one of the five cases in Los Angeles would be disqualified as an AIDS case, by virtue of chemotherapy and radiation treatments for Hodgkin's disease.
19. H. W. Jaffe et al., "National Case-Control Study of KS and PCP in Homosexual Men: Part 1," *Annals of Internal Medicine* 99(2), 1983: 145–151.
20. K. Leishman, "A Crisis in Public Health," *Atlantic,* October 1985: 20.
21. Centers for Disease Control, *Morbidity and Mortality Weekly Report,* September 24, 1982, and January 4, 1983; Centers for Disease Control, *Morbidity and Mortality Weekly Report,* "Possible Transfusion-Associated Acquired Immune Deficiency Syndrome (AIDS)—California," December 10, 1982.
22. Leishman, "A Crisis in Public Health," 20.
23. James Chin, "Memorandum to Local Health Officers re: The Reporting of AIDS Cases in California," State of California Department of Health Services, March 23, 1983.
24. James Chin, "The Use of Hepatitis B Vaccine," *New England Journal of Medicine,* September 9, 1982: 679.
25. Author's interview with Tim Piland, recorded in October 1994 at the San Francisco AIDS Office.
26. By the end of 1984 there were 876 cases logged in records at the offices of AIDS surveillance; all of the patients were homosexual/bisexual men (GM), or homosexual/bisexual men who used intravenous drugs (GIVDU), with the exception of two "no identifiable risk (NIR)" cases, four heterosexual IVDU cases, and one pediatric transfusion case (with two additional pediatric cases subsequently backdated to 1979). Moreover, although they were diagnosed and reported as AIDS cases in San Francisco, the sole pediatric transfusion case and several of the "heterosexual" cases were residents of other counties and therefore not rigorously investigated for risk or mode of acquiring the disease. For some of this general history of AIDS in San Francisco, see F. Fitzgerald, *Cities on a Hill,* New York: Simon & Schuster, 1986: 84–96, and Leishman, "A Crisis in Public Health," 18–40.
27. This was succeeded by the creation of the AIDS Office in 1985 under the direction of George Rutherford.
28. Project report, "Publications of the AIDS Epidemiology Group. San Francisco General Hospital," (July 1989) contains references to 41 articles on the cohort.
29. All quotes and figures from Andrew R. Moss et al., "Risk Factors for AIDS and HIV Seropositivity in Homosexual Men," *American Journal of Epidemiology,* 125(6), 1987: 1035–1047.
30. Ibid., 1035.
31. Of these men, 34 percent had more than 40 sexual partners in the preceding year yet remained HIV-negative. See Moss et al., "Risk Factors for AIDS," 1039.
32. Ibid., 1045.
33. Ibid.
34. Ibid., 1042, 1045.
35. Ibid., 1046.
36. Men who were older than 35 had a "relative hazard of 2.1[p=0.015]" compared with younger men. Andrew R. Moss et al., "Seropositivity for HIV and the Development of AIDS or AIDS Related Condition: Three Year Follow-up of the San Francisco General Hospital Cohort," *British Medical Journal* 296, March 12, 1988, 749.
37. A quote from Dr. Dennis Osmond, assistant adjunct professor, Department of Epidemiology and Biostatistics, University of California at San Francisco, during a lecture on the cohort studies and the epidemiology of HIV/AIDS in gay men at the Center for AIDS Prevention Studies (CAPS) fall 1993.

38. P. Bacchetti and A. R. Moss, "Incubation Period of AIDS in San Francisco," *Nature* 338, March 16, 1989: 253.

39. Ibid., 251.

40. Throughout this text, I use "homosexual and gay men" interchangeably to refer to men who have had sex with other men in or after 1978, which is synonymous with the way in which CDC categorizes male risk—referred to at various times as homosexual or gay/bisexual men, and most recently categorized as men who engage in "Male-to-Male Sex (MSM)." Until 1985, this category explicitly included men who injected drugs and also had sex with men.

41. "United Men's Health Study Publications," United Men's Health Study, Berkeley, Survey Research Center, September 20, 1993. The study's design and results were part of the public health curriculum taught by Dr. Winkelstein at the University of California at Berkeley in the mid-1990s: epidemiology 250 and PH 288: AIDS and Public Policy, required coursework for the Master's of public health degree in the School of Public Health.

42. For example see San Francisco Department of Public Health, Bureau of Communicable Disease Control, "Continued Sero-conversion for HIV Antibody among Homosexual and Bisexual Men," *San Francisco Epidemiologic Bulletin* 5(8), August 1989.

43. "United Men's Health Study Publications."

44. Prospective studies of disease sample a population that does not yet manifest the disease being investigated—subsequently following the cohort through time to gauge the incidence of the disease; in this case, researchers studied a cohort of men in San Francisco to determine how many of the men in the cohort went on to develop "AIDS" overtime. And as these studies progressed, they have also been used to assess risk factors associated with those who develop the disease (cases) versus those who do not (controls).

45. Original proposal from the files of Dr. W. Winkelstein Jr., principal investigator, *RFP-NIH-NIAID-MIDP-83-11.* "The Natural History of Acquired Immune Deficiency Syndrome (AIDS) in Homosexual Men," 1983.

46. Jay Levy's "AIDS related virus (ARV)," and Luc Montagnier's "lymphadenopathy associated virus (LAV)," and Robert Gallo's "human T-cell leukemia/lymphatrophic virus III (HTLV-III)" were all variants of the same retrovirus that was officially renamed "human immuno-deficiency virus (HIV)" after a negotiated legal settlement between Gallo and Montagnier in the spring of 1987. Since that time it has been established beyond doubt that LAV and HTLV-III are in fact identical isolates that came from the same patient. Jay Levy's isolate, however, was a separate viral strain. For an excellent review of the controversial history of the discovery of HIV, see Jamie Feldman's "Gallo, Montagnier, and the Debate over HIV."

47. Author's paraphrasing and comments noted by brackets. Also, I have deleted the number of months (three) cited by Winkelstein as this is a typographical error and should read "15 months." See Winkelstein's citation of the *Morbidity and Mortality Weekly Report* of September 1982 in Warren Winkelstein Jr. et al., "Homosexual Men," *The Epidemiology of AIDS,* ed. R. A. Kaslow and D. P. Francis, Oxford: Oxford University Press, 1989: 118.

48. Lecture by Dr. Warren Winkelstein, Epidemiology 250, University of California at Berkeley, fall 1993.

49. Winkelstein et al., "Sexual Practices and Risk of Infection," 321.

50. Although only half of the men answered questions regarding "ancillary sexual practices," douching and the use of sexual toys (referred to as sources of "rectal trauma") were significantly related to acquiring HIV. See Winkelstein et al., "Sexual Practices and Risk of Infection," 325.

51. Ibid., 321–322.

52. M. C. Samuel et al., "Factors Associated with HIV Seroconversion in Homosexual Men in Three San Francisco Cohort Studies, 1984–1989," *Journal of AIDS* 6 (1993): 308.

53. Warren Winkelstein Jr. et al., "The SFMHS: III. Reduction in HIV Transmission among Homosexual/Bisexual Men, 1982–1986," *American Journal of Public Health* 76(9), June 1987: 688.

54. None of the heterosexual cohort members tested positive for HIV antibodies. See Winkelstein et al., "Sexual Practices and Risk of Infection," 321.

55. For example, see "Help For Gays Who Feel Guilty Over Being Healthy," *San Francisco Examiner,* September 3, 1995: "With 50 percent of San Francisco's gay male population infected, many negatives have also reached the [conclusion] that they are somehow betraying the gay community by being virus-free."

56. See Table 1a and Figure 6 at the end of this chapter for a graphic depiction of these data.

57. Quotes are from Winkelstein et al., "The SFMHS: III," 685–689.

58. Ibid., 687.
59. Quite literally the same evidence as both researchers cite the same article in the journal *Mathematical Modeling* for their figures on rectal gonorrhea. J. Pickering et al., *Mathematical Modeling* 7 1986: 661–668.
60. Author's interview and both published and unpublished data from the Division of STD Control, 1360 Mission Street, Suite #401, San Francisco, California. See the tables at the end of this chapter for data on the incidence of sexually transmitted infections (rectal gonorrhea, etc.) among gay men in San Francisco from the late 1970s throughout the 1980s.
61. Michael S. Ascher et al., "Does Drug Use Cause AIDS?" *Nature* 362, March 11, 1993: 103.
62. This announcement of the decline in new AIDS cases was information that was "embargoed until February 15, 1994," then subsequently published in "AIDS News and Information," San Francisco Department of Public Health. It was immediately picked up by newspapers across the country: "The decline in AIDS cases is a direct consequence of a drop in new HIV infections that occurred after 1982 . . . but because the virus takes, on average, 10 years to wear down the victim's immune system and cause AIDS, the peak of AIDS diagnoses occurred a decade after prevention efforts began." "AIDS Cases Decline in S.F.," *San Francisco Chronicle*, February 16, 1994.
63. A comment made by the CDC's Harold Jaffe in the *Washington Post*, "Map of 'AIDS' Deadly March Evolves from Hepatitis Study: Blood Samples of Gay Men Prove Invaluable," February 1, 1987.
64. D. Osmond lecture attended by author at the Center for AIDS Prevention Studies, San Francisco, California, fall 1993.
65. Unless otherwise noted, my figures for this cohort will come from N. A. Hessol et al., "Incidence and Prevalence of HIV Infection among Homosexual and Bisexual Men, 1978–1988," a paper presented at the Fifth International Conference on AIDS, Montreal, Canada, June 5, 1989, and in other publications by Hessol. It is necessary to qualify the figures used for the number of men enrolled in this cohort, as publications vary widely in their cited figures. Although I have been unable to discover a consistent and reliable number for the men originally recruited into the SFCCC, the range appears to be between 6,697 to 6,875 men enrolled. See Winkelstein et al., "The SFMHS: III," 686, and W. W. Darrow et al., "The Gay Report on Sexually Transmitted Diseases," *Journal of American Medicine* 26(5), February 3, 1989: 725–727.
66. Centers for Disease Control, "Update: AIDS in the SF Cohort Study, 1978–1985," *Morbidity and Mortality Weekly Report*, September 27, 1985.
67. "Update: The SF City Clinic Cohort Study," *San Francisco Epidemiologic Bulletin*, November 1989: 47.
68. D. P. Francis et al., "The Prevention of Hepatitis B With Vaccine," *Annals of Internal Medicine* 97, 1982: 362–366.
69. Centers for Disease Control, "Inactivated Hepatitis B Virus Vaccine," *Morbidity and Mortality Weekly Report*, June 25, 1982: 317–330.
70. Centers for Disease Control, "Update: AIDS in the SF Cohort Study," 573.
71. *San Francisco Weekly*, April 12, 1995: 10.
72. E.g., conferring a relative risk of five. See Harold W. Jaffe, "AIDS in a Cohort of Homosexual Men: A Six-Year Follow-up Study," *Annals of Internal Medicine* 103, 1985: 210–214.
73. C. E. Stevens et al., "HTLV-III Infection in a Cohort of Homosexual Men in NYC," *Journal of the American Medical Association* 255(16), April 25, 1986: 2167–2172. See also G. W. Rutherford et al., "Course of HIV-I Infection in a Cohort of Homosexual and Bisexual Men: An 11 Year Follow-up Study," *British Medical Journal*, November 24, 1990: 1186 (Table V): "Cumulative risk of AIDS by time since HIV-1 seroconversion, San Francisco Clinic Cohort," wherein researchers concluded that exactly 1 percent of HIV-positives were projected to have developed AIDS in the second year following their "estimated date of HIV sero-conversion." This estimate carried a confidence interval of 0–2 percent, however, which means that possibly no one progressed to AIDS that rapidly.
74. Centers for Disease Control, "Update: AIDS in the SF Cohort Study," 574.
75. C. Russell, "Map of AIDS' Deadly March Evolves from Hepatitis Study," *Washington Post*, February 1, 1987. By 1987, members of the SFCC cohort accounted for one out of every five cumulatively reported cases of AIDS in San Francisco, and one out of every 50 cases in the United States.
76. Not until 1983 did any hepatitis B vaccine recipients develop AIDS in San Francisco, and these three men accounted for less than 1 percent of all cases reported that year, although

an additional 15 percent of the year's caseload occurred among *unvaccinated* members of the SFCCC who had been screened for the trials.

77. N. A. Hessol et al., "Prevalence, Incidence, and Progression of Human Immunodeficiency Virus Infection in Homosexual and Bisexual Men in Hepatitis B Vaccine Trials, 1978–1988," *American Journal of Epidemiology* 130(6), 1989: 1168.

78. Rutherford et al., "Course of HIV-I Infection," 1183.

79. See S. C. Hadler et al., "Outcome of Hepatitis B Virus Infection in Homosexual Men and Its Relation to Prior Human Immunodeficiency Virus Infection," *Journal of Infectious Diseases* 163, March 1991: 454–459. "Among HIV1-infected men, the risk of HBV carriage was increased in unvaccinated persons (21%), and those who failed to respond to vaccination (31%) and further increased in those who received vaccine doses at the time they developed new HBV infection (56%–80%), suggesting inactivated hepatitis B vaccine may temporarily impair the immune response to HBV infection in HIV-1 infected persons" (454, 458).

80. Steven B. Harris, Internet post, "Article 13454," *sci.med.aids.,* March 25, 1995.

81. "Update: The SF City Clinic Cohort Study," *San Francisco Epidemiologic Bulletin,* November 1989: 47.

82. Rutherford et al., "Course of HIV-I Infection," 1183–1188. This article is also unique for its claim that HIV was present in San Francisco in 1977, pushing the epidemic back in time yet an additional year.

83. For this method of estimating dates of HIV seroconversion, see Winkelstein et al., "Sexual Practices and Risk of Infection," 321.

84. Samuel et al., "Factors Associated with HIV Seroconversion," 303–312.

85. Ibid., 306.

86. Ibid., 308.

87. Ibid.

88. Ibid., 309.

89. Ibid., 310.

90. Walt Odets, "The Fatal Mistakes of AIDS Education," *Harper's,* May 1995: 13–17.

91. Although the city's public health director, Dr. M. Silverman, banned sex in gay bathhouses he did not close bathhouses frequented by heterosexuals because, he said, AIDS is "not likely to occur among heterosexuals." *San Francisco Chronicle,* "S.F. Orders Ban on Sex in Bathhouses," April 10, 1984: 1.

92. Shilts, "How AIDS Is Changing Gay Lifestyles," 1, 5, 7.

93. Quoted in Steven Seidman, "AIDS and the 'Homosexual' Question," *Embattled Eros: Sexual Politics and Ethics in Contemporary America,* New York: Routledge, 1992: 163.

94. Quoted in K. Ocamb, "Michael Callen, Entertainer, Activist, and Long-Term PWA, Dies," *Bay Area Reporter,* San Francisco, January 6, 1994: 1, 15. Callen's accomplishments as an AIDS dissident were legion: he coauthored the article cited above which created the guidelines for "safe sex"; he successfully lobbied the FDA to recommend PCP prophylaxis as standard practice in treating PWAs; he published *Surviving AIDS,* which documented various strategies for surviving and thriving with the disease; "co-founded the Community Research Initiative (CRI)—the first attempt by the gay community to conduct its own research"; "started and wrote the *PWA Newsline*"; and was a key player in many alternative AIDS organizations and underground buyer's clubs. See "Michael Callen, 1955–1993," *Village Voice,* January 11, 1994: 1, 22.

Chapter 3

1. In retrospect, it seems odd that PCP and KS were not noted earlier among members of San Francisco City Clinic Cohort (aka hepatitis B study) because: 1) the hepatitis B cohort comprised men considered to be at the greatest risk for AIDS; 2) stored serum samples show that some blood specimens from men enrolled in the hepatitis B vaccine study tested positive for HIV antibodies as early as 1978; and 3) officials at the SFDPH and CDC publicly acknowledge that six of the first ten AIDS cases reported in San Francisco after June 1981 were members of the HBV cohort.

2. Anywhere from 35,000 to 200,000 men, depending on which source you consult. See chapter 2 for a discussion of how these population parameters are estimated.

3. J. T. Murphy, G. E. Mueller, and S. Whitman, "Redefining the Growth of the Heterosexual HIV/AIDS Epidemic in Chicago." *Journal of Acquired Immune Deficiency Syndromes and*

Human Retrovirology 16 (122), 1997: 122–126. Cf. also D. Serraino et al., "The Classification of AIDS Cases Concordance between Two AIDS Surveillance Systems in Italy." *American Journal of Public Health* 85, 1995: 1112–1114 and O. C. Nwanyanwu et al., "Increasing Frequency of Heterosexually Transmitted AIDS in Southern Florida: Artifact or Reality?" *American Journal of Public Health* 83, 1993: 571–573.

4. "In fact, researchers later marked the spread of AIDS in concentric circles, pulsing out of the center of Manhattan to include larger and larger rings of land and population in the impoverished outlands of metropolitan New York City. [As of March 1983] this proliferation of AIDS through the East Coast corridors of poverty heralded the start of the second AIDS epidemic in the United States, distinct from epidemic in gay men." Shilts, *And the Band Played On,* 261.

5. There are numerous references I could cite in further evidence of this point, but I will limit myself to four. The first is an article on the resurgence in the Bay Area and Northern California of methamphetamines, characterized as a "white man's drug." Two of the three men profiled in the article were homosexual/bisexual, and two of the three injected the drug intravenously—both were HIV-positive. The IVDUs in this story supported their drug habits while in San Francisco by dealing drugs or engaging in prostitution. (S. Ferrias, "Rapid Rise of Speed: Fast Track to Nowhere," *San Francisco Examiner,* March 31, 1996: 1, 11.) A second article reported on a study from Yale which examined risk factors correlated with an AIDS diagnosis and concluded that "drug addicts and alcoholics on welfare in New York are 10 times more likely than other people their age in the city to get AIDS." (Cited in L. M. Krieger, "AIDSWEEK," *San Francisco Examiner,* April 3, 1996: 2.) Two additional epidemiological studies demonstrate a correlation between poverty and AIDS. According to the SFDPH, as of 1988, the "incidence of AIDS in the Tenderloin (1,753 cases per 100,000) . . . a high density, low income neighborhood on the southwestern edge of downtown San Francisco . . . is significantly higher than in the remainder of San Francisco, 649 cases per 100,000 (rate ratio = 2.7)." (SFDPH, *San Francisco Epidemiologic Bulletin* (9), September 1988.) Cf. also, P. A. Simon et al., "Income and AIDS rates in Los Angeles County," *AIDS* 9(3), 1995: 281–284 (I have added emphasis to the original text): "1990 US census data were used to classify LAC postal zones by median household income into low-, middle-, and high-income strata. AIDS rates were calculated for each income stratum based on 15,805 AIDS cases diagnosed from 1987 through 1992 and reported to the county health department. . . . *The AIDS rate was highest among residents of low-income areas (252.8 per 100,000),* intermediate among residents of middle-income areas (161.2 per 100,000), and lowest among residents of high-income areas (82.0 per 100,000). *This trend in rates was present in all racial/ethnic groups examined and was most pronounced among whites* (675.1, 226.7, and 88.4 per 100,000, respectively). Residents of low-income areas accounted for 78% of AIDS cases among blacks, 67% among Hispanics, and 47% among whites." As a caveat to this article's conclusions, it is impossible to eliminate a possible confounding factor of downward mobility from a higher income strata to a lower one *subsequent* to an individual's diagnosis with the disease, in which case poverty would be solely the consequence of an AIDS diagnosis and not a precursor.

6. Quoting "Harold Jaffe, author interview, April 30, 1987, Atlanta" cited in Etheridge, *Sentinel for Health,* 324. Despite his position as a physician with the Sexually Transmitted Disease Division of the Centers for Disease Control in Atlanta, Jaffe was apparently too afraid to enter the Ambush, a south-of-market gay leather bar, in order to buy bottles of poppers (amyl/butyl nitrites) to take back to Atlanta for toxicological testing in association with investigating the cause of AIDS. See Shilts, *And the Band Played On,* 86.

7. Jaffe et al., "National Case-Control Study," 145–151.

8. With very early epidemiological studies such as this one (prior to the use of the HIV antibody test in 1985/1986), the latency period for developing AIDS was poorly understood. Furthermore, research results can be confounded by the fact that it was impossible to know whether the homosexual men used as controls in this study were in fact healthy men who truly differed from reported AIDS cases, or whether they shared many of the same risk factors as AIDS cases but were asymptomatic and had yet to progress to full-blown disease.

9. Toxoplasmosis, cryptococcal meningitis, or cryptosporidiosis also occurred, but rarely.

10. Editing remarks, Kevin McKinney, ASSB, July 1996: "Median survival for the first couple of years was eight months." My own summary calculations for all 24 patients reported in 1981 refutes this official estimate, however, and I found that median survival differed for various

subsets of patients: median survival from diagnosis to death for the cohort as a whole was 15.8 months; but gay non-IV drug users (GM) survived on average 18.26 months, while gay IV drug users (GIVDUs) died on average only 4.7 months after their first AIDS diagnosis.

11. "During the past 30 months, Kaposi's sarcoma (KS), an uncommonly reported malignancy in the United States, has been diagnosed in 26 homosexual men (20 in New York City, 6 in California). The 26 patients range in age from 25–51 years (mean 39 years). Eight of these patients died (7 in NYC, 1 in California), all within 24 months after KS was diagnosed." Centers for Disease Control, "Kaposi's Sarcoma and *Pneumocystis* Pneumonia Among Homosexual Men."

12. Because my goal was to historically reconstruct the epidemic as it must have appeared to investigators, I used the unadjusted data from the SFDPH's chronological logbook to track the accretion of AIDS cases versus adjusted data from the department's AIDS Surveillance Reports (or other sources). As I discuss in later chapters, annual AIDS caseloads in surveillance reports are amended after the fact by adding AIDS cases reported in subsequent years of the epidemic to earlier years. For instance, AIDS cases captured in 1987 can be backdated to 1981/1982 dates of diagnosis. Backdating AIDS cases to earlier years of diagnosis has inflated the number of AIDS cases reported in 1981 from 24 cases (observed) to 34, thereby increasing the annual caseload by 42 percent. For adjusted data, see SFDPH AIDS Office, Seroepidemiology and Surveillance Branch, "AIDS Cases Reported through October, 1995," *AIDS Surveillance Report,* October 1995: 3, Table 4.

13. Risk is numerically ordered according to the CDC hierarchy of risk factors for acquiring the disease; the order 1 through 9 denotes a system whereby the highest risk for HIV/AIDS is (1), and designates male-to-male sexual intercourse as the mode of transmission. With the exception of risk (2), which connotes the combined risks of gay and injection drug use, the risk (1. gay sex) supersedes all lower-order risks (e.g., 4. hemophiliac; 6. transfusion).

14. For the 24 AIDS cases reported in San Francisco in 1981, only five of eleven interviews conducted by the CDC were still physically available for review during my fieldwork at the ASSB in 1994–1995. In addition, I thoroughly perused the medical charts for five cases, one of whom also had an interview extant in his file. In sum, I reconstructed extensive patient data for nine (38 percent) of the 24 AIDS cases reported in San Francisco between November 1980 (the earliest date at which a homosexual/bisexual AIDS case was diagnosed) and December 31, 1981. This percentage was similar for AIDS cases reported in San Francisco in 1982 (material not discussed in this text). Of the 94 AIDS cases reported in 1982, I reviewed 24 medical charts (including one patient who had also been interviewed), and found interview data for seven additional cases (thus extensive data for 30 of 94 patients, or 32 percent of the annual caseload).

15. This early description of AIDS comes from the "Case Consent Form for Interview and Specimen Collection" (CDC Protocol #577), a 25 page questionnaire used in the CDC's investigation of early AIDS patients. *OMB Number 0920–0008,* TF 73.10 (VD) 7–81.

16. Initially, officials at the SFDPH used an alphabetical system for assigning case numbers to AIDS patients. Because of this, the San Francisco case number of the first man reported with the disease (hypothetically 1020) is a higher number than that of the subsequent patient (hypothetically 1005). This arcane detail is only relevant because it meant that I could not rely upon the *sequence* of case numbers for discerning the chronological order of patients reported with the disease. To further complicate the matter, the fact that one AIDS case was reported a month prior to another AIDS case did not necessarily imply that the prior patient had developed the disease at an earlier date. Instead, it may have simply indicated that his doctor was more on-the-ball when it came to paperwork and phone calls. Therefore, in order to be absolutely certain about which patients developed the disease earlier than other reported patients I consulted either the AER (the earliest SFDPH AIDS case report form) or the patient's medical chart for date of diagnosis. This is the method that I relied upon in order to credibly substantiate my argument about which gay man in the city (among those reported to the SFDPH), was the first to develop symptoms of AIDS.

17. For my fieldwork only, these AIDS cases will be numbered consecutively from Case Numbers 1001–1024 (1981 cases).

18. The CDC questionnaire was revised after several months of use, and therefore my page estimate varies. The latter version contained disaggregated income categories, which I will note when it is available for an individual patient.

19. Two black pediatric patients (sisters born to the same injection-drug-using mother and diagnosed in 1978 and 1979) were in fact the first AIDS cases diagnosed in San Francisco.

This is evidenced by SFDPH AIDS case files and was well known by epidemiologists, such as Dr. Warren Winkelstein, as early as 1983 and cited in his initial proposal to the National Institutes of Health to study the natural history of the epidemic. See Dr. W. Winkelstein Jr., principal investigator, "The Natural History of Acquired Immune Deficiency Syndrome (AIDS) in Homosexual Men," *RFP-NIH-NIAID-MIDP-83-11*, 1983; proposal copy.

20. I can offer nothing to explain why only five of eleven interviews conducted by the CDC remain within SFDPH patient ACR files. Were these five interviews copies of the originals? If so, they did not appear to be. Moreover, were these five case interviews included in the statistical analysis for the CDC's subsequent National Case-Control Study on the disease published in 1983? If these interviews were elided from that analysis it could imply some selection or temporal bias in the methods by which CDC investigators selected interview subjects, and from among them, selected just a subset of completed interviews to analyze.

21. "To identify risk factors for the occurrence of Kaposi's sarcoma and *Pneumocystis carinii* pneumonia in homosexual men, we conducted a case-control study in New York City, San Francisco, Los Angeles, and Atlanta. . . . Histories of several infectious diseases, particularly sexually transmitted infections, were common for both cases and controls. However, compared with controls, cases were almost twice as likely to have reported a history of syphilis, and cases were also more likely to have a history of hepatitis other than hepatitis B. . . . The use of various illicit substances was also relatively common for both cases and controls. However, cases were somewhat more likely than controls to have reported use of one of various 'street' drugs. Almost all cases and controls reported use of nitrite inhalants for sexual stimulation, but the lifetime exposure to nitrites was greater for cases than controls. . . . For cases, the median lifetime use was 336 days, compared with 168 days and 264 days for clinic and private controls, respectively. Cases were also more likely than controls to have reported inhaling ethyl chloride, but the lifetime use of ethyl chloride by all groups was much lower than that of nitrites." Jaffe et al., "National Case-Control Study," 145, 147.

22. The questions which this patient declined to answer included how many sexual partners were women, men or boys, or natives of Africa. (Presumably, this African question was included in the CDC's early patient interviews because Kaposi's sarcoma is endemic to certain areas of tropical Africa and investigators were looking for some possibility of an infection being introduced via sex with persons from that continent). Other questions were: what was the frequency with which the patient had engaged in certain sexual acts (anal/oral intercourse and "fisting") and/or "paid for (or) accepted money from men or boys for sex." CDC interview with case #1001, author's notes, ASSB, July 13, 1994. Apparently, the CDC was wholly uninterested in the nature of the heterosexual sex these men may have engaged in because there are no parallel questions regarding the specifics of sexual acts with women or girls, nor are there any questions about accepting money from, nor giving money to, women or girls for sex.

23. Kaposi's sarcoma was neither well understood nor easily diagnosed in 1981, and recent research (1994–1996) has seriously problematized the issue of what causes this cancer. Some researchers have even debated whether Kaposi's sarcoma is truly a cancer. I have included the notes below, not only because they make the issue of diagnosis difficult, but also because the first two cases that I discuss were both Jewish and thus were members of a population that was previously known to be at increased risk for developing Kaposi's sarcoma. In a CDC publication from the early 1980s, investigators stated: "KS is a malignant neoplasm manifested primarily by multiple vascular nodules in the skin and other organs. The disease is multifocal, with a course ranging from indolent, with only skin manifestations, to fulminant, with extensive visceral involvement. Accurate incidence and mortality rates for KS are not available for the U.S. . . . It affects primarily elderly males [of Mediterranean or Jewish descent]. In a [previous study] 75% [of the patients] were male, and the mean age was 63 years (range 23–90 years) at the time of diagnosis. The disease in elderly men is usually manifested by skin lesions and a chronic clinical course (mean survival time is 8–13 years). Two exceptions to this epidemiological pattern have been noted previously. The first occurs in an endemic belt across equatorial Africa [associated with height above sea level], where KS commonly affects children and young adults and accounts for up to 9% of all cancers. Secondly, the disease appears to have a higher incidence in renal transplant recipients and in other receiving immunosuppressive therapy. . . . The histopathologic diagnosis of KS may be difficult for two reasons. Changes in some lesions

may be interpreted as nonspecific, and other cutaneous and soft tissue sarcomas, such as angiosarcoma of the skin, may be confused with KS." CDC, "Kaposi's Sarcoma and *Pneumocystis* Pneumonia," 306.

24.   PCP is not totally unexpected as a possible side effect of chemotherapy. In modern times, the occurrence of *Pneumocystis carinii* pneumonia is almost exclusively limited to severely malnourished hosts (especially children) and to individuals undergoing aggressive immunosuppressive medical treatments, with chemotherapy, radiation, steroids, or other drugs used to ameliorate the rejection of an organ transplant. This point was reiterated during a recent interview with Dr. Selma Dritz, the San Francisco public health official responsible for AIDS surveillance in 1981. Dr. Dritz begins by discussing the occurrence of PCP in San Francisco prior to AIDS: "Those patients who needed pentamidine almost invariably had had a renal transplant or were on chemotherapy or on radiation for cancer—kids with leukemia, persons whose immune systems had been depressed in order to keep them from rejecting the transplant. Without an immune system, the *Pneumocystis* could cause pneumonia. Two or three times a year, you'd have a case of *Pneumocystis*. . . . Now, we were finding *Pneumocystis* in apparently normally health young men, twenty-five, thirty, forty years old. These people shouldn't be getting it. So we began wondering, was something wrong with their immune systems? But we didn't have any evidence." Dritz, "Charting the Epidemiological Course of AIDS, 1981–1984," 12. Selma K. Dritz, "Charting the Epidemiological Course of AIDS, 1981–1984," an oral history conducted in 1992 by Sally Smith Hughes in *The AIDS Epidemic in San Francisco: The Medical Response, 1981–1984*. Volume I. Regional Oral History Office. Bancroft Library, University of California, Berkeley, 1995.

25.   To be fair, as the CDC initially reported the case to the SFDPH, whatever errors exist in this man's San Francisco file can be laid squarely at the feet of the CDC epidemiologist who investigated the case.

26.   Throughout the text I have added comments in brackets [ ] to clarify abbreviations or simplify medical terminology. As a further note, pancytopenia refers to a "deficiency of all cell elements of the blood; aplastic anemia," and is believed to be caused by "anatomically undeveloped . . . stem cells." In other words, the diagnosis implies that something has interfered with the production of red blood cells in this patient's bone marrow. See *Dorland's Illustrated Medical Dictionary*, 27th ed., Philadelphia: W. B. Saunders, 1988: 112, 1217.

27.   Centers for Disease Control, "*Pneumocystis* Pneumonia—Los Angeles," and "Kaposi's Sarcoma and *Pneumocystis* Pneumonia."

28.   Granuloma is "an imprecise term applied to 1) any small nodular delimited aggregation of mononuclear inflammatory cells, or 2) such a collection of modified macrophages resembling epithelial cells, usually surrounded by a rim of lymphocytes. . . . Granuloma formation represents a chronic inflammatory response initiated by various infectious and noninfectious agents." Acid-fast bacteria are "characteristic of certain bacteria, particularly Mycobacterium tuberculosis [TB and] Mycobacterium leprae [leprosy]." *Dorland's Illustrated Medical Dictionary*, 716, 16.

29.   This should read amyl nitrite, or "poppers" as they are known in the gay community—vials of volatile fluid that are inhaled as vasodilators to produce a high when dancing or having sex. The patient's ACR file at the SFDPH included a brief medical history documenting the May 1981 onset of dyspnea (shortness of breath) and the following comment: "history of excessive amyl use four-five times [per] week with sex. No history of intestinal parasites." As this brief handwritten medical history parallels what I found in the medical chart I presume that the additional drug/parasite information was relayed to the SFDPH by the CDC or by the patient's primary health care provider.

30.   PCP is present in normal lungs; however, a functioning immune system keeps the organism in check unless our immune system has been decimated by malnutrition (especially protein deficiencies), chemotherapy, radiation, congenital immune deficiencies, or pharmaceuticals that are designed to be immune-suppressive: for example, corticosteroids (to reduce inflammation, turn off the immune system's attack on "self") and medications prescribed to prevent the body's rejection of organ transplants.

31.   An alveolus refers to the little saclike pouches and ducts that exist in the lungs for the purpose of regulating "gas exchange . . . between alveolar gas and pulmonary capillary blood." See *Dorland's Illustrated Medical Dictionary*, 54.

32. "Sarcoidosis—a chronic, progressive, systemic granulomatous reticulosis [abnormal increase in cells] of unknown etiology, involving almost any organ, or tissue, including the skin, lungs, lymph nodes, liver, spleen, eyes, and small bones of the hands and feet." See *Dorland's Illustrated Medical Dictionary*, 1485.

33. "Lues" is from the Latin for "a plague."

34. Folinic acid is a "derivative of folic acid [a B vitamin]" whose derivatives in turn are "required for the synthesis of several amino acids." *Dorland's Illustrated Medical Dictionary*, 646. TMP-SMX "works by inhibiting folic acid synthesis."

35. According to the patient's medical history, the "roommate" was actually a sexual partner whom the patient had been seeing several days a week for the past year.

36. That a lengthy interview was taken by the CDC is clear: a signed consent form remains in the AIDS case file for patient #1003.

37. In contrast, the ACR form (noted as an AER form in 1980) completed by SFDPH investigators reported that the patient was diagnosed positive for both CMV and PCP as of June 1981; as a consequence of this error the SFDPH assessment of survival from the time of diagnosis to death for this patient was inaccurate by more than two months.

38. As there were no absolute CD4 T-cell values cited in this report it is impossible to know if the patient was absolutely deficient in these cells or just relatively deficient in CD4 T-cells vis-à-vis his CD8 cells.

39. Technically, the first and second AIDS cases diagnosed in San Francisco were African American infant girls from an HIV-positive mother who injected drugs. When the mother was diagnosed with AIDS in the early 1980s, these pediatric AIDS cases were retrospectively diagnosed and reported for 1978 and 1979 respectively; a third child born to the same woman died shortly after birth of non-AIDS-related congenital defects.

40. Per notes on the ARS form (San Francisco's local "AIDS reporting system") for Case #1005. The designation of a definitive census tract for a homeless AIDS patient potentially confounds SFDPH's analyses of the geographical incidence and prevalence of the disease. According to my review of early patients, census tract designations were ambiguous for fully half (12 of 24) of the AIDS cases reported in 1981. This finding has ramifications for interpreting several publications by the SFDPH that included "updates" on the incidence of AIDS in various neighborhoods in the city. See, for example, SFDPH AIDS Office, "Update: Acquired Immune-Deficiency Syndrome—The Tenderloin, San Francisco," *San Francisco Epidemiologic Bulletin* 4(9), September 1988. The SFDPH census tract data on early patients was also critically important for constructing methodologically relevant sampling strategies for early epidemiological research in the city; e.g., the census tract data used in the San Francisco Men's Health Study, which began in 1984. See original proposal from the files of Dr. W. Winkelstein, principal investigator, "Natural History of Acquired Immune-Deficiency Syndrome (AIDS) in Homosexual Men." Editing remarks of Kevin McKinney, ASSB, July 1996: "Our census tract information has about a 3% error rate. I think you can draw fairly safe conclusions about neighborhoods. In the early years there were a variety of methods used to assign a census tract to 'homeless individuals.'"

41. A protozoan "intracellular parasite of many organs and tissues of birds and mammals, including humans." *Dorland's Illustrated Medical Dictionary*, 1737.

42. Monilia pharyngitis is "a former name for a genus of fungi now called Candida." In this case, the physician believed that it was most likely that the patient's oral candida infection and elevated liver funtion tests were most likely attributable to the side effects of his antibiotic therapy [Bactrim] rather than to any underlying gay immunodeficiency syndrome. See *Dorland's Illustrated Medical Dictionary*, 1048.

43. Decadron is a trademark for a preparation of dexamethasone. "Dexamethasone—a synthetic glucocortoid 25 times as potent as cortisol." "Cortico-steroids have been by far the most important form of immunosuppressive therapy; these agents not only lead to the development of pneumocystosis by themselves but also potentiate the effects of chemotherapy protocols involving other cytotoxic drugs." See *Dorland's Illustrated Medical Dictionary*, 434, 458. For the discussion on PCP, see G. L. Mandell, R. G. Douglas, and J. E. Bennett, *Principles and Practice of Infectious Diseases*, New York: Churchill Livingstone, 1990: 2105.

44. On that basis alone, the patient was not technically an AIDS case as the very definition itself relied on the diagnosis of opportunistic infections "in a person with no known cause for diminished resistance." This exclusionary nature of an AIDS diagnosis was further codified in the CDC's Confidential Case Report form for the disease; under "Known Causes of Re-

duced Resistance" the CDC included: cancer, genetic immunodeficiencies, starvation, "systemic corticosteroid therapy within one month before diagnosis," and chemotherapy "within one year before diagnosis." CDC surveillance form, "AIDS Confidential Case Report," *CDC 50.42 Rev. 12–84.*

45. *Dorland's Illustrated Medical Dictionary,* 68.

46. This entry in his medical chart was imprinted with a hospital I.D. card that included a birthdate that validates the SFDPH when they identified patient #1008 as a 22 year old. As will shortly become clear, however, this patient had several hospital I.D. cards with different birthdates, which introduces considerable ambiguity vis-à-vis his age at the time of diagnosis with AIDS.

47. Census tract data from the San Francisco Department of City Planning show that the SFDPH designated the patient's residence as the bathhouse where he last resided.

48. The medical student also noted that this patient had no history of hepatitis, an odd conclusion given that this man was among those early AIDS cases who was reportedly enrolled in the hepatitis B study [ACR file] and given that the patient's roommate, with whom he shared needles, also reportedly had hepatitis. Although the patient's "lover" was identified by name in this entry, that individual was never reported as an AIDS case in San Francisco, either as a resident nor as an out-of-jurisdiction case.

49. According to this consultant, Kübler-Ross's five stages of dying are 1) denial ("there must be some mistake"); 2) anger ("why me?"); 3) bargaining ("please—I'll be a good person"); 4) depression; 5) acceptance.

50. Cytomegalovirus (CMV) is a member of the herpes family and, as such, was one of the first agents proposed as the cause of AIDS in the early 1980s before HIV was discovered. There were, and still are, compelling reasons to argue that CMV plays a crucial causative or co-factor role in AIDS. Most early AIDS patients were observed to have disseminated CMV infections (the virus is the leading cause of blindness in AIDS patients and a major cause of pneumonia); and the virus was readily cultured from semen, saliva, and urine of patients. In addition, CMV infection can and does cause an inversion of CD4 to CD8 T-cell ratios, the first immunological marker (or laboratory parameter) deemed indicative of AIDS. Furthermore, CMV "can infect any cell of the body, where it multiplies slowly and causes the host cell to swell in size—hence the prefix cytomegalo, which means 'an enlarged cell.' . . . In fatal cases, cell damage is seen in the gastrointestinal tract, lungs, liver, spleen, and kidneys. Normally, cytomegalovirus inclusion disease symptoms resemble those of infectious mononucleosis. . . . Epidemiologically, the virus has a worldwide distribution, especially in developing countries where infection is universal by childhood. *The prevalence of this disease increases with a lowering of socioeconomic status and hygienic practices.* The only drugs available, gancyclovir and foscarnet, are used only for high-risk patients. Infection can be prevented by avoiding close personal contact (including sexual) with an actively infected individual." (Prescott, L. M., J. P. Harley, and D. H. Klein, *Microbiology,* 2nd ed. Dubuque, Iowa: Wm. C. Brown Publishers, 1993: 730; my emphasis.) And as a final point, although CMV exposure and/or infection is very prevalent in the United States and the world (thus, a nearly ubiquitous organism that most individuals have been exposed to), CMV *disease* affects the same risk groups as does AIDS: gay men, infants of CMV-infected mothers, and recipients of blood products. "CMV (is) one of a group of highly host-specific herpes viruses that infect man, monkeys, or rodents. . . . Cytomegalic inclusion disease (is) any of a group of diseases caused by CMV infection. . . . The classic disease is congenital, being acquired in utero from the mother; infection can also be transmitted from mother to infant in passage through the birth canal or from ingestion of . . . mother's milk. Most infants are asymptomatic, but in some . . . sequelae resulting in blindness, deafness, quadriplegia, and mental retardation may occur. Acquired disease is transmitted via respiratory droplets or tissue or blood donation, or it may be sexually transmitted. The group also includes an infectious mononucleosis-like syndrome in previously well individuals and in those receiving multiple blood transfusions and a fatal disseminated infection in patients immunosuppressed or otherwise immuno-compromised." (*Dorland's Illustrated Medical Dictionary,* 428, 484.)

Chapter 4

1. I cannot be adamant about this point, however, because proportionally fewer interviews or medical charts were available for these 15 patients versus the nine AIDS cases reported dur-

ing July 1981. Thus, for some of these patients I was unable to cross-reference the accuracy of the SFDPH's files and had to rely instead on the ASSB's very limited case notes (which can and do err in attributing risk factors for AIDS and residence, and in accurately dating initial diagnoses or estimating survival).

2. "Interest intensified when many of the first AIDS cases in San Francisco—11 of the first 24 in 1981 (46%)—turned out to be participants in the HBV project." Russell, "Map of AIDS' Deadly March."

3. The earliest date for which I can document a KS diagnosis for patient #1010 is substantiated by a note in his AIDS case report (ACR) file that he was being treated for the cancer at Stanford as of July 1981. In contrast, the information on the patient's death certificate (never a reliable source as the information is usually anecdotally obtained) would place the KS diagnosis in January 1981. Nowhere, however, is there any evidence in this patient's ACR file that would support a diagnosis of KS in the summer of 1980. Per the editing remarks of Kevin McKinney, "A different date could have come from a match with the cancer registry." The earliest official surveillance form used to report cases of immune-deficiency was an AER form, and this was in use in 1981 at the San Francisco Department of Public Health. In order to avoid confusion, I have used a singular acronym in the text (i.e., ACR) to refer to official AIDS Case Report forms during this time; this seemingly picayune detail was methodologically relevant for my research, because it enabled me to reconstruct how errors were introduced into surveillance records when disease surveillance officers at the ASSB transcribed patient information from the AER to the ACR format in later years, and to determine what information was more contemporaneous with the patient's diagnosis and therefore presumably more reliable.

4. The CDC questionnaire asked a series of questions regarding sexual experience; but as there were no data provided for patient #1011 in response, I do not know how investigators arrived at the conclusion that he had had 1,844 sexual contacts during the preceding 16 years. Questions included: 1. If we define sexual intercourse as the entrance of your penis into another person's mouth, anus, or vagina, or the entrance of a penis into your mouth or anus, how old were you when you first had sexual intercourse? 2. If your first sexual partner was a woman, how old were you when you first had sexual intercourse with a man? 3. How old were you when you first began having regular sexual intercourse (at least monthly) with a man? 4. Now you are ____ years old, so in the past ____ years, how many different people have you had sexual intercourse with? 5. Of these different people, how many were men? How many were women? 6. Do you recall ever having sex with a person who was a native of Africa? If yes, give sex, country of origin, and date.

5. With respect to this particular case, designating his residence in census tract 164 would have placed him in an area with 0–9 AIDS cases; while a designation of census tract 163 or 203 would have placed him in an area with 10–19 cases. Only the assignment of census tract 203, however, places him near the Castro district. For instance, see the cartographical representation of the SFDPH's geographical analysis of "AIDS Cases per Census Tract of Residence, First 1,000 Cases (Figure 1)" in the article "Update: Acquired Immune-Deficiency Syndrome—The Tenderloin, San Francisco," *San Francisco Epidemiologic Bulletin.*

6. The man's HIV infection was presumed retrospectively of course, because he was diagnosed as an AIDS case before any HIV antibody test existed, and because there was no evidence in his medical chart to suggest that such a test was ever done once it became licensed for use in 1985. Although I was informed frequently during my fieldwork at ASSB that the results of an HIV antibody test were rarely included in medical charts because of concerns regarding patient confidentiality, I think it is unlikely that this particular patient was ever tested for HIV antibodies. I say this because patient #1018 had already been diagnosed with KS and PCP, and these diagnoses do not require documentation of an HIV-positive test in order to qualify as an AIDS case. Cf. chapter 2 for a discussion of cohort studies and estimates regarding the incubation period from HIV exposure to AIDS, and chapter 6 for further background regarding changing definitions of AIDS at different phases in the evolution of the epidemic, and the use of presumptive diagnoses.

7. This patient's "friend and lover" was identified by name in his records, but that individual had never been reported as an AIDS case in San Francisco as of 1994–1995.

8. Both of these latter complications are well-known side effects of chemotherapy.

9. For original report see Centers for Disease Control, "Possible Transfusion-Associated AIDS—California," 652–653. See also M. Cochrane, "The Social Construction of Knowl-

edge(s) on HIV and AIDS: With a Case Study of the History and Practices of AIDS Surveillance Activities in San Francisco," Ph.D. thesis, University of California at Berkeley, 1997, for further discussion of this infant's diagnosis of "failure to thrive" at birth, the ambiguity surrounding the date of his (A1) AIDS diagnosis (mycobacterium avium infection), and the subsequent unfounded diagnosis of *Pneumocystis carinii* pneumonia appended to his ACR case file at ASSB (this child was never diagnosed with PCP, but rather, the blood donor's PCP diagnosis in December 1981 was incorporated in error into his ACR case file).

10. Unless otherwise noted, words in brackets appeared so in the original publication.

11. The comment in brackets is my own and serves to orient the reader to Selma Dritz's previous comments regarding her contacts with Gaetan Dugas, an AIDS patient characterized in a 1982 CDC cluster study as "Patient Zero." See Centers for Disease Control, "A Cluster of Kaposi's Sarcoma and *Pneumocystis carinii* Pneumonia among Homosexual Male Residents of Los Angeles and Orange Counties, California," *Morbidity and Mortality Weekly Report*, June 18, 1982.

12. In fact, the CDC first developed the idea that the AIDS was an infectious disease being transmitted to infants and, based on a tip from New York clinicians, contacted Dr. Ammann regarding pediatric cases that he had treated in San Francisco. In turn, the CDC and Ammann contacted Dr. Dritz at the SFDPH to conduct further investigation of transfusion-associated AIDS cases.

13. Dritz, "Charting the Epidemiological Course of AIDS," 36–39.

14. According to the chronological logbook that listed AIDS cases as they were reported in San Francisco, *all* (not 98 percent) of the city's AIDS cases were either homosexual/bisexual men (GM) or gay intravenous drug users (GIVDU); in fact, after reviewing patient histories I established that fully one-fifth of the initial cohort of AIDS cases reported in 1981 were gay men who injected drugs (and no cross-reference, e.g. information other than the SFDPH case file, was available for 14 of these 24 men). In 1983, one heterosexual female (an intravenous drug user, IVDU) was reported during the summer, and nine heterosexual men were captured as AIDS cases (intravenous drugs users aside from two "no-identified-risk" cases and a couple of minority men who were non–San Francisco residents, and thus not investigated for risk factors).

15. Shilts, *And the Band Played On*, 195, 200.

16. This child has never been reported as a San Francisco resident with AIDS, nor was she captured in San Francisco health facilities as an out-of-jurisdiction AIDS case. And just as the male infant with Rh factor (pediatric TA-AIDS case) was captured and counted as an AIDS patient in San Francisco despite the fact the he lived in another county within California, this little girl would have been reported in one set of files or another at the ASSB if she had ever been diagnosed or treated with AIDS in this city.

17. In other words, to the best of my ability to trace AIDS cases reported in San Francisco as residents, as out-of-jurisdiction AIDS cases, and as AIDS cases reported in the epidemiological literature of the time.

18. Cf. Cochrane, "The Social Construction of Knowledge(s) on HIV and AIDS," 251–320 for a thorough discussion of transfusion-associated AIDS (TA-AIDS) cases, incubation periods for development of the disease, and the absence of evidence for large numbers of TA-AIDS cases in San Francisco despite seven years of an allegedly contaminated blood supply. Early reports on TA-AIDS suggested that the median incubation period was 28 months, with a range of 5 months to 5 years from the date of the transfusion to the onset of AIDS. This median 28-month incubation period continued to be used as a viable estimate for TA-AIDS cases through the mid-1980s. See M. E. Chamberland et al., "AIDS in the U.S.: An Analysis of Cases outside High-Incidence Groups," *Annals of Internal Medicine* 101(5), 1984: 619.

19. According to Shilts, this estimate was relayed to Selma Dritz by the head of San Francisco's Irwin Memorial Blood Bank in 1982. Shilts, *And the Band Played On*, 199. A lower estimate of 5 percent to 7 percent was cited by Dritz in a 1992 interview. Cf. Dritz, "Charting the Epidemiological Course of AIDS," 44.

20. M. P. Busch et al., "Risk of Human Immunodeficiency Virus (HIV) Transmission by Blood Transfusions before the Implementation of HIV-1 Antibody Screening," *Transfusion* 31(1), 1991: 9.

21. See R. Shilts, "Let It Bleed," *And the Band Played On*, 222. "Still, Dritz had the health of her city to tend to and a board of supervisors to answer to. Like so many health officials, her

data was hardly reassuring to the blood bankers. 'Of 140 [AIDS patients], 10 or 11 had donated whole blood in the previous few years,' she said. 'We don't know how many others
sold their blood or plasma at commercial centers.'"

22. Dritz, "Charting the Epidemiological Course of AIDS," 37.

23. Figures cited from R. H. Byers Jr. et al., "Estimating AIDS Infection Rates in the San Francisco Cohort," *AIDS* 2, 1988: 207–210. See also Chapter 2 of this text for a discussion of the
hepatitis B cohort data and a review of HIV seroprevalence rates among these men.

24. The study cited is R. M. Selik et al., "Trends in Transfusion-Associated Acquired Immune Deficiency Syndrome in the United States, 1982 through 1991," *Transfusion* 33(11), 1993: 891.

25. Editing remarks of Kevin McKinney, SFDPH AIDS Seroepidemiology and Surveillance
Branch, July 1996: "You don't have the medical expertise to conclude that these medical
problems and risk factors would manifest themselves as Kaposi's sarcoma (KS), *Pneumocystis carinii* pneumonia (PCP), and toxoplasmosis without the presence of a unifying underlying etiology."

26. While I have not included in this text an analysis for the additional 94 patients reported in
San Francisco in 1982, my conclusion after reviewing these case histories is that they do not
differ significantly from the patients I have described above, nor do they differ from AIDS
cases elsewhere in the nation as described in early epidemiological studies. Cf. for instance
Jaffe et al., "National Case-Control Study," 141–151.

Chapter 5

1. See Robert Root-Bernstein, *Rethinking AIDS: The Tragic Cost of Premature Consensus*, New
York: McMillan Free Press, 1993: 113. See also, Stephen O. Murray and Kenneth W. Payne,
"The Social Classification of AIDS in American Epidemiology," *Medical Anthropology* 10,
1989: 115–128, for their analysis of the CDC's characterization of Haitian risk factors and
gay men who used drugs.

2. E.g. HEAL in New York, San Francisco, and Los Angeles, and Continuum in London, England. LTS refers to long-term survivors, or those individuals who despite being diagnosed
with HIV or AIDS have lived many years; LTNPS refers to long-term non-progressors, those
individuals who are HIV-positive but have not clinically progressed to an AIDS diagnosis.

3. "Nukes" is the common parlance used among dissidents for all of the nucleoside analogue
compounds, such as AZT, DDI and DDC, that are chemically designed to disrupt DNA synthesis within all cells in the body which are actively replicating, not only those infected with HIV.

4. Author's interview, anonymous informant.

5. "Federally funded testing programs alone, which primarily serve low-risk groups, account
for roughly 20% of the entire budget." A. Bennett and A. Sharpe, "Health Hazard: AIDS
Fight Is Skewed by Federal Campaign Exaggerating Risks," *Wall Street Journal*, May 1, 1996.
Cited at californ@netcom.com, May 8, 1996.

6. Fewer than 200 CD4 T-cells or CD4 T-cell counts equal to or less than 14 percent of total
lymphocytes (CDC's 1993 AIDS surveillance case definition).

7. It is ironic that the City Clinic does not have a large AIDS caseload, given that the majority
of the earliest AIDS cases in San Francisco were clients of the clinic. Frozen serum samples
from the hepatitis B cohort, collected from gay/bisexual men attending this municipal STD
clinic, showed that nearly 70 percent of these men were HIV-antibody-positive as of 1985.
If few clients of the City Clinic are currently being diagnosed with AIDS, this implies that
there has been a quantum shift in the sites that gay men have chosen for their health care.
This fact alone could also explain some of the observed decline in the incidence of reported
STDs in San Francisco, if men are being treated elsewhere by their personal physicians, who
may be less likely to report common sexually transmitted diseases to the Department of
Public Health.

8. Cited by Kevin McKinney, AIDS surveillance field unit coordinator, in September 1994.

9. The original 1981 AIDS surveillance case definition was previously modified in 1985 and
1987. Centers for Disease Control, *HIV/AIDS Surveillance Report* 5(4), 1994.

10. As of 1998, there were 24 states in the United States that did have mandatory HIV reporting
and thus conduct surveillance on HIV-antibody-positive persons. As of January 2000, however, the CDC was planning to implement a new policy of mandatory HIV reporting in all
50 states.

11. In reality, and in AIDS surveillance practice, some of these OI's can also be *presumptively* diagnosed and yet still qualify as an AIDS diagnosis, especially when the patient is a member of a population considered to be at high risk for contracting the disease.

12. Department of Public Health, "1993 Revision of the HIV Infection Classification System and the AIDS Surveillance Definition," *San Francisco Epidemiologic Bulletin* 9(1), January 1993: 2–3.

13. Pediatric AIDS patients are the sole exception to this method of capturing cases as they are only reported after being diagnosed with an AIDS-defining opportunistic infection. And the definition for pediatric AIDS diagnosis has been invariable from the earliest days of the epidemic: "It has always been 'failure to thrive.' 'Failure to thrive' and developmental deficits are unique ways that pediatric AIDS differs from wasting and HIV encephalopathy in adults. In addition, *Pneumocystis carinii* pneumonia and lymphoid interstitial pneumonia are diagnoses that are sufficient to diagnose pediatric AIDS in the absence of an HIV test if the child is linked to a mother with a known HIV-risk factor [e.g., IV drug use or a transfusion history], and if the child has never been diagnosed with cancer or a genetic immune disorder." The latter would eliminate any consideration of an AIDS diagnosis. Quotes from author's interview of Kevin McKinney, AIDS surveillance field unit coordinator, ASSB, July 1994.

14. Author interview with anonymous San Francisco disease control investigator, ASSB, July 1994.

15. San Francisco Department of Public Health AIDS Office, *Quarterly AIDS Surveillance Report,* March 31, 2002: 1. These data are cumulative from 1981 through March 31, 2002, and include all persons diagnosed in San Francisco and San Francisco residents diagnosed in other jurisdictions.

16. Opportunistic infections are only noted the first time they occur in a patient's medical history—for example, the initial diagnosis of PCP will be noted on a patient's ACR, but not subsequent PCP events. CD4 counts have only recently been noted in patients' charts and are updated every six months if these are available.

17. If an ACR exists the DCI records an HSU (health status update), adding recent CD4 counts or new opportunistic infections to the ACR. At six-month intervals the most recent CD4 count is entered into the HARS computer database (e.g., CD4 = 50 [15%]).

18. NIR ("no identifiable risk") is the appellation given to AIDS cases for which a DCI and subsequent investigators are unable to establish a recognized HIV transmission risk factor: the patient does not acknowledge being a homosexual, hemophiliac, IV drug user, transfusion or transplant recipient, etc.

19. For instance, is this a male patient who had sexual intercourse with another man after 1978, is the patient a hemophiliac, did this patient inject drugs or receive a transfusion after 1978, or has this patient had sexual intercourse with a person belonging to a risk group for AIDS (i.e., someone who is known to have one or more of the above-mentioned risk factors for HIV infection)?

20. During my fieldwork at SFGH, I found that a patient's chart commonly comprised two or three volumes, and it was not uncommon to discover that a patient from the first year of the epidemic had medical charts as long as five to nine volumes. In my experience, reading each and every page required an hour or more per volume of staff time (a patient's chart consisting of three volumes would require an unrealistic three to four hours of work for a surveillance officer).

21. More than 4,500 AIDS cases were reported in San Francisco in 1993, nearly triple the number reported during the preceding year, and twice the caseload reported in 1995.

22. CDC surveillance criteria say that an AIDS case is classified as an IVDU if he or she ever injected drugs.

23. Author interview with Kevin McKinney, ASSB, July 25, 1994.

24. The CDC's hierarchy of risk factors "de-emphasizes and under-represents every patient characteristic except homosexuality. One cannot help but suspect a theological mindset behind this statistical misrepresentation of reality: that which is most 'sinful' is presumed to be most dangerous." John Lauritsen as quoted in Murray and Payne, "The Social Classification of AIDS," 119.

25. "One hundred thirty-eight gay and bisexual men had other risk factors: 131 (13%) were also intravenous drug users, 6 (1%) had received blood transfusions since 1978, and 1 (<1%) had haemophilia [*sic*]." San Francisco Department of Public Health, Bureau of Communicable Disease Control, "AIDS in San Francisco: The First 1,000 Cases," *San Francisco Epidemiologic Bulletin* 1(2), October 1985.

26. Ibid.
27. At first blush, the CDC's statistics may appear to be free of the biases inherent to San Francisco's surveillance statistics, as the Centers for Disease Control has a more extensive computer database and software which enables it to record AIDS cases under a primary risk category, and then subsequently under secondary and tertiary risk factors. As I discussed previously, the CDC did fail to disaggregate GIVDU's from the homosexual-bisexual category until 1985, but presumably, after that time, its statistics should be devoid of major distortions. And it is true that the CDC publishes both an annual national surveillance report on the basis of the primary risk categories for HIV/AIDS, and quarterly abbreviated reports enumerating those cases of AIDS with multiple risk categories, e.g., a gay male with a transfusion or a hemophiliac IVDU. However, since the CDC derives its data on multiple risks from information provided to it by cities and states, if those jurisdictions do not investigate or record a patient's secondary and tertiary HIV risk factors, then the CDC cannot collate and publish those risks. Thus, jurisdictional biases are reproduced at the national level.
28. California State Department of Health, "Report on Duplicate AIDS Cases," San Francisco AIDS Surveillance Branch, unpublished document, August 17, 1994.
29. Communication Technologies in association with The San Francisco AIDS Foundation, "A report on HIV-Related Knowledge, Attitudes, and Behaviours Among San Francisco Gay and Bisexual Men: Results from the Fifth Population-Based Survey," Unpublished report, San Francisco AIDS Surveillance Branch, January 31, 1990. Ibid., 10–13: "The following are more likely to say they have used intravenous drugs at some point in their life: . . . those who have tested positive for the HIV-antibody (26%). Those who have tested negative and those who have not taken the test are less likely to have ever used intravenous drugs (10% and 5% respectively)."
30. San Francisco Department of Public Health AIDS Office, AIDS Seroepidemiology and Surveillance Branch, "AIDS Cases Reported through September, 1995," AIDS Surveillance Report 1995: 2 (Table 1). As of this date there was a cumulative total of 20,036 homosexual/bisexual men reported as AIDS cases in San Francisco; 2,022 of these men—10 percent of the total—were reported as GIVU.
31. See also San Francisco Department of Public Health AIDS Office, AIDS Seroepidemiology and Surveillance Branch, "HIV Incidence and Prevalence in San Francisco in 1992: Summary Report from an HIV Consensus Meeting," February 22, 1992. This report estimates IVDU populations in the city as follows: Non-gay IVDUs (male and female) equal 13,000 persons out of a total population of 724,000 residents. Gay male intravenous drug users are estimated at 3,000 persons; thus the total number of IVDUs in the city equals 16,000 (or approximately 11 percent of the total population in San Francisco). See also the comments of G. Lemp in 1994 that 12 percent of gay men in the 17–22 age group injected drugs in the past year in San Francisco ("AIDSWEEK," San Francisco Examiner, August 10, 1994).
32. I actually ran a computer list of the number of AIDS cases in San Francisco who died of AIDS with a sole diagnosis of "wasting" or a low CD4 count; as of April 14, 1994, 634 San Francisco AIDS cases had died of these two ambiguous "AIDS-related conditions"—and a handful of these cases had more than 200 T-cells, albeit qualifying for an AIDS diagnosis by virtue of a low percentage of CD4 T-cells.
33. Author interview with Kevin McKinney, ASSB, July 1994.
34. Ibid.
35. The city of New York Department of Health, Office of AIDS Surveillance, AIDS Surveillance Update, Fourth Quarter 1992, January 1993: 6 (Table 6).
36. It was especially difficult to obtain and document this interview; I was shuffled from one receptionist to another, told to come back next week when the surveillance supervisor responsible for this data would be back to work, and eventually taken to a private conference room where an AIDS surveillance coordinator who will remain anonymous insisted that I turn off my tape recorder. Answers to my questions about the rise in male heterosexual cases in NYC seemed to be vague and only reluctantly acknowledged and raised further questions about the degree to which contending political forces within the Department of Health and the city at large influence reliable documentation on HIV/AIDS risk factors in New York City.
37. In other words, NYC AIDS surveillance was lax in resolving the risk for HIV/AIDS among 4,000 no-identified-risk cases that it reported.
38. I question whether New York City was ever rigorous in investigating risk factors for its reported AIDS cases. Laxity in this regard is alluded to in one of the department's publica-

tions in 1993, wherein Dr. P. A. Thomas et al. of the NYC Office of AIDS Surveillance stated: "Trends in [AIDS] incidence by risk factor are approximated. Risk assignment is inexact, based on medical chart review and not a thorough personal assessment of each case. Although more than one risk factor is recorded for 5% of cases, for the most part a complete set of risk factors for each case is not sought." P. A. Thomas et al., "Trends in the First Ten Years of AIDS in New York City," *American Journal of Epidemiology* 137(2), January 15, 1993: 130.

39. Quoting Kevin McKinney, San Francisco, ASSB, January, 1995.

40. Thomas et al., "Trends in the First Ten Years," 123: "a relatively constant proportion of cases—approximately 10%—are reported without risk factors."

41. The nature of the association between Kaposi's sarcoma and the use of poppers has been at the center of vehement debates between dissidents such as Peter Duesberg, Bryan Ellison, and John Lauritsen, who, on the one hand, assert that poppers are carcinogens, and, on the other hand, orthodox AIDS researchers such as W. Winkelstein, H. Sheppard, and M. Ascher who assert that these drugs are merely "surrogate markers" of sexual risk behavior.

42. This individual's "gender" (a culturally variable, socially constructed category of personal attributes, mannerisms, and perhaps position vis-à-vis a sexual division of labor) is not at issue here; the person's original genitalia (i.e., the "sex") is what concerns the CDC.

43. The new term "transgendered" now encompasses both pre-op and post-op transsexuals.

44. Prophylaxis for *Pneumocystis carinii* pneumonia (PCP) refers to the use of aerosolized pentamidine, TMP-SMX (Bactrim, Septra), dapsone, or atovaquone to prevent this opportunistic infection. The exact cause of PCP itself is poorly understood; it is thought to be caused by a protozoan, but may possibly be caused by fungi. Historically, PCP has been the leading cause of death for Persons With AIDS (PWAs) in the United States.

45. I heartily agree with this point, as do many AIDS dissidents. The initiation of PCP prophylaxis as a standard treatment for AIDS patients came about, as a matter of fact, from the research and clinical practice of Dr. Joseph Sonnabend, the AIDS dissident who first promoted a multifactorial theory of the disease. It was established AIDS researchers who neglected to advocate the use of PCP prophylaxis, and it was not until Michael Callen, a patient of Dr. Sonnabend's and a longtime AIDS dissident, vigorously implored the FDA to support these therapies that aerosolized pentamidine (and subsequently dapsone, Septra, and Bactrim) were codified as standard AIDS therapies in the United States in 1989. Had this prophylaxis been rigorously promoted in previous years of the epidemic, Callen estimated, more than 30,000 premature AIDS deaths could have been prevented. There is some poetic license associated with Callen's estimate. Treatment with PCP prophylaxis has greater than 90 percent efficacy in preventing the recurrence of PCP in people with AIDS, though an unknown number of these individuals may have gone on to die from other opportunistic infections associated with the disease. See M. Callen, "AIDS and Passive Genocide: 30,534 Unnecessary Deaths From PCP Due to a Scandalous Failure to Prophylax. Testimony Given at FDA Hearing Concerning the Approval of Aerosol Pentamidine as Prophylaxis Against PCP," *AIDS Forum* 2(1), May 1989: 13–16.

46. Although three AIDS patients with >1000 T-cells *and* a diagnosis of PCP is hardly a trend, it is intriguing that there are reported symptomatic AIDS patients in San Francisco who defy the very clinical *essence* of AIDS; that is, they do not suffer from a depletion of CD4 T-helper cells nor are they technically "immune deficient" according to the parameters by which immune deficiency is defined.

47. Author interview of anonymous San Francisco disease control investigator, ASSB, August 1994.

48. Quotes from San Francisco Department of Health AIDS Office, AIDS Seroepidemiology and Surveillance Branch, "Utilization of PCP prophylaxis and Antiviral Agents. Summary Report," Unpublished rough draft, October 4, 1994. The published report was titled "Prevention of *Pneumocystis carinii* pneumonia: Who is not receiving recommended prophylaxis?" *San Francisco Epidemiologic Bulletin* 10(11–12), November/December 1994.

Chapter 6

1. See N. Krieger, "The Making of Public Health Data," and Tesh, *Hidden Arguments.* See also, T. May, *Social Research: Issues, Methods and Process,* Bristol, Pa.: Open University Press, 1993:

52. "Official statistics . . . often employ unexamined assumptions about social life which, if researchers are not cautious, they can inherit and reproduce in their studies. They are not simply 'social facts,' but also social and political constructions which may be based upon the interests of those who commissioned the research in the first instance. Before using such statistics, the researcher therefore needs to understand how they were constructed."

2. N. Krieger, "The Making of Public Health Data," 412, 427.

3. This is not the case for AIDS cases reported from Africa, as clinical criteria (the "Bangui" African AIDS case definition) based on nonspecific symptoms of illness alone (loss of 10 percent of body weight, fever for more than one month, herpes, or a persistent cough) have traditionally been used for AIDS case surveillance in African countries since 1986.

4. San Francisco Department of Public Health AIDS Office, Seroepidemiology and Surveillance Branch. "AIDS Cases Reported through March 2002," *AIDS Surveillance Report*, San Francisco, California, 2002: 1 (San Francisco as of March 31, 2002).

5. Dr. Harvey Bialey, science editor of the journal *Biotechnology*, quoted in Peter H. Duesberg, *Infectious AIDS: Have We Been Misled?*, Berkeley, Calif.: North Atlantic Books, 1995: back cover.

6. Author interview Kevin McKinney, AIDS surveillance field coordinator at the ASSB between November 1990 and June 1996, on July 6, 1994.

7. Ibid. "We keep it in our registry if the case was first diagnosed in San Francisco, or a San Francisco resident wherever they were diagnosed," McKinney said.

8. It is also not uncommon that a single AIDS patient is reported more than once under different names (regardless of residency). According to McKinney, these discrepancies in official data are usually resolved, however, as "a lot of time, at death the real data catches up." McKinney, 1994.

9. Soundex Coding System: When disease control investigators in San Francisco report an AIDS case to CDC, they do not use the patient's name as identification. Instead, the last name is entered by code into the CDC soundex database along with date of birth. The CDC operator then responds whether or not there is a match, indicating that this particular soundex code and date of birth is a duplicate of an AIDS case previously reported elsewhere. If the patient is a duplicate, information on the specifics of the case are filed as out-of-jurisdiction, and the individual is no longer followed by surveillance staff in San Francisco.

10. Author's interviews with Kevin McKinney, ASSB, July 6, 21, 1994; August 2, 1994; and September 6, 1994.

11. Author interview with anonymous disease control investigator, ASSB, July 19, 1994.

12. Author's interview with Kevin McKinney, ASSB, August 1994.

13. At the risk of being redundant, San Francisco's ASSB *does not* count nonresidents when it submits AIDS caseloads for Ryan White Care funding. That calculation is made solely on the basis of actual residency as per previous quotes by Kevin McKinney. For confirmed nonresidents, San Francisco's ASSB refers these case reports back to the relevant jurisdiction (albeit without divulging the individual's name), to ensure that the patient's actual city of residence receives funds necessary for care and support services.

14. While AIDS surveillance reports in San Francisco do include homeless and/or transient patients, there are no prisons within the county so the former point does not affect the city's cumulative caseload or mortality.

15. Information provided by Kevin McKinney, AIDS surveillance field unit coordinator at San Francisco's ASSB, August 1994.

16. And this is no minor point, as fatal side effects of current therapies, such as the use of "AIDS cocktails" including protease inhibitors, are increasingly seen among persons with AIDS. For example, in the spring of 2001, the SFDPH AIDS Office announced that "non AIDS-related mortality" was now the primary cause of death for PWAs in San Francisco, accounting for 55 percent of all deaths, while traditional opportunistic infections associated with the disease accounted for only 45 percent of reported mortality. Cf. also the "comprehensive retrospective review of more than 10,000 adult AIDS patients participating in 21 different AIDS Clinical Trials Group (ACTG) studies" which confirmed that there was significant drug toxicity associated with AIDS-related medications across the board; "High Rate of Severe Liver Toxicity Associated with Antiretroviral Therapy," BiGoldberg@aol.com, May 24, 2001.

17. Jaffe et al., "The Acquired Immunodeficiency Syndrome in a Cohort of Homosexual Men," 211. "Of the 166 patients with the syndrome, 147 (88.6%) lived in the San Francisco Stan-

dard Metropolitan Statistical Area (SMSA) at the time of the onset of the disease; the remaining 19 had moved to ten other American cities." The authors reported that "86 (approximately 52%) of the 166 reported patients in the cohort were known to have died."

18. Ibid., 212.

19. Dr. David Ho, head of the Aaron Diamond AIDS Research Center, summarized this view in 1993 (at the Frontiers in HIV Pathogenesis conference) in the pithy epigram, "It's the Virus, Stupid." See "AIDS Research. Keystone's Blunt Message: It's the Virus, Stupid," *Science* 260, April 16, 1993: 292–293.

20. Jaffe et al., "The Acquired Immunodeficiency Syndrome in a Cohort of Homosexual Men," 211.

21. Ibid., 212.

22. Etheridge, *Sentinel for Health.*

23. Centers for Disease Control, "Update on Acquired Immune Deficiency Syndrome," 507, 513. The CDC added an interesting footnote to this exclusion to the AIDS case definition: "The CDC encourages reports of any cancer among persons with AIDS and of selected rare lymphomas among persons with a risk factor for AIDS. This differs from the request for reports of AIDS cases regardless of the absence of risk factors." In other words, for homosexuals or persons already diagnosed with AIDS the CDC is requesting reports of cancer that may be related to the new syndrome of immune deficiency; however, if a person does not have a known risk factor for AIDS and develops "cancer or selected rare lymphomas" then the CDC will not consider this a case of AIDS. By this logic, a gay man with Burkitt's lymphoma would be of interest to the CDC as a potential AIDS case; but a non–IV-drug-using heterosexual man or woman with Burkitt's lymphoma would be of no interest to the CDC.

24. Ibid., 507.

25. San Francisco Department of Public Health, October 1995. These figures are based on my review of the chronological logbook for AIDS cases at the ASSB that documented patients as they were reported to the Department of Health. However, because of the ASSB's policy of backdating individuals to the initial date when they were diagnosed, the official number of AIDS cases published by the San Francisco ASSB is constantly in flux. Therefore, when I speak of 118 AIDS patients reported in the city between 1980 and 1982, I am not including any patients who were subsequently added to this roster via backdating.

26. For children under 13 years of age, regardless of the presence or absence of viral antibodies, a diagnosis of lymphoid interstitial pneumonia was a diagnosis of AIDS. Opportunistic infections have also been removed from the surveillance definition of AIDS; in 1985, strongyloidosis was eliminated as an AIDS-defining OI.

27. San Francisco Department of Public Health, Bureau of Communicable Disease Control, "Revision of the CDC Surveillance Case Definition for Acquired Immunodeficiency Syndrome," *San Francisco Epidemiological Bulletin* 3, 8 (August 1987): 38.

28. Ibid.

29. R. M. Selik et al., "Impact of the 1987 Revision of the Case Definition of AIDS in the U.S.," *Journal of Acquired Immune Deficiency Syndrome* 3, 1 (1990): 73, 75.

30. Ibid., 75.

31. Centers for Disease Control, "Update on Acquired Immune Deficiency Syndrome," 508.

32. Selik et al., "Impact of the 1987 Revision," 76.

33. These other previously recognized causes of immune deficiency are: 1) previous treatment with corticosteroids or "immunosuppressive/cytotoxic" therapies; 2) previous diagnosis with some cancers, such as Hodgkin's disease, lymphocytic leukemia, etc.; and 3) genetic (congenital) immunodeficiency syndromes. See *San Francisco Epidemiologic Bulletin,* August 1987.

34. *San Francisco Epidemiologic Bulletin,* August 1987: 36.

35. S. F. Payne et al., "Effect of the Revised AIDS Case Definition on AIDS Reporting in San Francisco," *AIDS* 4, 1990: 336.

36. Ibid.; Selik et al., "Impact of the 1987 Revision," 75, 76.

37. "We found a greater proportion of presumptive diagnoses and a smaller proportion of definitively diagnosed opportunistic infections among homosexual and bisexual men without histories of intravenous drug use, due primarily to a larger percentage with presumptively diagnosed PCP. Among IVDUs, on the other hand, a greater proportion of cases had definitively diagnosed opportunistic infections meeting the revised case definition." Payne et al., "Effect of the Revised AIDS Case Definition," 338.

38. Selik et al., "Impact of the 1987 Revision," 77–78.
39. Ibid., 78, 81.
40. Ibid., 78.
41. It was sometimes too easy to be diagnosed with AIDS if you are a homosexual or bisexual man. San Francisco newspapers have chronicled two separate cases of individuals diagnosed in error with HIV/AIDS. In the first example, "Raymond Machesney, 57, a former Catholic priest, was diagnosed with the HIV virus that causes AIDS two separate times in 1985. . . . After seven years of experimental (AIDS) drug treatments . . . he was told he had never been infected with the virus. . . . he was awarded $4.1 million in damages by a federal jury" (*San Francisco Sentinel*, "Man Wins $4.1 Million in HIV Suit," June 28, 1995: 22.) In a similar case, "Lon Blatteau . . . a San Mateo County man who was misdiagnosed with HIV infection in 1988 and put on AZT—even though he had a t-cell count of more than 1,000— has filed a million dollar lawsuit against his former healthcare providers (in Tacoma, Washington)" (*Bay Area Reporter*, "Lawsuit Filed over HIV Misdiagnosis, AZT Regimen," June 15, 1995). Although I do not think these cases are common, I also do not think they are singular occurrences. During my own fieldwork at Bay Area hospitals, I reviewed the medical chart of one gay man who had tested HIV-negative on two occasions and yet was receiving chemotherapy at the hospital's AIDS clinic. Although it is possible that this patient had recently seroconverted with HIV, it was not noted in his chart, and he was not yet reported as an AIDS case at the ASSB. The patient was considered a high-risk individual, however, because his lover had AIDS.
42. CDC, "U.S. HIV and AIDS Cases Reported through December 1998: Year-End Edition," *Morbidity and Mortality Weekly Report*, 10, 2 (December 1998): 14 (Table 5).
43. R. S. Root-Bernstein, *Rethinking AIDS: The Tragic Cost of Premature Consensus*, New York: Macmillan Free Press, 1993: 24.
44. B. Nussbaum, *Good Intentions: How Big Business and the Medical Establishment Are Corrupting the Fight Against AIDS*, New York: Atlantic Monthly Press, 1990: 176.
45. Centers for Disease Control, "Current Trends. Estimates of HIV Prevalence and Projected AIDS Cases," *Morbidity and Mortality Report*, February 23, 1990: 118.
46. Payne et al., "Effect of the Revised AIDS Case Definition," 336.
47. McKinney added the caveat that the SFDPH surveillance report figures cannot be taken literally, as they are based on initial diagnoses that patients presented with, and therefore do not tell us how many patients subsequently developed additional opportunistic infections that met later AIDS case definitions. See San Francisco Department of Public Health AIDS Office, Seroepidemiology and Surveillance Branch, "AIDS Cases Reported through October 1995," *AIDS Surveillance Report*, 1995: 7 ("Table 11: Cases meeting the 1985 and earlier case definitions for AIDS; Cases meeting the 1987 case definition of AIDS; Cases meeting the 1993 case definition of AIDS").
48. This number is only an approximation of the magnitude of difference expected, as an unknown number of patients reported under the 1987 or 1993 case definition may subsequently develop opportunistic infections that meet previous AIDS case definitions.
49. "SFDPH, "AIDS Cases Reported through October 1995," 8.
50. See H. W. Haverkos, "Reported Cases of AIDS: An Update," *New England Journal of Medicine* 329 (7), August 12, 1993: 511. In order to determine the percentage change in AIDS cases from 1989 to 1992, Haverkos "calculated by subtracting the 1989 figure from the 1992 figure and dividing the difference by the 1989 figure." I have used the same methodology for figures published in San Francisco's October 31, 1995 monthly *AIDS Surveillance Report*: (1981) n = 23; (1982) n = 92. 92 − 23 = 69. 69 divided by 23 = 3. Three times 100 = 300% change in AIDS cases between 1981 and 1982 in San Francisco.
51. Chang et al., "The New AIDS Case Definition: Implications for San Francisco," *Journal of the American Medical Association* 267(7), February 19, 1992: 973.
52. E. Burkett, *The Gravest Show on Earth: America in the Age of AIDS*, New York: Houghton Mifflin, 1995: 142–143.
53. "San Francisco Comment," *San Francisco Epidemiologic Bulletin* 9(1), January 1993: 4.
54. Burkett, *The Gravest Show on Earth*, 142.
55. As of December 1993, San Francisco had the highest annual rate of AIDS cases in the United States (284.2 per 100,000 population); this was more than twice that of Jersey City, N.J. (131 per 100,000) and greater than New York (171 per 100,000 population). However, the absolute number of new AIDS cases in San Francisco (4,555) in 1993 paled in compari-

son to New York City's 14,665 new diagnoses that same year; see CDC, *HIV/AIDS Surveillance Report* 5, 4 (December 1994): 8–9.

56. San Francisco Department of Public Health AIDS Office. Testimony to the National Commission on AIDS Regarding the Proposed Expansion of the AIDS Surveillance Case Definition, December 9–10, 1991: 2–3.

57. Ibid., 3. $340,000 was allocated for this very project in the CDC's annual renewal of San Francisco's AIDS Surveillance budget for 1994.

58. San Francisco Department of Public Health. "Revision of the HIV Infection Classification System and the AIDS Surveillance Definition," *San Francisco Epidemiologic Bulletin* 9, 1 (January 1993): 1.

59. Centers for Disease Control, "Update: Impact of the Expanded AIDS Surveillance Case Definition for Adolescents and Adults on Case Reporting—U.S. 1993," *Morbidity and Mortality Weekly Report,* March 11, 1994: 167.

60. L. M. Krieger, "AIDSWEEK," 2.

61. *Washington Post,* "AIDS: Apples, Oranges . . ." March 12, 1994: A20.

62. Burkett, *The Gravest Show on Earth,* 192.

63. Ibid., 194–196.

64. Some of the increase in heterosexual AIDS cases can also be attributed to contingent and local surveillance policies, such as those in New York City that I documented previously. For instance, because of increasing caseloads after 1993 of AIDS patients with no identified risk, the NYC AIDS Office stopped categorizing men who claimed they were infected via heterosexual intercourse as NIRs and, without further investigation, reported them en masse as "male heterosexual" AIDS cases. Consequently, NIR cases declined, and reports of male heterosexual AIDS cases increased. Unfortunately, flawed surveillance practices such as these are not confined to New York City, but have also artificially inflated estimates of heterosexual AIDS in Chicago, in southern Florida, and in Italy. In the Chicago study, the authors conducted their own retrospective analysis of risk for 395 "heterosexual AIDS cases" using a methodology similar to my own, cross-referencing medical charts and interviewing health-care providers and/or family members. As a result, "85% were re-classified into different transmission categories. Most notably, *69% were re-classified into transmission categories that did not involve heterosexual contact,* including NIR" (J. T. Murphy et al., "Redefining the Growth of the Heterosexual HIV/AIDS Epidemic in Chicago," *Journal of Acquired Immune Deficiency Syndromes and Human Retrovirology,* 16(2), 1997: 122). See also Nwanyanwu et al., "Increasing Frequency of Heterosexually Transmitted AIDS in Southern Florida: Artifact or Reality?" 571–573; and Serraino et al., "The Classification of AIDS Cases: Concordance between Two AIDS Surveillance Systems in Italy," 1112–1114.

65. "If the old definition were still in use, and the statisticians had compared apples with apples, instead of oranges, the number of reported [AIDS] cases would actually have been lower [in 1993] than in recent years—just a little over 48,000 new cases instead of about 50,000;" *Washington Post,* "AIDS: Apples, Oranges . . . ," A20. See also D. R. Boldt, "AIDING AIDS: The Story of a Media Virus." Forbes Media Critic, Volume 4, Number 1. Fall 1996: pp. 48–57.

66. From 1991 on, AIDS surveillance departments throughout the country were integrally involved in constructing the revised case definition. Public health officials in San Francisco were thus forewarned about the imminent changes in surveillance practice and, as early as 1992, local surveillance departments and DCIs began making note of patients who would qualify as new AIDS cases after January 1, 1993. An *MMWR* article assessing the impact of the revised definition alludes to this fact by noting that "56% (of the 1993 caseload) had been diagnosed in earlier years, compared with 42% of cases reported in 1992." See Centers for Disease Control, "Update: Impact of the Expanded AIDS Surveillance Case Definition for Adolescents and Adults on Case Reporting—U.S., 1993," 161.

67. See also "The New AIDS Case Definition: Implications for San Francisco," *Journal of the American Medical Association* 267(7), February 19, 1992: 973.

68. Predictions of living PWAs and projected data are from San Francisco Department of Public Health, AIDS Office Seroepidemiology and Surveillance Branch, "Projections of the AIDS Epidemic in San Francisco through 1997," July 14, 1992.

69. While reviewing computer-generated CD4 printouts at the ASSB, I captured one patient with 760 T-cells who qualified as an AIDS case by virtue of the fact that his total number of CD4 T-cells (albeit within a normal range) comprised only 13 percent of his total lympho-

cytes. Despite a subsequent test of >14 percent T-cells, this patient remains an AIDS case because he once met 1993 AIDS case surveillance criteria.

70. As of October 31, 1995, "homosexual/bisexual" men and "gay IVDUs" still comprised 94 percent of all cumulative AIDS cases in San Francisco; males (straight and gay) account for 97 percent of all persons reported with AIDS in the city (SFDPH, "AIDS Cases Reported through October 1995," Table 1).

71. Author interview with Kevin McKinney, ASSB, July 1994. This change in AIDS definition has also affected mortality statistics. Because CD4 counts were used as an AIDS indicator "disease" after 1993, some AIDS patients in San Francisco have died without ever developing any other clinical opportunistic infection historically associated with the immune-deficiency syndrome; in fact, a total of 634 AIDS deaths resulted from the "wasting" or a low CD4 count according to a computer list generated in August 1994 from the SF database detailing all AIDS deaths.

72. Centers for Disease Control, "Current Trends: Heterosexually Acquired AIDS—United States 1993," *Morbidity and Mortality Weekly Report* 43(9), March 11, 1994: 155–160.

73. Author interview with Kevin McKinney, ASSB, July 1994. McKinney's intuition is corroborated by a retrospective review of heterosexual cases reported in Chicago that suggested that "the rise in the number of reported heterosexually transmitted cases [in Chicago from 1989 to 1994] may be an artifact of inaccurate surveillance by AIDS case reporting sources." The review by Murphy et al. (see note 65 above) of 395 AIDS cases originally reported as acquired via "heterosexual exposure" led to a reclassification in which "the cumulative percentage of cases attributable to heterosexual contact declined from 8% to 5% as a result." See Murphy, Mueller, and Whitman, "Redefining the Growth of the Heterosexual HIV/AIDS Epidemic in Chicago," 122.

74. Kevin McKinney: "We were reporting 2,000 cases [annually] from the 1980s [until] 1992; then, with the CDC's change in the AIDS clinical definition on January 1, 1993, AIDS cases reported in San Francisco increased to 4934 cases annually." Author interview with Kevin McKinney, ASSB, July 1994. According to an internal report on the San Francisco AIDS Surveillance Program, for the six-month period from January 1 through June 30, 1994, "a total of 1,342 cases had been reported" in the city, a figure approximately 30 percent larger than the monthly average prior to the 1993 change in case definition. Figures are taken from San Francisco Department of Public Health, "III. Surveillance Report," unpublished document, ASSB, August 1994: 1, 2.

75. Thereby, presumably, increasing San Francisco's allocation of Ryan White monies under Title II criteria.

76. G. F. Lemp, "Testimony to the National Commission on AIDS Regarding the Proposed Expansion of the AIDS Surveillance Case Definition," SFDPH AIDS Office, December 9 and 10, 1991: 1–5.

77. Chang et al., "The New AIDS Case Definition," 975.

78. Lemp, "Testimony to the National Commission on AIDS," 3.

79. See P. Bacchetti and A. R. Moss, "Letters to Nature: Incubation Period of AIDS in San Francisco," *Nature* 338, March 16, 1989: 251–253. I discussed these projections in a previous chapter examining cohort data from the early 1980s. Bacchetti and Moss projected a sharp decline in HIV seroconversions between early 1983 and throughout 1984, "which manifested itself as a much more gradual drop in AIDS diagnoses six to eight years after the drop in seroconversions" [thus between 1989 and 1991]. Their projection for the number of AIDS cases expected in future years matched their curve for HIV seroconversions *only after* including all of the additional AIDS cases (17 percent–30 percent of the cumulative caseload) included by virtue of the 1987 expansion in the case surveillance definition.

80. SFDPH AIDS Office, "Projections of the AIDS Epidemic in San Francisco through 1997," unpublished document, July 14, 1992: 2. See also, A. M. Hirozawa et al., "Projections of the AIDS Epidemic in San Francisco through 1997: Impact of the New Case Definition," paper presented at the Eighth International Conference on AIDS, Amsterdam, The Netherlands, July 19–24, 1992.

81. SFDPH AIDS Office, "Projections of the AIDS Epidemic in San Francisco through 1997," Tables 1–7.

82. Hirozawa et al., "Projections of the AIDS Epidemic," unnumbered pages titled "Conclusions."

83. SFDPH, "New AIDS Cases Have Peaked in San Francisco," press release, February 15, 1994.

84. SFDPH AIDS Office, "AIDS Cases Reported through January 1994," *AIDS Surveillance Report* 1994: 8 (Table 12).

85. SFDPH, AIDS Office, "Projections of the AIDS Epidemic in San Francisco: 1994–1997," February 15, 1994: (Figure 1. "Projected and Observed AIDS Cases by Year of Diagnosis").

86. See SFDPH AIDS Office, "AIDS Cases Reported through October 1995," *AIDS Surveillance Report,* October 31, 1995: 8 ("Table 12: AIDS Cases By Year and Month of Primary Diagnosis, SF, 1981–1995").

87. City and County of San Francisco Department of Public Health, "New AIDS Cases Have Peaked in San Francisco," press release, February 15, 1994.

88. Ibid.

89. From 9,109 PWAs projected in 1992 to 6,460 PWAs projected in 1997. See SFDPH AIDS Office, "Projections of the AIDS Epidemic in San Francisco: 1994–1997," February 15, 1994: Table 26: "Persons Living With AIDS in San Francisco through 1997—All Persons."

90. SFDPH AIDS Office, "Projections of the AIDS Epidemic in San Francisco: 1994–1997," February 15, 1994: Table 21: "Persons Living With AIDS in San Francisco Through 1997. Injection Drug Users—All."

91. These projections of PWAs in San Francisco are themselves generous estimates and include fudge factors for underreporting, delays in reporting, and underestimates of the sizes of populations at risk (e.g., gay men and injection-drug users in the city). See the 39-page report by the SFDPH from which the press release was derived for the methods of calculating "projected" versus actual "observed" numbers of PWAs SFDPH AIDS Office, ("Projections of the AIDS Epidemic in San Francisco: 1994–1997," February 15, 1994).

92. Comments in parentheses are in the original text: M. Colebruno, "Differences Abound over AIDS Report," *San Francisco Sentinel,* March 30, 1994.

93. The quotes on the "second wave" of HIV infections are from the coverage of the press release in "HIV News: Public Health Release New AIDS Figures," *San Francisco Sentinel,* February 23, 1994. Dr. Katz's argument to the Board of Supervisors is from M. Colebruno, "Differences Abound over AIDS Report," *San Francisco Sentinel,* March 30, 1994. Cf. SFDPH AIDS Office, "HIV Incidence and Prevalence in San Francisco in 1992: Summary Report from an HIV Consensus Meeting," February 12, 1992: 1–13, which is the original source for these often-cited population estimates of HIV seroprevalence and HIV seroincidence. The estimate of 1,000 new HIV infections annually remained in use in department documents throughout the 1990s. Similarly unchanged since the consensus meeting in September 1991 is the statement that "28,000 men, women, and children" in San Francisco are HIV infected. The population estimate was originally determined by the consensus among these researchers that there were 58,000 homosexual/bisexual men in the city (in the fall of 1991), and that 25,000 (43 percent) of them were HIV-positive. This estimate for the size of the gay male population was in turn derived from a Communications Technologies Survey (1990) wherein survey researchers originally produced an estimate of approximately 36,000 homosexual/bisexual men in the city, but increased the number by 60 percent after consulting AIDS surveillance figures at the SFDPH. Therefore, the Communication Technologies Survey reciprocally validated projections for HIV/AIDS by the HIV consensus meeting; and in turn, data from the AIDS Office reciprocally corroborated the use of a multiplier to estimate the number of gay men in the Communications Technologies report. Cf. Communication Technologies in Association with the San Francisco AIDS Foundation, "A Report on HIV-Related Knowledge, Attitudes, and Behaviors among San Francisco Gay and Bisexual Men: Results from the Fifth Population-Based Survey," San Francisco AIDS Surveillance Branch, unpublished report, January 31, 1990.

94. Which is tantamount to "changing the goalposts" in the middle of the game, according to AIDS dissident Dr. Peter H. Duesberg, a molecular biologist at the University of California at Berkeley. Cf. P. H. Duesberg, *Inventing the AIDS Virus,* Washington, D.C.: Regnery Publishing, 1996.

95. SFDPH AIDS Office, "AIDS Cases Reported through October 1995," *AIDS Surveillance Report,* October 1995: 7–8. These figures are only broad estimates as they refer solely to the presenting diagnoses of patients; throughout the course of their illness, some individuals who initially met the 1987 or 1993 definitions of AIDS may subsequently progress to develop opportunistic infections that meet the 1985 criteria.

96. Another even greater elaboration of the epidemic is imminent in the near future as mandatory reporting of HIV-positive persons transmogrifies AIDS into "HIV disease." See J. Marquis, "Bill OK'd to track HIV cases but not names," *Los Angeles Times,* August 29, 1998: A1, A21.

97. For geographical analyses of these trends, see A. K. Dutt et al., "Geographical Patterns of AIDS in the United States," *Geographical Review* 77(4), 1987; W. B. Wood, "AIDS North and South"; Shannon et al., *The Geography of AIDS;* Gould, *The Slow Plague.*

98. M. H. Gail et al., "Therapy May Explain Recent Deficits in AIDS Incidence," *Journal of Acquired Immune Deficiency Syndromes and Human Retrovirology* 3, 1990: 296–306; G. F. Lemp et al., "Projected Incidence of AIDS in San Francisco," *Journal of Acquired Immune Deficiency Syndromes and Human Retrovirology* 16(3), 1997: 182–189.

Chapter 7

The epigraph is taken from p. 322 of Jones and Moon's book, published in 1987 by Routledge & Kegan Paul.

1. J. Golinski, *Making Natural Knowledge: Constructivism and the History of Science,* Cambridge: Cambridge University Press, 1998: ix.

2. "Historical instances of controversy over natural phenomena or intellectual practices have two advantages . . . 1) they often involve disagreements over the reality of entities or propriety of practices whose existence or value are subsequently taken to be unproblematic or settled. In H. M. Collins' metaphor, institutionalized beliefs about the natural world are like the ship in the bottle, whereas instances of scientific controversy offer us the opportunity to see that the ship was once a pile of sticks and string, and that it was once outside the bottle . . . and 2) in the course of controversy [historical actors] attempt to deconstruct the taken-for-granted quality of their antagonists' preferred beliefs and practices, and they do this by trying to display the artifactual and conventional status of those beliefs and practices." Shapin and Schaffer, *Leviathan and the Air-Pump,* 6–7, citing H. M Collins, "The Seven Sexes: A Study in the Sociology of a Phenomenon, or the Replication of Experiments in Physics," *Sociology* 9, 1975: 205–224.

3. Epstein has written on the sociology of knowledge regarding the cause of AIDS, debates regarding treatments for HIV/AIDS, and the politics surrounding the construction of AIDS risk groups. See Epstein, *Impure Science,* and "Nature vs. Nurture and the Politics of AIDS Organizing," *Out/Look,* fall 1988: 46–53. Also see J. H. Fujimura and D. Y. Chou, "Dissent in Science: Styles of Scientific Practice and the Controversy over the Cause of AIDS," *Social Science and Medicine* 38(8), 1994: 1017–1036.

4. Epstein, "Impure Science," Ph.D. diss., 64, 143–152.

5. Fujimura and Chou, "Dissent in Science," 1023.

6. "AIDS" as we understand the term could not exist without several recent theoretical developments in the fields of retrovirology, molecular biology, and immunology, or without the invention of several "tools" for apprehending or quantifying this new knowledge—for instance the discovery of monoclonal antibodies in the 1970s. Secondarily, the clinical "facts" of AIDS are inseparable from the technological development of FACS (fluorescence-activated cell sorters), machines that aid in the characterization and quantification of different types of T-cell populations. See A. Cambrosio and P. Keating, "A Matter of FACS: Constituting Novel Entities in Immunology," *Medical Anthropology Quarterly* 6(4), December 1992: 362–384, and P. Keating, "The Tools of the Discipline: Standards, Models, and Measures in the Affinity/Avidity Controversy in Immunology," in *The Right Tools for the Job: At Work in Twentieth-Century Life Sciences,* ed. A. E. Clarke and J. H. Fujimura, Princeton, N.J.: Princeton University Press, 1992: 312–354.

7. This latter point, while widely acknowledged by orthodox AIDS researchers, does not, in their opinion, reflect a poor understanding of the etiology of the disease, but rather constitutes an agenda for further research on the way in which HIV induces immune suppression. "(AIDS) is characterized by the progressive loss of the CD4+ helper/inducer subset of T lymphocytes, leading to severe immunosuppression and constitutional disease, neurological complications, and opportunistic infections and neoplasms that rarely occur in persons with intact immune function. Although the precise mechanisms leading to the destruction of the immune system have not been fully delineated, abundant epidemiologic, virologic and immunologic data support the conclusion that infection with the human immunodeficiency virus (HIV) is the underlying cause of AIDS." National Institute of Allergy and Infectious Diseases, "The Relationship between the Human Immunodeficiency Virus and the Acquired Immunodeficiency Syndrome," Bethesda, Md.: National Institutes of Health, September 1995: 1.

8. Epstein, "Impure Science," Ph.D. diss., 5.
9. Fujimura and Chou, "Dissent in Science," 1017.
10. Ibid., 1020.
11. In this same period, epidemiological evidence came to light of AIDS cases among hemophiliacs, Haitians, transfusion recipients, as well as sexual partners of intravenous drug users and their children. Further evidence for the argument that research on the cause of AIDS clearly diminished subsequent to 1983, when Gallo published an article on the discovery of the first retrovirus associated with AIDS (HTLV-I), and Montagnier published on LAV, is found in a 1991 article by Elford et al. examining the growth of scientific literature on the disease. "More than 30,000 papers on HIV and AIDS were indexed by Medline between 1981 and 1990. . . . The percentage of papers discussing the aetiology of AIDS fell from 25 to 3% between 1983 and 1990. During the same period, papers concerned with HIV increased from 2 to 37% of the HIV/AIDS total." In conclusion the authors argued that "the discovery of HIV . . . has seen a relative decline in aetiological research, coupled with a rapid growth of interest in the virus itself. Although it is generally accepted that HIV is the cause of AIDS, cofactors responsible for differences in disease progression clearly require further investigation. Research into aetiology may therefore need to be granted greater priority in the 1990s than it has received during the last few years." J. Elford et al., "Research into HIV and AIDS between 1981 and 1990: The Epidemic Curve," AIDS 5, 1991: 1515, 1518.
12. For instance, Grmek locates the "paradigmatic" moment in the search for the cause of AIDS as occurring in June 1982, exactly 12 months after the "discovery" of the epidemic, when the CDC published the results of an epidemiological study of a "cluster" of men in Los Angeles who had developed the disease. Of 19 reported cases of PCP and KS from the Los Angeles area, the CDC obtained "data on sexual partners" for 13 cases, and determined that "within five years of the onset of symptoms, 9 patients had had sexual contact with other patients with KS or PCP . . . the other 4 patients in the group of 13 had no known sexual contact with reported cases." In conclusion, the CDC determined that the probability "would seem to be remote" that such an association between cases could have occurred by chance, suggesting that "one hypothesis consistent with the observations reported here is that . . . infectious agents are being sexually transmitted among homosexually active males. Infectious agents not yet identified may cause the acquired cellular immuno-deficiency that appears to underlie KS and/or PCP." While the CDC investigators also concluded that alternative hypotheses, such as the use of nitrate inhalants, or a "certain style of life," remained viable explanations for this "cluster of cases," this *MMWR* report, which was followed immediately by reports of "Opportunistic Infections and Kaposi's Sarcoma among Haitians" (July 9, 1982) and "PCP among Persons with Hemophilia A" (July 16, 1982) are frequently cited as the definitive epidemiological evidence implicating a viral agent as the cause of AIDS. See M. D. Grmek, "In Search of Patient Zero," *History of AIDS: Emergence and Origin of a Pandemic*, 18–20; and Centers for Disease Control, "A Cluster of Kaposi's Sarcoma and *Pneumocystis carinii* Pneumonia."
13. Others have divided hypotheses about AIDS differently; for instance, J. A. Sonnabend has identified the following theories to explain the emergence of the AIDS epidemic: 1) a new agent was recently introduced into these populations; 2) a new agent was introduced, but it requires a co-factor for disease to appear; and 3) old infectious and noninfectious agents are being combined in unprecedented ways, driven by the quantitative increase of new opportunities for being exposed to these agents. (J. A. Sonnabend, "Why AIDS Research Has Left So Many Promising Leads Unexplored," unpublished article, 1991/1992). More recent hypotheses include revisiting the theory that AIDS was caused by contaminated polio vaccines used for immunizing populations throughout Central Africa in the 1950s. See E. Hooper's best-seller, *The River: A Journey to the Source of HIV and AIDS*, Boston: Little, Brown, 1999.
14. Latour and Woolgar, postscript to second edition (1986), *Laboratory Life*, 273–286.
15. Golinski, *Making Natural Knowledge*, xi (italics in the original).
16. Isaacs was credited with the discovery of interferon in 1957. See Nussbaum, *Good Intentions*, 76.
17. Sonnabend discovered while working in the laboratory of Jan Vilcek at New York University in 1981 that people with AIDS had large amounts of interferon in circulation. See O. T. Preble et al., "Role of Interferon in AIDS," *Annals of the New York Academy of Science* 437 (1984); and Nussbaum, *Good Intentions*, 76. Despite this finding, AIDS clinicians in San Francisco

treated some of the earliest AIDS patients with massive doses of intravenous interferon in an attempt to arrest Kaposi's sarcoma lesions. See Sally Smith Hughes's interview with Dr. Marcus Conant: (Hughes) "There were several interferon trials at San Francisco General, beginning in 1982. Could you tell me about them?" (Conant) "It was a very interesting trial, because they were using massive doses of Interferon, much higher than we use today. I believe one of the arms of that trial had ninety million units of interferon three times a week, which is just astoundingly high. A reasonable dose of interferon might be something like three million units three times a week. Paul Dague, the psychologist that I loved so much, was in that trial. I can remember him coming to my office on Parnassus [Avenue] one day, and he described what the side effects were like. He looked up and he said, 'I'd rather die of Kaposi's sarcoma than stay in this trial.' I realized how really sick it was making him. It was making him sicker than hell." Marcus A Conant, "Founding the KS Clinic, and Continued AIDS Activism," An oral history conducted in 1992 by Sally Smith Hughes, *The AIDS Epidemic in San Francisco: The Medical Response, 1981–1984*, Volume 2, Regional Oral History Office, Bancroft Library, University of California, Berkeley, 1996: 165.

18. B. Adkins, "Looking at AIDS in Totality: A Conversation with Joseph Sonnabend," *New York Native*, October 7–13, 1985: 22.

19. "In the cities in which AIDS did occur, there certainly were quite . . . extensive changes. And these were changes of . . . a quantitative nature rather than a qualitative nature. And this simply means that the opportunities for promiscuous sex increased enormously. As a result, the prevalence of different pathogens, different pathogenic organisms increased so that even single exposures would be associated with the acquisition of some infection." Joseph Sonnabend quoted in "The AIDS Catch," Meditel Productions, Producer Joan Shenton, London: 1990. See also J. A. Sonnabend, S. S. Witkin, and D. T. Purtillo, "A Multifactorial Model for the Development of AIDS in Homosexual Men," *Annals of the New York Academy of Science* 437 (1984): 177–183.

20. D'Adesky, "The Man Who Invented Safer Sex Returns," 33.

21. J. A. Sonnabend, "The Etiology of AIDS," *AIDS Research* 1(1), 1983: 1–3; J. A. Sonnabend and S. Saadoun, "The Acquired Immunodeficiency Syndrome: A Discussion of Etiologic Hypotheses," *AIDS Research* 1(2), 1984: 107–120; J. A. Sonnabend, S. S. Witkin, and D. T. Purtillo, "Acquired Immune Deficiency Syndrome (AIDS)—An Explanation for Its Occurrence among Homosexual Men," in *The Acquired Immune Deficiency Syndrome and Infections in Homosexual Men*, ed. P. Ma and D. Armstrong, New York: Yorke Medical Books, 1984: 409–425.

22. J. I. Wallace et al., "T-cell Ratios in Homosexuals," *Lancet*, April 17, 1982: 908.

23. CICS or "immune complex–mediated inflammation refers to the inflammatory responses that occur when an antibody binds to antigen and activates the complement cascade." See D. P. Stites, A. I. Terr, and T. G. Parslow, *Basic and Clinical Immunology*, 8th ed., East Norwalk, Conn.: Appleton & Lange, 1994: 147. "Cell-mediated immunity" is the arm of the immune system associated with the production of lymphocytes, such as specialized CD4 T-cells, and CD8 T-cells, and natural killer cells that target infected cells within a host's body and destroy them and the pathogens that have colonized them.

24. "Humoral immunity" is the arm of the immune system associated with producing antibodies to fend off disease and invading pathogens.

25. "The best documented example of autoimmunity in AIDS is athrombocytopenia associated with anti-platelet antibodies. It is possible that the leukopenia frequently observed in AIDS patients also results, at least in part, from autoimmunity. Additional evidence that AIDS includes an autoimmune component comes from the finding of an unusual acid-labile form of interferon alpha in the sera of some patients. This type of interferon is found in systemic lupus erythematosis and some other autoimmune diseases." Sonnabend, "The Etiology of AIDS," 7.

26. Ibid., 11.

27. However, Sonnabend has elaborated upon the multifactorial theory to account for HIV's apparent greater infectivity in sub-Sahara Africa, and suggested mechanisms by which heterosexual transmission (and possibly disease progression itself) appears to be enhanced among populations in the developing world, especially Africa. See J. A. Sonnabend, "The Debate of HIV in Africa," letter, *Lancet* 355, June 2000: 2163, and "Epidemiological Differences in the HIV Epidemic in Africa Compared to the US and Europe," *Proceedings of the*

Mbeki AIDS Panel, May 2000, paper presented at the Twelfth International Conference on AIDS in Durban, South Africa, July 2000.

28. Fujimura and Chou, "Dissent in Science," 1024.

29. "They have shown beyond a doubt that HIV is associated with AIDS, you can't deny that. But it might even be benign. My point is, in the absence of knowledge, you keep an open mind. It wasn't just me—others were saying it. The government supported people like Bob Gallo and Tony Fauci, but we were locked out of the debate." Sonnabend quoted in D'Adesky, "The Man Who Invented Safer Sex Returns," 34.

30. Thus Sonnabend argues that the "risks for infection" with HIV may differ from the "risk for sero-conversion" to HIV-antibody-positive status, a hypothesis that appeared to have some merit when Gene Shearer of the NIH announced in 1992 that, in one study, approximately 5 percent of the cohort (consisting of people in high-risk groups) showed immune responses specific to HIV, although they had not produced antibodies to the virus. See M. Callen, "AIDS Inside: A Dangerous Talk with Dr. Sonnabend," *QW,* September 27, 1992: 42–46, 71–72.

31. Sonnabend has also published numerous theoretical papers explaining how the burden of infectious disease in developing countries, such as those of sub-Sahara Africa, could enhance both the vulnerability for HIV infection and the likelihood of transmitting HIV during heterosexual intercourse, thereby generating and sustaining HIV/AIDS epidemics among both men and women in these countries.

32. As of the late 1980s, even established AIDS researchers were willing to concede this point, as HIV infected too few lymphocytes to produce the massive destruction of the CD4 T-cell population that they once alleged. For Sonnabend's quote, see D'Adesky, "The Man Who Invented Safer Sex Returns," 34. The theory that HIV was directly cytotoxic to CD4 T-cell lymphocytes was always problematic as the small number of T-cells directly infected with HIV could easily be replaced by the immune system in a matter of days. Therefore, as early as 1988, even orthodox AIDS researchers such as Anthony Fauci of the National Institutes of Health were seeking indirect mechanisms by which HIV caused the destruction of CD4 helper cells. Cf. A. S. Fauci, "The Human Immunodeficiency Virus: Infectivity and Mechanisms of Pathogenesis," *Science* 239, February 5, 1988: 617–622, for Fauci's hypothesis that HIV-infected T-cells may fuse with uninfected T-cells, or that a reaction by the immune system to HIV-infected cells may precipitate "autoimmune phenomena," whereby natural killer cells and CD8 suppressors cells target uninfected T-cells for destruction. Other AIDS researchers have proposed that HIV causes uninfected T-cells to commit suicide (apoptosis), or that the virus "picks on naive immune cells," especially CD8 T-cells, that make up the host's ability to ward off new infections, or that some HIV strains are especially prone to clumping together (synciatia). For examples of theories of "indirect pathogenesis" see G. Strobel and S. Dickman, "Does HIV Pick on Naive Immune Cells," *New Scientist,* May 6, 1995: 16.

33. Callen, "Who's Afraid of Joe Sonnabend?" 43.

34. Sonnabend, "The Etiology of AIDS," 10.

35. Ibid., 9, 10.

36. D'Adesky, "The Man Who Invented Safer Sex Returns," 29.

37. Adkins, "Looking at AIDS in Totality," 22.

38. Sonnabend, "The Etiology of AIDS," 11.

39. N. Hodgkinson, *AIDS: The Failure of Contemporary Science,* 63.

40. D. Hopkins, "Dr. Joseph Sonnabend," *Interview* 12(12), December 1992: 142. See also Callen, "Who's Afraid of Joe Sonnabend?" 42–43, 68–69. "What mystifies me is that gay people—whose lives depend upon this information and who have so much at stake—are so willing to swallow everything said by what is, in fact, a pretty mediocre research leadership—instead of actually demanding better research . . . accepting without question the information coming from those academic centers with, in effect, the best media-relations departments."

41. Shapin and Schaffer, *Leviathan and the Air-Pump,* 342.

42. The term is from Shapin and Schaffer, *Leviathan and the Air-Pump,* 333–334, and describes both the "cultural domain" of professional scientific communities—their distinct scientific disciplines, their methodologies for generating accrediting valid knowledge, and the means of authority by which they maintain social order among their professional members—and their physical places and apparatuses of experimental and laboratory research.

43. I could cite many examples; a recent corroboration of this point can be found in M. Robain et al., "Cytomegalovirus Seroconversion as a Cofactor for Progression to AIDS," *AIDS* 15(2), 2001: 251–256. "The risk of progression to AIDS was increased two-fold in CMV seroconverters compared with subjects who remained CMV-seronegative. . . . This analysis of 61 CMV seroconversions, the largest study in the literature, confirms the impact of recent CMV infection on progression to AIDS."

44. Sonnabend, "Fact and Speculation about the Cause of AIDS," *AIDS Forum* 2(1), May 1989: 4.

45. SFDPH, "Receipt of Recommended Medical Care in HIV-Infected and At-Risk Persons," *San Francisco Epidemiologic Bulletin* 10 (5-6), May–June 1994: 20.

46. Italics in the original, Callen, "Who's Afraid of Joe Sonnabend?"

47. Shapin and Schaffer, *Leviathan and the Air-Pump*, 6. See also Nussbaum, *Good Intentions*, 74. Additional examples of the personal and professional price Joseph Sonnabend has paid for positing an alternative theory for AIDS and challenging various tenets of orthodox AIDS science and discourse include the following: 1) Sonnabend, Callen, and Berkowitz were pilloried in the gay press as homophobes and attacked by the Gay Men's Health Crisis and other AIDS research and service organizations when they initially articulated their multifactorial hypothesis in the gay press and cautioned gay men to avoid unprotected anal sex and the exchange of body fluids with multiple partners. See M. Callen and R. Berkowitz, "We Know Who We Are: Two Gay Men Declare War on Promiscuity," *New York Native*, November 8–21, 1982, and subsequent responses to this article. Despite the criticism, Sonnabend's guidelines for "safe sex" in the midst of an epidemic were adopted by GMHC shortly thereafter, and served as the cornerstone of AIDS prevention and education programs in the United States—even though these rejected Sonnabend's multifactorial theory of disease and favored Gallo's theory that HIV causes AIDS; 2) When Sonnabend became the first scientist to publicly suggest that Robert Gallo's HTLV-III retrovirus was actually the same retrovirus that the French had isolated one year previously (February 1985), he became persona non grata in established AIDS research circles, lost funding opportunities, and lost control of his journal *AIDS Research*, which was reconstituted as the *AIDS Research and Human Retroviruses* in 1986 with Gallo and fellow retrovirologists at the editorial helm. "Nobody really knew what I was talking about at the time, but now they do," Sonnabend is quoted as saying by B. Deer ("A Life in the Day of Joseph Sonnabend," *Sunday Times Magazine*, London, 1992: 3). And when Sonnabend refused to acquiesce to an AIDS Medical Foundation press release that claimed HIV was an equal-opportunity virus that presaged an heterosexual AIDS epidemic, he felt obliged to resign from the research organization, which was subsequently reconstituted as AMFAR (American Foundation for AIDS Research) in 1995/1996. "I . . . discovered that my foundation had hired a publicist as a fund-raiser, someone who came from radio. He . . . orchestrated the whole [heterosexual AIDS] campaign. There were cover stories in the international magazines saying this explosion into the general population was about to happen. . . . I was appalled. There was certainly no evidence for such claims, and I felt the consequences would be absolutely dreadful. . . . There would be general hysteria, and if people felt a fatal disease was spreading from homosexual men, there could be violence against them as a visible group. . . . In effect, I was fired, on the issue of heterosexual spread. I didn't think I could fight this, so I resigned." (Sonnabend, quoted by Hodgkinson, *AIDS: The Failure of Contemporary Science*, 50).

48. For a review of Sonnabend's clinical management of PWAs, as well as a critique of established AIDS research and treatments, see Sonnabend, "Fact and Speculation about the Cause of AIDS," and Callen's three-part interview series in *QW* magazine.

49. Sonnabend, "Fact and Speculation about the Cause of AIDS," 6–7.

50. Callen, "AIDS and Passive Genocide: 30,534 Unnecessary Deaths From PCP," 13–16. The larger number in the title is the total number of AIDS deaths from PCP since the beginning of the epidemic, which Callen argued were unnecessary as it was widely known, as early as 1977, that prophylaxis with sulfa drugs such as Bactrim, could prevent this form of pneumonia. The more conservative number of 16,929 PWA deaths cited in my text is the number of PCP deaths that Callen argued occurred after May of 1987, when he and other AIDS activists "begged" Dr. Anthony Fauci, the head of the government's AIDS research program, to "issue interim guidelines urging physicians to prophylax those patients deemed at high risk for PCP." Those guidelines were issued (on the basis of community-led research in San Francisco and New York's CRIA) as a result of Callen's testimony in May 1989; how-

ever, in the interim (approximately two years) "nearly 17,000 Americans died of a disease they probably shouldn't have gotten in the first place" (14). In his final article, written shortly before his death, Callen claimed that this widely publicized quantification of unnecessary deaths from PCP cost CRIA $8 million in research funds because the NIH resented the bad publicity Callen had fostered and retaliated against the community organization that he and Sonnabend were associated with. See M. Callen, "The Finale," *Genre*, March 1994: 46.

51. Guidelines for the practice of "safe sex" (the use of condoms to limit one's exposure to semen during anal intercourse) were conceived on the basis of Sonnabend's multifactorial thesis, and first articulated in a November 1982 publication by two of Sonnabend's early AIDS patients and in a subsequent booklet. See Callen and Berkowitz, "We Know Who We Are," and *How to Have Sex in an Epidemic: One Approach*, New York: News from the Front Publications, May 1983. See also R. Berkowitz, *Staying Alive: A Personal History. The Invention of Safe Sex.* Boulder, Colo.: Westview Press, 2003.

52. Sonnabend's reasoning was as follows: "Early in the AIDS epidemic it was rapidly known that for people at risk for PCP, there was a 60 percent risk of recurrence of PCP within a year of the initial diagnosis. Despite this fact, the 'AIDS leadership' in this country would not approve the use of prophylaxis without a massive trial, despite the fact that pentamidine had been approved as prophylaxis for children with leukemia and renal transplant recipients in the 1970s. All that was needed was for the 'AIDS leadership' to issue interim guidelines for the use of pentamidine while a trial was conducted to validate these clinical guidelines; but AMFAR wouldn't do it, and people were denied this treatment." Author interview with Joseph Sonnabend, New York City, March 30, 1997.

53. Chaired by Mathilde Krim, the AIDS Medical Foundation (AMF) was the precursor to the American Foundation for AIDS Research (AMFAR).

54. Renamed *AIDS Research and Human Retroviruses* in 1986 with editors R. Gallo and D. Bolognesi.

55. Renamed the Community Research Initiative on AIDS (CRIA), and newly funded by private donors.

56. Sonnabend resigned this position in the spring of 1996.

57. For a relatively comprehensive biographical account of Sonnabend, see D'Adesky, "The Man Who Invented Safer Sex Returns."

58. "In my original criticism of the trial that lead to AZT's approval, I said that the use of AZT for more than 12 weeks was not justified by the evidence presented. The trial was so ineptly conceived and run that it was even uncertain that it should be used at all. That uncertainty was not at all resolved by subsequent trials, and I find that there is still no compelling reason to justify its use. That is, apart from its effect on interferon." (J. A. Sonnabend, quoted in Callen, "Sonnabend's Last Round," 44). See also J. A. Sonnabend, "Review of AZT Multicenter Trial Data Obtained under the Freedom of Information Act by Project Inform and ACT-UP," *AIDS Forum* 1(1), January 1989: 9–15. However, vis-à-vis combination therapy with protease inhibitors and so on, Sonnabend does treat patients with antiretroviral drugs. With such treatment, he says, he has seen patients improve "and have their lives returned. I advocate for the judicious use of these drugs in people I deem need them. It is the intervention that has had the greatest beneficial impact on sicker patients." Author interview, J. A. Sonnabend, 2003.

59. M. Callen, " 'Not Everyone Dies of AIDS': I Will Survive," *Village Voice*, May 3, 1988: unpaginated copy.

60. D'Adesky, "The Man Who Invented Safer Sex Returns," 33.

61. Joseph Sonnabend, author's interview, New York City, December 1994. While addressing the AIDS epidemic in sub-Sahara Africa is another book, the multifactorial theory anticipates recent research on the role of autoimmunity and cytokines (e.g., tumor necrosis factor) in promoting disease progression, and antedates studies demonstrating that poverty, ubiquitous infectious diseases, and overactive immune responses increase patients' (HIV) viral loads, and enhance both an individual's susceptibility to primary HIV infection and the likelihood that he or she will transmit the virus during sex or during childbirth. See recent research among Africans suggesting that a host with an overactive immune system (constantly assaulted by various pathogens or burdened with chronic infections) is "more susceptible to HIV transmission." Zvi Bentwich et al., "Immune Activation is a Dominant Factor in the Pathogenesis of African AIDS," *Immunology Today* 16(4), 1995: 187–191. The

hypothesis that disease progression is associated with an overstimulated immune system is also the thrust behind recent experimental therapy of PWAs with cyclosporine and thalidomide, potent immunosuppressive drugs. See popular coverage of thalidomide (it "appears to heal mouth ulcers in AIDS patients"), Good News/Bad News: Health Report, *Time*, November 13, 1995: unpaginated.

62. Tesh, *Hidden Arguments*, 47.
63. N. Kreiger and Fee, "Public Health Then and Now. Understanding AIDS: Historical Interpretations and The Limits of Biomedical Individualism," *American Journal of Public Health* 83(10), 1993: 1482.
64. In this regard, see also Tesh, *Hidden Arguments*, 65.
65. N. Kreiger and Fee, "Public Health Then and Now," 1481–1482.
66. Tesh, *Hidden Arguments*, 82.
67. Ibid., 72, 75; Meredith Turshen voiced a similar argument in her study of the eradication of smallpox in Africa in the 1970s—though the smallpox virus was successfully eradicated (vindicating theories of specific etiology), there was no corresponding change in the morbidity or mortality of populations in sub-Sahara Africa; people simply died from other causes. "The smallpox eradication campaign . . . alleviated a specific form of suffering and eliminated a particular way of death, but one cannot claim that it improved world health . . . all the old problems that cause poverty and ill health were left untouched, and the health services functioned no better afterward." M. Turshen, "Disease Eradication," *The Politics of Public Health*, New Brunswick, N.J.: Rutgers University Press, 1989: 155.
68. M. J. Schmerin et al., "Amebiasis: An Increasing Problem among Homosexuals in New York City," *Journal of the American Medical Association* 238(13), September 26, 1977: 1386–1389; and L. Corey and K. K. Holmes, "Sexual Transmission of Hepatitis A in Homosexual Men," *New England Journal of Medicine* 302(8), February 21, 1980: 435–438.
69. I. Hacking, *Representing and Intervening: Introductory Topics in the Philosophy of Natural Science*, Cambridge: Cambridge University Press, 1983: 46. "There are—in the extremes of reading Kuhn—no criteria for saying which representation of reality is best. Representations get chosen by social pressures. What Hertz had held up as a possibility too scary to discuss, Kuhn said was brute fact . . . we shall count as real what we can use to intervene in the world to affect something else, or what the world can use to affect us. Reality as intervention does not even begin to mesh with reality as representation until modern science."
70. J. Cohen, "Special News Report: The Duesberg Phenomenon," *Science* 266, December 9, 1994: 1642–1649.
71. "The younger a person, the slower the progression to AIDS" (J. Maddox, citing C. Lee et al., *British Medical Journal* 303, 1991: 1093, in "Has Duesberg A Right of Reply," *Nature* 363, May 13, 1993: 109). "What is surprising is how few cofactors are apparent in AIDS so far, among them HLA and age" (R. A. Weiss and H. W. Jaffe, "Commentary: Duesberg, HIV, and AIDS," *Nature* 345, June 21, 1990: 660).
72. Despite empirical evidence that seems to suggest otherwise, orthodox AIDS epidemiologists and public health officials continue to argue that multiple lifestyle and behavioral risk factors observed among AIDS patients are merely surrogate markers and/or coincidental correlates of "unsafe sex." See D. Perlman, "Biologist's Theory on AIDS Attacked: Conventional View on HIV Supported," *San Francisco Chronicle*, March 11, 1993. See also D. Swirsky and J. N. Weber, "HIV and AIDS," *Nature* 347, September 27, 1991: 324; "Rebuttal to Duesberg," *San Francisco Examiner*, July 23, 1992: A13; and W. Winkelstein Jr., "Dissenting Scientists: Earth Is Not Flat," *Daily Californian*, April 13, 1993: 4 for the following: "After controlling for HIV serostatus, we found (in our study of 767 men in the SFMHS cohort) no difference in the occurrence of AIDS between heavy users of recreational drugs, light users and non-users." Citing M. S. Ascher, H. W. Sheppard, W. Winkelstein Jr., and E. Vittinghoff, "Does Drug Use Cause AIDS?" *Nature* 362, March 11, 1993: 103–104.
73. The entire quote read as follows: "unemployment, lack of warm relationship, socially isolated, being 'used' for sex, lowered need or desire for sex." This patient had an estimated 1,100 sexual partners in the previous 10 years, 90 percent of whom were one-night stands; he died early the next year, shortly before his thirty-sixth birthday.

Glossary

A1 dx   Initial AIDS diagnosis for patients reported by surveillance departments

AIDS   Acquired immune deficiency syndrome

ACRs   AIDS case reports

ASSB   AIDS Office Seroepidemiology and Surveillance Branch in San Francisco

ASU   AIDS Surveillance Unit, the initial name of the ASSB in 1985

ARV   AIDS-related virus, the name of Dr. Jay Levy's independent isolate of LAV/HTLV-III discovered at the University of California at San Francisco in 1983

AZT   Azidothymidine, also known as zidovudine—the first antiviral drug approved to treat persons with clinical symptoms of AIDS

BCDC   Bureau of Communicable Disease Control, the division of the SFDPH that was initially responsible for reporting AIDS cases in the early 1980s

CD4   T-helper lymphocytes, the white blood cells that respond to infection in the body and signal other cells of the immune system to find, contain, and destroy pathogens.

CDC   The Centers for Disease Control, located in Atlanta

CAPS   Center for AIDS Prevention Studies, located in San Francisco

CMV   Cytomegalovirus, a large herpes virus ubiquitous among AIDS cases and often responsible for pneumonia and blindness among patients

DCI   Disease control investigator; the official title for AIDS surveillance officers at the ASSB

DNCB   1-chloro-2,4-dinitrobenzene, a photochemical applied topically to the skin and promoted for its immune-restorative properties by certain alternative AIDS activists organizations

DOA   An acronym used at hospitals signifying that the patient was dead on arrival

DOE   Dypsnea upon exertion, a term in medical charts signifying shortness of breath

EIS   Epidemiological Intelligence Service, an elite investigative unit at the Centers for Disease Control. EIS officers were the first investigators to study clusters of AIDS patients in 1981.

EBV   Epstein-Barr virus, a herpes virus

FOUR H's   Homosexuals, Haitians, heroin addicts, and hemophiliacs, the first populations considered at high risk for acquiring AIDS

GAY BOWEL SYNDROME
                Or "gay bowel disease," a term coined in the late 1970s to encompass a constellation of gastrointestinal problems among urban gay men who were very sexually active with multiple partners and experienced frequent infections with a variety of microorganisms, such as amebiasis, shigella, and giardia

GAY CANCER
An early vernacular name for Kaposi's sarcoma, a skin cancer that was one of the opportunistic infections that first defined AIDS as a clinical syndrome

GAY IVDU   Or GIVDU; a term used in official AIDS surveillance practice that denotes a homosexual or bisexual man who is also an intravenous drug user and thereby has two separate but compounding risks for contracting AIDS

GRID   Gay-related immune deficiency was one of the earliest acronyms for AIDS, and in use until approximately July 1982

HARS   The acronym for the computerized registry of AIDS patients at the ASSB in San Francisco

HBV   The hepatitis B virus or the hepatitis B (virus) vaccine, depending on the context in which the acronym is used

HIV   The human immunodeficiency virus; as of 1986–1987, the official name for the novel retrovirus that was discovered by Dr. Luc Montagnier at Pasteur Institute in 1983 and announced as "the probable cause of AIDS" in 1984 by the U.S. secretary of Health and Human Services

HSU   Health status update; in AIDS surveillance departments this term refers to the process whereby disease control investigators update the current health status of AIDS patients they have previously reported and whom they continue to monitor until notice of the patient's death is received

HTLV-I   Human T-cell leukemia virus; a retrovirus isolated by Robert Gallo at the National Cancer Institute that he initially claimed was the retrovirus associated with immune deficiency among gay men

HTLV-III   Human T-cell lymphatrophic virus, the name that Robert Gallo at the National Cancer Institute used to refer to a retrovirus that was first isolated in the spring of 1983 by Luc Montagnier at the Pasteur Institute in Paris. In contrast, Dr. Montagnier argued that his retrovirus was not in the HTLV family, but rather a distinct family of lentiviruses, and he referred to the identical retrovirus as lymphadenopathy associated virus or LAV. This same virus is referred to as the human immunodeficiency virus, HIV, or HIV-1, and before 1986–1987 was referred to as LAV, HTLV-III, or ARV.

ICL   Idiopathic CD4 T-cell lymphocytopenia

IDUs   Injection drug users

IVDAs   Intravenous drug abusers

IVDU   Intravenous drug users

KOCH POSTULATES
Guidelines for establishing the cause of a disease as articulated by physician/bacteriologist/microbiologist Robert Koch in the late 1800s:

1) the germ must be present in all cases of the disease;

2) the germ must not occur in other diseases or as a nonpathogenic agent;

3) the germ must be isolated in pure form from an infected host; and

4) the pure isolate must induce the same disease when inoculated into a naive host

KS	Kaposi's sarcoma, also known in the early days of the AIDS epidemic as "gay cancer"
LAV	Luc Montagnier's lymphadenopathy associated virus or LAV, a retrovirus initially isolated from an AIDS patient in the spring of 1983 at the Pasteur Institute in Paris. This same virus is referred to as the human immunodeficiency virus, HIV, or HIV-1, or HTLV-III, or ARV.
MAI	Mycobacterium avium infection, one of many possible opportunistic infections found in AIDS patients
MMWR	The *Morbidity and Mortality Weekly Report,* an epidemiological bulletin published by the CDC and the first publication to announce the discovery of AIDS, on June 5, 1981
NCI	National Cancer Institute
NDI	National Death Index
NIH	National Institutes of Health
NIRs	No identified risk, an appellation for AIDS cases in which the risk for HIV infection has not yet been established
NK	Natural killer cells, a type of lymphocyte (or white blood cell) that is stimulated when the host's body is invaded by a pathogen
OIs	Opportunistic infections
OR	Operating room
OOJ files	Out-of-jurisdiction AIDS case reports; files for ASSB cases that are not aggressively followed up by disease control investigators in San Francisco because they are being actively monitored by other municipalities
PCP	*Pneumocystis carinii* pneumonia, one of the most common opportunistic infections among AIDS patients; accounted for the vast majority of AIDS deaths (more than 70 percent) in the first decade of the epidemic in the United States
PRODROMAL	"A premonitory symptom," used often in medical parlance, in medical charts, and in surveillance practice to denote the symptom that immediately preceded a more significant clinical diagnosis
PWAs	Persons with AIDS or persons living with AIDS
ROHO	The Regional Oral History Office at Bancroft Library at the University of California at Berkeley
SFAF	The San Francisco AIDS Foundation, initially founded in 1981 by Marcus Conant as the Kaposi's Sarcoma Research and Education Foundation with a $50,000 grant from the American Cancer Society
SFCCC	The San Francisco City Clinic Cohort, the hepatitis B epidemiology and vaccine study. This cohort subsequently developed into a follow-up study of early AIDS patients in the city.
SFDPH	The San Francisco Department of Public Health
SFGH	San Francisco General Hospital
SFGHS	The San Francisco General Hospital Study, one of three AIDS cohort studies in San Francisco during the 1980s
SFMHS	The San Francisco Men's Health Study, a prospective "natural history" cohort study of gay men in San Francisco

SMSA	San Francisco standard metropolitan statistical area
STDs	Sexually transmitted diseases; venereal diseases including gonorrhea, syphilis, chlamydia, and the usual suspects
SSA	Social Security Administration
TA-AIDS	Transfusion-associated AIDS cases
TB	Tuberculosis
UCB	University of California at Berkeley
UCSF	University of California at San Francisco

Works Cited

AIDS Oral History Series. Bancroft Library's Regional Oral History Office (ROHO). University of California at Berkeley. Oral Histories in Biomedical Science and Public Health Collection.

"The AIDS Catch." Meditel Productions. Channel 4 TV. Joan Shenton, Producer. London, 1990.

Abramson, P. R. "Sex, Lies, and Ethnography." In *The Time of AIDS: Social Analysis, Theory, and Method*, ed. G. Herdt and S. Lindenbaum. London: Sage Publications, 1992: 101–123.

Abu-Lughod, J. "On the Re-Making of History: How to Re-invent the Past." *Remaking History*. Dia Art Foundation: Discussing Contemporary Culture, Number 4. Eds. B. Druger and P. Mariani. Seattle: Bay Press, 1989: 111–129.

Adams, J. *AIDS: The HIV Myth*. New York: St. Martin's Press, 1989.

Adkins, B. "Looking at AIDS in Totality: A Conversation with Joseph Sonnabend." *New York Native*. October 7–13, 1985.

Aggleton, P, G. Hart, and P. Davis. *AIDS: Social Representations, Social Practices*. New York: Falmer Press, 1989.

"AIDS Forum." *Skeptic* 3, 2, (1995): 24–30.

"AIDS Research. Keystone's Blunt Message: It's the Virus, Stupid." *Science* 260 (April 16, 1993): 292–293.

"AIDS Research: The Story So Far." KTEH-TV. Broadcast April 24, 1994.

"Alternative AIDS Hypotheses." Special issue, *Genetica: An International Journal of Genetics* 95, 1–3 (March 1995).

Altman, L. K. "Virus Linked to a Cancer Is Identified: Malignancy Is Found in Gay AIDS Patients." *New York Times*, March 1, 1996: A7.

Angier, N. "The Science of Desire: The Search for the Gay Gene and the Biology of Behavior." *New York Times Book Review*, October 16, 1994: 9.

Armenian, H. K., et al. "Composite Risk Score for Kaposi's Sarcoma Based on a Case-Control and Longitudinal Study in the Multicenter AIDS Cohort Study (MACS) Population." *American Journal of Epidemiology* 138, 4 (1993): 256–265.

Ascher, M. S., et al. "Does Drug Use Cause AIDS?" *Nature* 362 (March 11, 1993): 103–104.

Auerbach, D., et al. "Cluster of Cases of the Acquired Immune Deficiency Syndrome: Patients Linked by Sexual Contact." *American Journal of Medicine* 76 (March 1984): 487–492.

Bacchetti, P., and A. R. Moss. "Incubation Period of AIDS in San Francisco." Letter to the editor. *Nature* 338 (March 16, 1989): 251–253.

Barnes, B. *Interests and the Growth of Knowledge*. London: Routledge & Kegan Paul, 1977.

Bay Area Reporter. "AIDS Epidemic Growth Slows," November 23, 1994: 1, 14.

———. "Lawsuit Filed over HIV Misdiagnosis, AZT Regimen," June 15, 1995.

Bayer, R., and D. L. Kirp. "The United States: At the Center of the Storm." In *AIDS in the Industrialized Democracies: Passions, Politics, and Policies*, ed. D. L. Kirp and R. Bayer. New Brunswick: Rutgers University Press, 1992: 7–40.

Bell, R. *Impure Science: Fraud, Compromise, and Political Influence in Scientific Research*. New York: John Wiley & Sons, 1992.

Bennett, A., and A. Sharpe. "Health Hazard: AIDS Fight Is Skewed by Federal Campaign Exaggerating Risks." *Wall Street Journal*, May 1, 1996.

Bentwich, Z., A. Kalinkovich, and Z. Weisman. "Immune Activation Is a Dominant Factor in the Pathogenesis of African AIDS." *Immunology Today* 16, 4 (1995): 187–191.

Berger, P. L., and T. Luckmann. *The Social Construction of Reality: A Treatise in the Sociology of Knowledge*. New York: Anchor Books, 1966.

Berkeley Survey Research Center. "United Men's Health Study Publications." Distributed by the United Men's Health Study. Berkeley, California. September 20, 1993.

Berkowitz, R. "The Co-Factor Factor: A New Strain of Herpes Is Being Touted as the Missing Link Between HIV and AIDS." *Spin*, March 1996: 103–104.

———. *Stayin' Alive: A Personal History. The Invention of Safe Sex*. Boulder, Colo.: Westview Press, 2003.

Berlant, J. L. *Profession and Monopoly: A Study of Medicine in the United States and Great Britain.* Berkeley: University of California Press, 1975.

Berridge, V., and P. Strong. "AIDS Policies in the United Kingdom: A Preliminary Analysis." In *AIDS: The Making of a Chronic Disease,* ed. E. Fee and D. M. Fox. Berkeley: University of California Press, 1992: 299–325.

Bersani, L. "Is the Rectum a Grave?" In *AIDS: Cultural Analysis, Cultural Activism,* ed. D. Crimp. Cambridge: MIT Press, 1988.

Bethell, T. "Open Forum: Is Duesberg Right about AIDS?" *San Francisco Chronicle,* September 3, 1992: A29.

Black, N., et al. *Health and Disease: A Reader.* Milton Keynes, England: Open University Press, 1984.

Bleys, R. C. *The Geography of Perversion: Male-to-Male Sexual Behavior outside the West and the Ethnographic Imagination, 1750–1918.* New York: New York University Press, 1995.

Bloor, D. *Knowledge and Social Imagery.* Chicago: University of Chicago Press, 1976, 1991.

Boffin, T., and S. Gupta. *Ecstatic Antibodies: Resisting the AIDS Mythology.* London: Rivers Oram Press, 1990.

Boldt, D. R. "AIDING AIDS: The Story of a Media Virus." Forbes Media Critic. Volume 4. Number 1. Fall 1996: 48–57.

Botkin, M. "Queer Watch: Big Gay Brain." *Bay Area Reporter,* November 23, 1994: 22.

Brody, J. E. "The Continuing Spread of Herpes." *New York Times,* November 26, 1980.

Burkett, E. *The Gravest Show on Earth: America in the Age of AIDS.* New York: Houghton Mifflin, 1995.

Burr, C. "Homosexuality and Biology." *Atlantic,* March 1993: 47–65.

Busch, M. P., et al. "Risk of Human Immunodeficiency Virus (HIV) Transmission by Blood Transfusions before the Implementation of HIV-1 Antibody Screening." *Transfusion* 31, 1 (1991): 4–21.

Byers, R. H., Jr. et al. "Estimating AIDS Infection Rates in the San Francisco Cohort." *AIDS* 2 (1988): 207–210.

Callen, M. " 'Not Everyone Dies of AIDS': I Will Survive." *Village Voice,* May 3, 1988: unpaginated copy.

———. "AIDS and Passive Genocide: 30,534 Unnecessary Deaths from PCP Due to a Scandalous Failure to Prophylax. Testimony Given at FDA Hearing Concerning the Approval of Aerosol Pentamidine as Prophylaxis against PCP." *AIDS Forum* 2, 1 (May 1989).

———. *Surviving AIDS.* New York: Harper Collins Publishers, 1990.

———. "AIDS Inside: A Dangerous Talk with Dr. Sonnabend." *QW,* September 27, 1992: 42–46, 71–72 (Part one of three-part series).

———. "Who's Afraid of Joe Sonnabend?" *QW,* October 4, 1992: 42–44, 68–69 (Part two of three).

———. "Sonnabend's Last Round: The Renegade Researcher Plots the Triumph of HIV Heresy." *QW,* October 11, 1992: 43–45, 72–73 (Part three of three).

———. "The Finale." *Genre,* March 1994.

Callen, M., and R. Berkowitz. "We Know Who We Are: Two Gay Men Declare War on Promiscuity." *New York Native,* November 8–21, 1982.

———. *How to Have Sex in an Epidemic: One Approach.* New York: News from the Front Publications, May 1983.

———. Reply to "We Know Who We Are." Unpublished manuscript dated 1983. From the files of R. Berkowitz, December 1994.

Cambrosio, A., and P. Keating. "A Matter of FACS: Constituting Novel Entities in Immunology." *Medical Anthropology Quarterly* 6,4 (December 1992): 362–384.

Cantwell, A., Jr. *AIDS and the Doctors of Death.* Los Angeles: Aries Rising Press, 1988.

Castells, M. "Cultural Identity, Sexual Liberation, and Urban Structure: The Gay Community of San Francisco." *The City and the Grassroots.* Berkeley: University of California Press, 1983: 138–169.

Centers for Disease Control (CDC). "*Pneumocystis* Pneumonia—Los Angeles." *Morbidity and Mortality Report,* June 5, 1981: 250–252.

———. "Kaposi's Sarcoma and Pneumocystis Pneumonia Among Homosexual Men—New York City and California." *Morbidity and Mortality Weekly Report,* July 3, 1981: 305–308.

———. "Follow-up on Kaposi's Sarcoma and Pneumocystis carinii Pneumonia." *Morbidity and Mortality Weekly Report,* August 28, 1981: 409–410.

———. "A Cluster of Kaposi's Sarcoma and *Pneumocystis carinii* Pneumonia among Homosexual Male Residents of Los Angeles and Orange Counties, California." *Morbidity and Mortality Weekly Report* 31, 23 (June 18, 1982): 305–307.

———. "Inactivated Hepatitis B Virus Vaccine." *Morbidity and Mortality Weekly Report,* June 25, 1982: 317–330.

————. "*Pneumocystis carinii* Pneumonia among Persons with Hemophilia A." *Morbidity and Mortality Weekly Report,* July 16, 1982: 365–367.

————. "Update on Acquired Immune Deficiency Syndrome (AIDS)—United States." *Morbidity and Mortality Weekly Report,* 31, 37 (September 24, 1982): 507–514.

————. "Possible Transfusion-Associated AIDS—California." *Morbidity and Mortality Weekly Report,* December 10, 1982: 652–653.

————. "Update on AIDS among Patients with Hemophilia A." *Morbidity and Mortality Weekly Report,* December 10, 1982.

————. "Hepatitis B Vaccine: Evidence Confirming Lack of AIDS Transmission." *Morbidity and Mortality Weekly Report,* December 14, 1982: 685–687.

————. "Unexplained Immunodeficiency and Opportunistic Infections in Infants—New York, New Jersey, California." *Morbidity and Mortality Weekly Report,* December 17, 1982: 665–667.

————. "Acquired Immune Deficiency Syndrome (AIDS) in Prison Inmates—New York, New Jersey." *Morbidity and Mortality Weekly Report,* January 7, 1983: 700–701.

————. "Immunodeficiency among Female Sexual Partners of Males with Acquired Immune Deficiency Syndrome (AIDS)—New York." *Morbidity and Mortality Weekly Report,* January 7, 1983: 697–698.

————. "Update: AIDS in the SF Cohort Study, 1978–1985." *Morbidity and Mortality Weekly Report* 34, 38 (September 27, 1985): 573–575.

————. "Progress toward Achieving the National 1990 Objectives for Sexually Transmitted Diseases." *Morbidity and Mortality Weekly Report* 36, 12 (April 3, 1987): 173–176.

————. "Current Trends. Estimates of HIV Prevalence and Projected AIDS Cases: Summary of a Workshop, October 31–November 1, 1989." *Morbidity and Mortality Weekly Report,* February 23, 1990: 118.

————. "UCSF: Few Cases of Female-to-Male HIV Transmission." *CDC AIDS Weekly,* July 2, 1990: 18.

————. "Current Trends: Heterosexually Acquired AIDS—United States 1993." *Morbidity and Mortality Weekly Report* 43, 9 (March 11, 1994): 155–160.

————. "Update: Impact of the Expanded AIDS Surveillance Case Definition for Adolescents and Adults on Case Reporting—U.S., 1993." *Morbidity and Mortality Weekly Report,* March 11, 1994: 160–161, 167–170.

————. "U.S. HIV and AIDS Cases Reported through December 1994." *HIV/AIDS Surveillance Report* 5, 4 (December 1994).

————. "U.S. HIV and AIDS Cases Reported through June 1997." *HIV/AIDS Surveillance Report* 9, 1 (June 1997).

————. "U.S. HIV and AIDS Cases Reported through December 1998." *HIV/AIDS Surveillance Report* 10, 2 (December 1998).

Chamberland, M. E., et al. "AIDS in the U.S.: An Analysis of Cases outside High-Incidence Groups." *Annals of Internal Medicine* 101, 5 (1984).

Chang, S. W., M. H. Kate, and S. R. Hernandez. "The New AIDS Case Definition: Implications For San Francisco." *Journal of the American Medical Association* 267, 7 (February 19, 1992): 973–975.

Chicago Tribune. " 'Gay Gene' Findings Come under Fire: Study's Author Faces Allegations on Data," June 25, 1995: 1.

Chin, J. "The Use of Hepatitis B Vaccine." *New England Journal of Medicine,* September 9, 1982: 679.

————. "Memorandum to Local Health Officers re: The Reporting of AIDS Cases in California." State of California. Department of Health Services. Unpublished document, March 23, 1983.

Chirimuuta, R. C., and R. J. Chirimuuta. *AIDS, Africa, and Racism.* London: Free Association Books, 1989.

Clarke, L. K., and M. Potts, eds. *The AIDS Reader: Documentary History of a Modern Epidemic.* Boston: Branden Publishing, 1988.

Coates. T. J., et al. "Does HIV Prevention Work for Men Who Have Sex With Men (MSM)." Report prepared for the Office of Technology Assessment, U.S. Congress, August 1995.

Cohen, J. "Special News Report: The Duesberg Phenomenon." *Science* 266 (December 9, 1994): 1642–1649.

Cole, L. "The Restraint of Science, Historical Perspectives. Why Scientists Acquiesced to Politically Imposed Truth." *Politics and the Restraint of Science.* Totowa, N.J.: Rowman & Allenhead Publishers, 1983.

Cole, S. *Making Science: Between Nature and Society.* Boston: Harvard University Press, 1992.

Colebruno, M. "Differences Abound over AIDS Report." *San Francisco Sentinel,* March 30, 1994.

Comaroff, J. L., and J. Comaroff. "Medicine, Colonialism, and the Black Body." *Ethnography and the Historical Imagination.* San Francisco: Westview Press, 1992: 215–233.

———. *Ethnography and the Historical Imagination.* San Francisco: Westview Press, 1992.

Communication Technologies and the San Francisco AIDS Foundation. "A Report on HIV-Related Knowledge, Attitudes, and Behaviors among San Francisco Gay and Bisexual Men: Results from the Fifth Population-Based Survey." San Francisco AIDS Surveillance Branch. Unpublished report. January 31, 1990.

Conant, M. A. "Founding the KS Clinic, and Continued AIDS Activism." An oral history conducted in 1992 by Sally Smith Hughes. *The AIDS Epidemic in San Francisco: The Medical Response, 1981–1984. Volume II.* Regional Oral History Office. The Bancroft Library, University of California, Berkeley, 1996.

Connor, S. "Homosexuality Linked to Genes: Ethical Dilemmas Loom as Genetic Study of Gays' Families Suggests Predisposition Is Inherited through Men's Mothers." *Independent,* July 16, 1993: 1.

Connor, S., and S. Kingman. *The Search for the Virus: The Scientific Discovery of AIDS and the Quest for a Cure.* 2nd ed. London: Penguin Books, 1989.

Conrad, P., and Schneider, J. W. *Deviance and Medicalization: From Badness to Sickness.* Philadelphia: Temple University Press, 1980.

Cooper, D. *Sexing the City: Lesbian and Gay Politics within the Activist State.* London: Oram Rivers Press, 1994.

Corey, L., and K. K. Holmes. "Sexual Transmission of Hepatitis A in Homosexual Men." *New England Journal of Medicine* 302, 8 (February 21, 1980): 435–438.

Crewdson, J. "Inquiry Rejects Gallo's Claim to AIDS Test: Leaves Little Doubt French Scientists Discovered Virus." *San Francisco Examiner,* June 19, 1994.

Crimp, D., ed. *AIDS: Cultural Analysis, Cultural Activism.* Cambridge: MIT Press, 1989.

D'Adesky, A-C. "The Man Who Invented Safer Sex Returns: Dr. Joseph Sonnabend's Once Maligned Ideas about HIV Are Finding Broader Scientific Support—But Few Will Admit It." *Out* (Issue 1), summer 1992.

———. "Blame It on Herpes?" *Out,* October 1995: 122–124.

Darrow, W. W., et al. "The Gay Report on Sexually Transmitted Diseases." *American Journal of Public Health* 71, 9 (September 1981): 1004–1011.

Davidson, K. "Psychiatrists Debate Biology's Role in Sexuality." *San Francisco Examiner,* May 28, 1993: A5.

Deer, B. "A Life in the Day of Joseph Sonnabend." *Sunday Times Magazine* (London) 1992 (date unknown).

Delaney, M. "Part One: Is HIV the Cause of AIDS? Part Two: How Does HIV Cause AIDS?" *Project Inform Discussion Paper #5.* June 25, 1992: 1–6.

———. "Open Forum: Evidence Does Not Back Duesberg's AIDS Views." *San Francisco Chronicle,* September 4, 1992: A29.

Demeritt, D. Social Theory and the Reconstruction of Science and Geography. *Transactions of the Institute of British Geographers* 21, 3 (1996): 484–503.

Donovan, A. L. Laudan, and R. Laudan, eds. *Scrutinizing Science: Empirical Studies of Scientific Change.* Baltimore: Johns Hopkins University Press, 1988.

Dorland's Illustrated Medical Dictionary. 27th ed. Philadelphia: W. B. Saunders, 1988.

Dritz, S. K. "Medical Aspects of Homosexuality." *New England Journal of Medicine* 302, 8 (February 21, 1980): 463–464.

———. "Charting the Epidemiological Course of AIDS, 1981–1984." An oral history conducted in 1992 by Sally Smith Hughes. *The AIDS Epidemic in San Francisco: The Medical Response, 1981–1984. Volume I.* Regional Oral History Office. The Bancroft Library, University of California, Berkeley, 1995.

Duesberg, P. H. "Retroviruses as Carcinogens and Pathogens: Expectations and Reality." *Cancer Research* 47 (March 1, 1987).

———. "Correspondence: Duesberg Replies." *Nature* 346 (August 30, 1990): 788.

———. "Human Immunodeficiency Virus and Acquired Immunodeficiency Syndrome: Correlation but Not Causation." *The AIDS Reader: Social, Political, Ethical Issues,* ed. N. F. McKenzie. New York: Meridian, 1991: 42–73.

———. "The Role of Drugs in the Origin of AIDS." *Biomedicine and Pharmacotherapy* 46 (1992).

———. "Duesberg Replies." *San Francisco Chronicle,* September 17, 1992: A26.

———. "HIV and the Aetiology of AIDS." *Lancet* 341 (April 10, 1993): 957–958.

————. "AIDS Theories." *Daily Californian,* April 20, 1993: 5.

————. "Can Epidemiology Determine Whether Drugs or HIV Cause AIDS?" AIDS-Forschung, December 1993: 627–635.

————. *Infectious AIDS: Have We Been Misled?* Berkeley, Calif.: North Atlantic Books, 1995.

————. *Inventing the AIDS Virus.* Washington, D.C.: Regnery Publishing, 1996.

————, ed. *AIDS: Virus or Drug Induced?* Boston: Kluwer Academic Publishers, 1995.

Duesberg, P. H., and B. J. Ellison. "Is the AIDS Virus a Science Fiction? Immunosuppressive Behavior, Not HIV, May Be the Cause of AIDS." *Policy Review* 53 (summer 1990).

Duesberg, P. H., and J. Yiamouyiannis. *AIDS: The Good News Is HIV Doesn't Cause It.* Delaware, Ohio: Health Action Press, 1995.

Dutt, A. K., et al. "Geographical Patterns of AIDS in the United States." *Geographical Review* 77, 4 (1987).

Elford, J., R. Bor, and P. Summers. "Research into HIV and AIDS between 1981 and 1990: The Epidemic Curve." *AIDS* 5, 12 (1991): 1515–1519.

Ellison, B. J., and P. H. Duesberg. *Why We Will Never Win the War on AIDS.* El Cerrito, Calif.: Inside Story Communications, 1994.

Engelhardt, H. T., Jr. and A. L. Caplan, eds. *Scientific Controversies: Case Studies in the Resolution and Closure of Disputes in Science and Technology.* Cambridge: Cambridge University Press, 1987.

English Collective of Prostitutes. *Prostitute Women and AIDS: Resisting the Virus of Repression.* London: Crossroads Books, 1992.

Epstein, S. "Nature vs. Nurture and the Politics of AIDS Organizing." *Out/Look,* fall 1988: 46–53.

————. "Democratic Science? AIDS Activism and the Contested Construction of Knowledge." *Socialist Review* 21, 2 (April–June 1991).

————. "Impure Science: AIDS, Activism, and the Politics of Knowledge." Ph.D. diss., department of sociology, University of California at Berkeley, 1993.

————. *Impure Science: AIDS, Activism, and the Politics of Knowledge.* Berkeley: University of California Press, 1996.

erni, j. n. *Unstable Frontiers: Technomedicine and the Cultural Politics of "Curing" AIDS.* Minneapolis: University of Minnesota Press, 1994.

Etheridge, E. W. *Sentinel for Health: A History of the Centers for Disease Control.* Berkeley: University of California Press, 1992.

European Study Group on Heterosexual Transmission of HIV. "Comparison of Female to Male and Male to Female Transmission of HIV in 563 Stable Couples." *British Medical Journal* 304 (March 28, 1992): 809–813.

Evans, A. S. "Does HIV Cause AIDS? An Historical Perspective." *Journal of Acquired Immune Deficiency Syndrome* 2 (1989): 107–113.

————. *Causation and Disease: A Chronological Journey.* New York: Plenum Medical Book Company, 1993.

Farber, C. "AIDS: Words from the Front." *Spin,* January 1988.

Farmer, P. *AIDS and Accusation: Haiti and the Geography of Blame.* Berkeley: University of California Press, 1992.

Fauci, A. S. "The Human Immunodeficiency Virus: Infectivity and Mechanisms of Pathogenesis." In *The AIDS Reader: Social, Political and Ethical Issues,* ed. N. F. McKenzie. New York: Penguin Books, 1991. First published in *Science* 239 (February 5, 1988): 617–622.

Fee, E., and D. M. Fox, eds. *AIDS: The Burdens of History.* Berkeley: University of California Press, 1988.

————. *AIDS: The Making of a Chronic Disease.* Berkeley: University of California Press, 1992.

Fee, E., and N. Krieger. "Public Health Then and Now. Understanding AIDS: Historical Interpretations and the Limits of Biomedical Individualism." *American Journal of Public Health* 83, 10 (1993): 1477–1486.

Feldman, J. L. "Gallo, Montagnier, and the Debate over HIV: A Narrative Analysis." *Camera Obscura: A Journal of Feminism and Film Theory* 28. Special Issue. Ed. P. A. Treichler and L. Cartwright. Bloomington: Indiana University Press, 1992: 101–134.

————. "French and American Medical Perspectives on AIDS: Discourse and Practice." Ph.D. dissertation. Department of anthropology, University of Illinois at Urbana-Champaign, 1993.

Ferrias, S. "Rapid Rise of Speed: Fast Track to Nowhere." *San Francisco Examiner,* March 31, 1996: 1, 11.

Fitzgerald, F. *Cities on a Hill: A Journey through Contemporary Cultures.* 3rd ed. New York: Simon & Schuster, 1986.

Fleck, L. *Genesis and Development of a Scientific Fact.* Ed. T. J. Trenn and R. K. Merton. Trans. F. Bradley and T. J. Trenn. Chicago: University of Chicago Press, 1979.

Fleming, A., et al., eds. *The Global Impact of AIDS: Proceedings of the First International Conference on the Global Impact of AIDS.* New York: Alan R. Liss, 1988.

Foster, D. R. "Back to the Future: Dr. Robert Gallo Seeks to Put His Controversial Past Behind Him with Plans for a Major New AIDS Research Initiative." *Advocate,* January 23, 1996: 56–58.

Foucault, M. *Birth of the Clinic: An Archaeology of Medical Perception.* New York: Random House, 1975.

———. *The History of Sexuality. Volume 1.* New York: Random House, 1978.

Francis, D. P., et al. "The Prevention of Hepatitis B with Vaccine." *Annals of Internal Medicine* 97 (1982): 362–366.

Fujimura, J. H., and D. Y. Chou. "Dissent in Science: Styles of Scientific Practice and the Controversy over the Cause of AIDS." *Social Science and Medicine* 38, 8 (1994): 1017–1036.

Fumento, M. *The Myth of Heterosexual AIDS: How a Tragedy Has Been Distorted by the Media and Partisan Politics.* New York: Basic Books, 1988.

Gagnon, J. H. "Epidemics and Researchers: AIDS and the Practice of Social Studies." In *The Time of AIDS: Social Analysis, Theory, and Method,* ed. G. Herdt and S. Lindenbaum. London: Sage Publications, 1992: 27–40.

Gail, M. H., P. S. Rosenberg, and J. J. Goedert. "Therapy May Explain Recent Deficits in AIDS Incidence," *Journal of Acquired Immune Deficiency Syndromes and Human Retrovirology* 3 (1990): 296–306.

Gallo, R. *Virus Hunting. AIDS, Cancer, and the Human Retrovirus: A Story of Scientific Discovery.* New York: Basic Books, 1991.

Gardner, L. I., Jr. "Spatial Diffusion of the Human Immunodeficiency Virus Infection Epidemic in the United States, 1985–87." *Annals of the Association of American Geographers* 79, 1 (March 1989): 25–43.

Geertz, C. "Thick Description: Toward an Interpretive Theory of Culture." *The Interpretation of Cultures.* New York: Basic Books, 1973.

Gilman, S. L. *Disease and Representation: Images of Illness from Madness to AIDS.* Ithaca: Cornell University Press, 1988.

Goldman, B. "Profile of the Gay STD Patient." Paper presented at the 105th Annual Meeting of the American Public Health Association. Washington, D.C., October 30–November 3, 1977.

Golinski, J. "The Theory of Practice and the Practice of Theory: Sociological Approaches in the History of Science." *ISIS* 81 (1990): 492–505.

———. *Making Natural Knowledge: Constructivism and the History of Science.* Cambridge: Cambridge University Press, 1998.

Gould, P. *The Slow Plague: A Geography of the AIDS Epidemic.* Cambridge, Mass.: Blackwell Publishers, 1993.

Gregory, D. *Geographical Imaginations.* Cambridge, Mass.: Blackwell Publishers, 1994.

Grmek, M. D. *History of AIDS: Emergence and Origin of a Pandemic.* Princeton, N.J.: Princeton University Press, 1990.

Groopman, J. "A Dangerous Delusion About AIDS." Op-ed, *New York Times,* September 10, 1992: A19.

Group for the Scientific Re-appraisal of the HIV-AIDS Hypothesis. Publishers of the monthly newsletter renamed "Reappraising AIDS." 7514 Girard Avenue, #1-331, La Jolla, CA 92037. philpott@wwnet.com publisher/editor.

Hacking, I. *Scientific Revolutions.* Oxford Readings in Philosophy. Oxford: Oxford University Press, 1981.

———. *Representing and Intervening: Introductory Topics in the Philosophy of Natural Science.* Cambridge: Cambridge University Press, 1983.

Hadler, S. C., et al. "Outcome of Hepatitis B Virus Infection in Homosexual Men and Its Relation to Prior Human Immunodeficiency Virus Infection." *Journal of Infectious Diseases* 163 (March 1991): 454–459.

Hamer, D., and P. Coperland. *The Science of Desire.* New York: Simon & Schuster, 1994.

Haraway, D. "Teddy Bear Patriarchy: Taxidermy in the Garden of Eden, New York City, 1908–1936." *Primate Visions: Gender, Race, and Nature in the World of Modern Science.* New York: Routledge, Chapman & Hall, 1989: 26–58.

————. "The Biopolitics of Postmodern Bodies: Constitutions of Self in Immune System Discourse." *Simians, Cyborgs, and Women: The Reinvention of Nature.* New York: Routledge, Chapman & Hall, 1991: 203–230.

Harding, S. *The Racial Economy of Knowledge.* Bloomington: Indiana University Press, 1993.

Harris, S. "Special Section: The AIDS Heresies: Does HIV Really Cause AIDS?—A Case Study in Skepticism Taken Too Far." *Skeptic* 3, 2 (1995): 42–79.

Harvey, D. "Population, Resources, and the Ideology of Science." *Economic Geography* 50, 3 (July 1974).

Haverkos, H. W. "Reported Cases of AIDS: An Update." *New England Journal of Medicine* 329, 7 (August 12, 1993): 511.

Herdt, G., and S. Lindenbaum, eds. *The Time of AIDS: Social Analysis, Theory, and Method.* London: Sage Publications, 1992.

Hermans, P., et al. "Epidemiology of AIDS-Related Kaposi's Sarcoma in Europe over 10 Years." *AIDS* 10 (1996): 911–917.

Hessol, N. A., et al. "Incidence and Prevalence of HIV Infection among Homosexual and Bisexual Men, 1978–1988." Presented at the Fifth International Conference on AIDS. Montreal, Quebec, Canada, June 5, 1989.

————. "Prevalence, Incidence, and Progression of Human Immunodeficiency Virus Infection in Homosexual and Bisexual Men in Hepatitis B Vaccine Trials, 1978–1988." *American Journal of Epidemiology* 130, 6 (1989): 1167–1175.

Hirozawa, A. M. "Projections of the AIDS Epidemic in San Francisco through 1997: Impact of the New Case Definition." Presented at the Eighth International Conference on AIDS. Amsterdam, The Netherlands, July 19–24, 1992.

Hodgkinson, N. *AIDS: The Failure of Contemporary Science.* London: Fourth Estate Limited, 1996.

Hooper, E. *The River: A Journey to the Source of HIV and AIDS.* Boston: Little, Brown, 1999.

Hopkins, D. "Dr. Joseph Sonnabend." *Interview* 12, 12 (December 1992).

Horgan, J. "Hierarchy of Worthlessness." *Scientific American,* June 1993: 123–131.

Horton, M., and P. Aggleton. "Perverts, Inverts, and Experts: The Cultural Production of an AIDS Research Paradigm." In *AIDS: Social Representations. Social Practices,* ed. P. Aggleton, G. Hart, and P. Davies. New York: Falmer Press, 1989: 74–100.

"How the Virus Attacks, and How to Attack the Virus," *Newsweek,* June 25, 1990: 22.

Hunt, C. W. "Africa and The AIDS Pandemic: Migrant Labor and STDs." Master's thesis, University of Oregon, 1989.

Hunter, J. D. *Culture Wars: The Struggle To Define America. Making Sense of the Battles over the Family, Art, Education, Law, and Politics.* New York: Basic Books, 1990.

"Is There a 'Gay Gene'? Why New Findings Are Causing a Storm—Especially among Homosexuals." *U.S. News and World Report,* November 13, 1995: 93.

Jackson, P. "Gender and Sexuality: The Spatial Basis of Gay Identity." *Maps of Meaning.* London: Unwin Hyman, 1989: 123–131.

Jaffe, H. W., W. W. Darrow, et al. "AIDS in a Cohort of Homosexual Men: A Six-Year Follow-up Study." *Annals of Internal Medicine* 103 (1985): 210–214.

Jaffe, H. W., K. Choi, et al. "National Case-Control Study of Kaposi's Sarcoma and *Pneumocystis carinii* Pneumonia in Homosexual Men: Part 1, Epidemiologic Results." *Annals of Internal Medicine* 99, 2 (1983): 145–151.

Jones, K., and G. Moon. *Health, Disease and Society: A Critical Medical Geography.* London: Routledge & Kegan Paul, 1987.

Jones, M. "Why Do Doctors Hate This Man? Scientist Peter Duesberg Blasts the Theory That HIV Causes AIDS." *Genre,* June 1994: 39–43, 97–100.

Journal of the American Medical Association. "The New AIDS Case Definition: Implications for San Francisco." 267, 7 (February 19, 1992): 973–975.

Katz, M. H., et al. "Temporal Trends of Opportunistic Infections and Malignancies in Homosexual Men with AIDS." *Journal of Infectious Diseases* 170 (1994): 198–202.

Kearns, R. A., and W. M. Gesler. *Putting Health into Place: Landscape, Identity, and Well-Being.* New York: Syracuse University Press, 1998.

Keating, P. "The Tools of the Discipline: Standards, Models, and Measures in the Affinity/Avidity Controversy in Immunology." In *The Right Tools for the Job: At Work in Twentieth-Century Life Sciences,* ed. A. E. Clarke and J. H. Fujimura. Princeton, N.J.: Princeton University Press, 1992: 312–354.

Kellog, T., et al. "Notification of Recipients of HIV-Infected Transfusions: A Health Department's Role in Look-Back." Paper presented at the 116th Annual Meeting of the American Public Health Association. Boston, Massachusetts, November, 1988.

Kirp, D. L., and R. Bayer, eds. *AIDS in the Industrialized Democracies.* New Brunswick, N.J.: Rutgers University Press, 1992.

Knorr-Cetina, K. D. *The Manufacture of Knowledge: An Essay on the Constructivist and Contextual Nature of Science.* Oxford: Pergamon, 1981.

Kohn, A. "Criticism and Challenge—AIDS on Trial." *False Prophets: Fraud and Error in Science and Medicine.* Oxford: Blackwell, 1986.

Kolata, G. "Debunking Doubts That HIV Causes AIDS: Researchers Try to Destroy an Unorthodox View." *New York Times,* March 11, 1993.

———. "AIDS in San Francisco Hit Peak in '92, Officials Say." *New York Times,* February 16, 1994.

Krieg, J. P. *Epidemics in the Modern World.* New York: Maxwell Macmillan International, 1992.

Krieger, L. M. "Kaposi's Sarcoma, AIDS Link Questioned: Experts Now View Them as Separate, Though Related." *San Francisco Examiner,* June 5, 1992.

———. "AIDSWEEK: Study Backs Harm to T-cells by Poppers." *San Francisco Examiner,* September 9, 1992.

———. "Losses Exacted by AIDS Probe: With Leading Scientist Exonerated, Researchers Look Back at 4-Year Distraction." *San Francisco Examiner,* November 14, 1993.

———. "Skin Disease Emerges in Those without AIDS: Another Cause to Kaposi's Sarcoma?" *San Francisco Examiner,* December 14, 1993: A1, A16.

———. "AIDSWEEK." *San Francisco Examiner,* December 6, 1995: 2.

———. "Virus Linked to AIDS Isolated: UCSF Captures Source of Deadly Kaposi's Sarcoma." *San Francisco Examiner,* March 1, 1996: A1, A20.

———. "AIDSWEEK." *San Francisco Examiner,* April 3, 1996: 2.

———. "Kaposi's Sarcoma Microbe: Common Virus Causes AIDS-Related Illness. Germ Is Found in Semen of Most Healthy Men, but It's Usually Harmless." *San Francisco Examiner,* May 1, 1996: A1, A10.

Krieger, N. "The Making of Public Health Data: Paradigms, Politics, and Policy." *Journal of Public Health Policy* 13 (1992): 412–427.

Krieger, N., and G. Margo, eds. *AIDS: The Politics of Survival.* Amityville, N.Y.: Baywood Publishing, 1994.

Kuby, J. *Immunology.* 2nd ed. New York: W. H. Freeman, 1994.

Kuhn, T. S. *The Structure of Scientific Revolutions.* Vol. 2, no. 2 of the *International Encyclopedia of Science.* Chicago: University of Chicago Press, 1970.

Langmuir, A. D. "William Farr: Founder of Modern Concepts of Surveillance." *International Journal of Epidemiology* 5, 1 (1976): 16.

Latour, B. *Science in Action: How to Follow Scientists and Engineers through Society.* Cambridge, Mass.: Harvard University Press, 1987.

Latour, B., and S. Woolgar. *Laboratory Life: The Construction of Scientific Facts.* 2nd ed. Princeton, N.J.: Princeton University Press, 1986.

Laudan, L. *Progress and Its Problems: Toward a Theory of Scientific Growth.* Berkeley: University of California Press, 1977.

Lauritsen, J. "CDC's Tables Obscure AIDS/Drug Connection." *Coming Up!* 6, 7 (1985): 6–18.

———. *Poison by Prescription: The AZT Story.* New York: Asklepios, 1990.

———. *The AIDS War: Propaganda, Profiteering, and Genocide from the Medical-Industrial Complex.* New York: Asklepios, 1993.

Lauritsen, J., and H. Wilson. *Death Rush: Poppers and AIDS.* New York: Asklepios, 1986.

Lee, C., et al. "Progression of HIV in a Haemophilic Cohort Followed for 11 years and the Effect of Treatment." *British Medical Journal* 303 (November 2, 1991): 1093–1096.

Leishman, K. "A Crisis in Public Health." *Atlantic,* October 1985: 18–40.

Lemp, G. F. "Testimony to the National Commission on AIDS Regarding the Proposed Expansion of the AIDS Surveillance Case Definition." AIDS Office Seroepidemiology and Surveillance Branch. December 9 and 10, 1991.

LeVay, S. *The Sexual Brain.* Boston: MIT Press, 1993.

Liverside, A. "Heresy! 3 Modern Galileos: Linus Pauling, Peter Duesberg, Thomas Gold." *Omni,* June 1993: 43–51.

Los Angeles Times. "Key Protein in Attack of AIDS Virus Discovered." Associated Press article, May 10, 1996.

Lowy, I. "Ludwick Fleck on the Social Construction of Medical Knowledge." *Sociology of Health and Illness* 10, 2 (1988): 133–155.

Loytonen, M. "The Spatial Diffusion of Human Immunodeficiency Virus Type 1 in Finland, 1982–1997." *Annals of the Association of American Geographers,* 81, 1 (March 1991): 127–151.

Ludlam, C. A., et al. "Disordered Immune Regulation in Haemophiliacs Not Exposed to Commercial Factor VIII." *Lancet,* May 28, 1983.

Mack, A. *In Time of Plague: The History and Social Consequences of Lethal Epidemic Disease.* New York: New York University Press, 1991.

Maddox, J. "AIDS Research Turned Upside Down." *Nature* 353 (September 26, 1991): 297.

———. "Rage and Confusion Hide Role of HIV." *Nature* 357 (May 21, 1992): 188–189.

Mandell, G. L., R. G. Douglas, and J. E. Bennett. *Principles and Practice of Infectious Diseases.* 3rd ed. New York: Churchill Livingstone, 1990.

Mann, J., D. J. M. Tarantola, and T. W. Netter, eds. *A Global Report: AIDS in the World.* Cambridge, Mass.: Harvard University Press, 1992.

Marmor, M., et al. "Risk Factors for Kaposi's Sarcoma in Homosexual Men." *Lancet* 1 (1982): 1083–1087.

Marquis, J. "Bill OK'd to Track HIV Cases but Not Names." *Los Angeles Times,* August 29, 1998: A1, A21.

Martin, E. *The Woman in the Body: A Cultural Analysis of Reproduction.* Boston: Beacon Press, 1987.

———. "Toward an Anthropology of Immunology: The Body as Nation-State." *Medical Anthropology Quarterly* 4, 4 (December 1990): 410–426.

May, T. *Social Research: Issues, Methods and Process.* Bristol, Pa.: Open University Press, 1993.

McKenzie, N. F., ed. *The AIDS Reader: Social, Political, Ethical Issues.* New York: Penguin Books, 1991.

Meade, M. S., J. W. Floring, and W. M. Gesler. *Medical Geography.* New York: Guilford Press, 1988.

Medical Staff Conference. "Venereal Aspects of Gastroenterology." *Western Journal of Medicine* 130 (March 1979): 236–246.

Meyer, J. "County's AIDS Program Is Mismanaged, Audit Says." *Los Angeles Times,* May 14, 1998: B3, B5.

Miller, H. *Medicine and Society.* Oxford: Oxford University Press, 1973.

Miller, J. A. "Jeremy Bentham's Panoptic Device." *October* 41 (1987).

Moss, A. R., et al. "Risk Factors for AIDS and HIV Seropositivity in Homosexual Men." *American Journal of Epidemiology* 125, 6 (1987): 1035–1047.

———. "Seropositivity for HIV and the Development of AIDS or AIDS Related Condition: Three Year Follow-up of the San Francisco General Hospital Cohort." *British Medical Journal* 296 (March 12, 1988): 745–750.

Murphy, J. T., G. E. Mueller, and S. Whitman. "Redefining the Growth of the Heterosexual HIV/AIDS Epidemic in Chicago." *Journal of Acquired Immune Deficiency Syndromes and Human Retrovirology* 16, 2 (1997): 122–126.

Murray, S. O., and K. W. Payne. "The Social Classification of AIDS in American Epidemiology." *Medical Anthropology* 10 (1989): 115–128.

National Institute of Allergy and Infectious Diseases. *The Relationship between the Human Immunodeficiency Virus and the Acquired Immunodeficiency Syndrome.* Bethesda, Md.: National Institutes of Health, 1995.

"New AIDS Advances Mean Bright Future for AIDS Patients." *CNN: News,* June 13, 1996. Transcript cited by Philip Johnson, rethinkaids.uclink.berkeley.edu. June 14, 1996 06:38.

New York Department of Health Office of AIDS Surveillance. "The City of New York: AIDS Surveillance Update. Fourth Quarter 1992." January 1993: 6.

———. "AIDS Surveillance Update: Second Quarter 1995." July 1995: 7.

New York Times. "Debunking Doubts That HIV Causes AIDS." March 11, 1993.

———. "Forecasting the Future of AIDS." February 16, 1994.

Nussbaum, B. *Good Intentions: How Big Business and the Medical Establishment Are Corrupting the Fight against AIDS.* New York: Atlantic Monthly Press, 1990.

Nwanyanwu, O. C., et al. "Increasing Frequency of Heterosexually Transmitted AIDS in Southern Florida: Artifact or Reality?" *American Journal of Public Health* 83, 4 (April 1993): 571–573.

Ocamb, K. "Michael Callen, Entertainer, Activist, and Long-Term PWA, Dies." *Bay Area Reporter,* January 6, 1994: 1, 15.

Odets, W. "The Fatal Mistakes of AIDS Education." *Harper's,* May 1995: 13–17.

Oppenheimer, G. "Causes, Cases, and Cohorts: The Role Of Epidemiology in the Historical Construction of AIDS." In *AIDS: The Making of a Chronic Disease,* ed. E. Fee and D. M. Fox. Berkeley: University of California Press, 1992: 49–83.

Ormiston, G. L., and R. Sassower. *Narrative Experiments: The Discursive Authority of Science and Technology.* Minneapolis: University of Minnesota Press, 1989.

Ortleb, C. L. "Peter Duesberg Accuses Berkeley Scientists of Fabricating Data on Drug-"AIDS' Link: He Charges That Colleagues' Article Contains Unsupported Conclusions." *New York Native,* April 26, 1993: 4–5.

Osmond, D., et al. "Time of Exposure and Risk of HIV Infection in Homosexual Partners of Men with AIDS." *American Journal of Public Health* 78, 8 (August 1988): 944.

Ostrow, D. G. "A Case-Control Study of HIV Type 1 Seroconversion and Risk-Related Behaviors in the Chicago MACS/CCS Cohort, 1984–1992." *American Journal of Epidemiology* 142, 8 (1995): 875–883.

Packard, R. M., and P. Epstein. "Medical Research on AIDS in Africa: A Historical Perspective." In *AIDS: The Making of a Chronic Disease,* ed. E. Fee and D. M. Fox. Berkeley: University of California Press, 1992: 346–376.

Padian, N., et al. "Male-to-female Transmission of Human Immunodeficiency Virus." *Journal of the American Medical Association* 258 (1987): 788–790.

Palca, J. "Duesberg Vindicated? Not Yet." *Science* 254 (October 18, 1991): 376.

Patton, B. "Cell Wars: Military Metaphors and the Crisis of Authority in the AIDS Epidemic." In *Fluid Exchanges: Artists and Critics in the AIDS Crisis,* ed. J. Miller. Toronto: University of Toronto Press, 1992: 272–286.

Patton, C. *Sex and Germs: The Politics of AIDS.* Boston: South End Press, 1985.

———. *Inventing AIDS.* London: Routledge, Chapman, & Hall, 1990.

———. *Last Served? Gendering the AIDS Epidemic.* London: Taylor & Francis, 1994.

Payer, L. *Medicine and Culture.* New York: Penguin, 1988.

Payne, S. F., G. W. Rutherford, G. F. Lemp, and A. C. Clevenger. "Effect of the Revised AIDS Case Definition on AIDS Reporting in San Francisco: Evidence of Increased Reporting in IVDUs." *AIDS* 4 (1990): 335–339.

Phair, J., et al. "Acquired Immune Deficiency Syndrome Occurring within 5 Years of Infection with Human Immunodeficiency Virus Type-1: The Multicenter AIDS Cohort Study." *Journal of Acquired Immune Deficiency Syndromes* 5 (1992): 290–496.

Pickering, J., et al. "Modelling the Incidence of the Acquired Immunodeficiency Syndrome in San Francisco, Los Angeles, and New York." *Mathematical Modelling* 7 (1986): 661–688.

Preble, O. T., et al. "Role of Interferon in AIDS." *Annals of the New York Academy of Sciences* 437 (1984).

Prescott, L. M., J. P. Harley, and D. A. Klein. *Microbiology.* 2nd ed. Dubuque, Iowa: William C. Brown Publishers, 1993.

Ranger, T., and P. Slack. *Epidemics and Ideas: Essays on the Historical Perception of Pestilence.* Cambridge: Cambridge University Press, 1992.

"Research: Citation Analysis Reveals Leading Institutions, Scientists Researching AIDS." *Scientist,* July 22, 1996.

Ritter, M. "New Chemical Footholds Identified for HIV in Cells: Research on How Killer Virus Invades." *San Francisco Examiner,* June 19, 1996.

Robain, M., et al. "Cytomegalovirus Seroconversion as a Cofactor for Progression to AIDS." *AIDS* 15, 2 (January 26, 2001): 251–256.

Root-Bernstein, R. *Rethinking AIDS: The Tragic Cost of Premature Consensus.* New York: Macmillan Free Press, 1993.

Rosenberg, C. E., and J. Golden, eds. *Framing Disease: Studies in Cultural History.* New Brunswick, N.J.: Rutgers University Press, 1992.

Rouse, J. *Knowledge and Power: Toward a Political Philosophy of Science.* Ithaca: Cornell University Press, 1987.

Rushing, W. A. *The AIDS Epidemic: Social Dimensions of an Infectious Disease.* Boulder: Westview Press, 1995.

Russell, C. " 'Map of AIDS' Deadly March Evolves from Hepatitis Study." *Washington Post,* February 1, 1987.

Rutherford, G. W., et al.. "Course of HIV-I Infection in a Cohort of Homosexual and Bisexual Men: An 11 year follow up study." *British Medical Journal* (November 24, 1990): 1183–1188.

Rutledge, L. W. *The Gay Decades: From Stonewall to the Present.* New York: Penguin Books, 1992.

Samuel, M. C., et al. "Factors Associated with HIV Seroconversion in Homosexual Men in Three San Francisco Cohort Studies, 1984–1989." *Journal of AIDS* 6 (1993): 303–312.

San Francisco AIDS Foundation. *Bulletin of Experimental Treatments for AIDS*. March 1995: 92.

San Francisco Chronicle. "Riot coverage." May 23, 1979: 46

———. "Probe of riot." May 30, 1979: 6.

———. "Gay Visitor Wins Mental Test Delay." June 27, 1979: 3.

———. "San Francisco District Attorney Regarding the Bathhouses." June 27, 1979: 5.

———. "FBI Probe of Police Raid." July 17, 1979: 2.

———. "U.S. Representatives." July 26, 1979: 14.

———. "U.S. Immigration Versus Gays." August 7, 1979: 5B.

———. "San Francisco Mayoral Race." November 21, 1979: 5.

———. "Preparing to Fight in the Gay-Christian War." February 23, 1981: 4.

———. "Judge Blocks Health Fund Cuts For Poor, Seamen." June 5, 1981: 12.

———. "A Pneumonia That Strikes Gay Males." June 6, 1981: 4.

———. " 'High Risk' Reported: US Surveys Gays and Disease." September 1, 1981: 6.

———. "Five Years That Shook The City." Special supplement, November 22, 1981.

———. "S.F. Orders Ban on Sex in Bathhouses." April 10, 1984: 1.

———. "Biologist's Theory on AIDS Attacked: Conventional View on HIV supported." March 11, 1993.

———. "AIDS Cases Decline in S.F." February 16, 1994.

San Francisco Department of Public Health. "AIDS in San Francisco: The First 1,000 Cases." *San Francisco Epidemiologic Bulletin* 1, 2 (October 1985).

———. "Antibody to Human Immunodeficiency Virus in Female Prostitutes." *San Francisco Epidemiologic Bulletin* 3, 4 (April 1987): 11–15.

———. "Revision of the CDC Surveillance Case Definition for AIDS." *San Francisco Epidemiologic Bulletin* 3, 8 (August 1987): 33–43.

———. "Hepatitis B in San Francisco, 1983–1989." *San Francisco Epidemiologic Bulletin* 3, 12 (December 1987): 58, Figure 3.

———."Update: Acquired Immune-deficiency Syndrome—The Tenderloin, San Francisco." *San Francisco Epidemiologic Bulletin* 4, 9 (September 1988).

———. "Continued Sero-conversion for HIV Antibody among Homosexual and Bisexual Men." *San Francisco Epidemiologic Bulletin* 5, 8 (August 1989).

———. "Update: The SF City Clinic Cohort Study." *San Francisco Epidemiologic Bulletin*, November 1989.

———. "Hepatitis B in San Francisco." *San Francisco Epidemiologic Bulletin* 6, 4 (April 1990).

———. "Revision of the HIV Infection Classification System and the AIDS Surveillance Definition." *San Francisco Epidemiologic Bulletin* 9, 1 (January 1993): 1–6.

———. "San Francisco Comment." *San Francisco Epidemiologic Bulletin* 9, 1 (January 1993): 4.

———. "New AIDS Cases Have Peaked in San Francisco." Press release. February 15, 1994.

———. "Receipt of Recommended Medical Care in HIV-Infected and At-Risk Persons." *San Francisco Epidemiologic Bulletin* 10, 5–6 (May–June 1994): 19–26.

———. "Prevention of *Pneumocystis carinii* pneumonia: Who Is Not Receiving Recommended Prophylaxis?" *San Francisco Epidemiologic Bulletin* 10, 11–12 (November–December 1994).

San Francisco Department of Public Health AIDS Office. AIDS Seroepidemiology and Surveillance Branch. "HIV Incidence and Prevalence in San Francisco in 1992: Summary Report from an HIV Consensus Meeting." February 12, 1992.

———. "Projections of the AIDS Epidemic in San Francisco through 1997." Unpublished document. July 14, 1992.

———. "AIDS Cases Reported through January 1994." *AIDS Surveillance Report*, January 1994.

———. "AIDS Cases Reported through February 1994." *AIDS Surveillance Report*, February 1994.

———. "Projections of the AIDS Epidemic in San Francisco: 1994–1997." February 15, 1994.

———. "Report on Duplicate AIDS Cases." California State Department of Health. Unpublished document. August 17, 1994.

———. "III. Surveillance Report." Unpublished document. August 1994.

———. "Summary Report." Unpublished document. October 4, 1994.

———. "Utilization of PCP Prophylaxis and Antiviral Agents." Summary report. October 4, 1994.

———. "AIDS Cases Reported through December 1994." *AIDS Surveillance Report*, December 1994.

———. "AIDS Cases Reported through July 31, 1995." *AIDS Surveillance Report*, July 1995.

————. "AIDS Cases Reported through September, 1995." *AIDS Surveillance Report,* September 1995.

————. "AIDS Cases Reported through October 1995." *AIDS Surveillance Report,* October 1995.

————. "AIDS Cases Reported through June, 1998." *AIDS Surveillance Report,* June 1998.

————. "AIDS Cases Reported through June 30, 2000." *AIDS Surveillance Report,* June 2000.

————. "AIDS Cases Reported through March 2002." *AIDS Surveillance Report,* March 31, 2002.

San Francisco Examiner. "Rebuttal to Duesberg." July 25, 1992: A13.

————. "AIDSWEEK." August 10, 1994.

————. "Report on How HIV Got in the Blood Supply: Committee Cites Mistakes, Failure of Leadership in '80s." July 14, 1995.

————. "Help For Gays Who Feel Guilty over Being Healthy." September 3, 1995.

San Francisco Men's Health Study. "Publications of the AIDS Epidemiology Group. San Francisco General Hospital." Project report containing references to 41 articles regarding the SFMHS cohort, July 1989.

San Francisco Sentinel. "HIV News: K.S. Cases Found in HIV-Negative Gay Men." December 1, 1993: 18.

————. "HIV News." March 29, 1995.

————. "Man Wins $4.1 Million in HIV Suit." June 28, 1995: 22–23.

Schechter, M. T., et al. "Aetiology of AIDS." *Lancet* 341 (May 8, 1993): 1222–1223.

Schecter, S. *The AIDS Notebooks.* Albany: State University of New York Press, 1990.

Schmerin, M. J., A. Gelston, and T. C. Jones. "Amebiasis: An Increasing Problem among Homosexuals in New York City." *Journal of the American Medical Association* 238, 13 (September 26, 1977): 1386–1387.

Schoub, B. D. *AIDS and HIV in Perspective: A Guide to Understanding the Virus and Its Consequences.* Cambridge: Cambridge University Press, 1994.

Schultz, T. F., and R. A. Weiss. "News and Views: Kaposi's Sarcoma: A Finger on the Culprit." *Nature* 373 (January 5, 1995): 1718.

Schuster, L. "Scientist: Herpesvirus Is Likely Cause of AIDS." *Bay Area Reporter.* February 9, 1995.

Schwartz, J. *The Creative Moment: How Science Made Itself Alien to Modern Culture.* New York: Harper Collins, 1992.

Seidman, S. "AIDS and the 'Homosexual' Question: The Gay Sexuality Debates." *Embattled Eros: Sexual Politics and Ethics in Contemporary America.* New York: Routledge, 1992: 145–186.

Selik, R. M., et al. "Acquired Immune Deficiency Syndrome (AIDS) Trends in the United States, 1978–1982." *American Journal of Medicine* 76 (March 1984): 493–500.

Selik, R. M., J. W. Buehler, et al. "Impact of the 1987 Revision of the Case Definition of AIDS in the U.S." *Journal of Acquired Immune Deficiency Syndromes* 3 (1990): 73–82.

Selik, R. M., H. Haverkos, and J. W. Curran. "Acquired Immune Deficiency Syndrome (AIDS) Trends in the United States, 1978–1982." *American Journal of Medicine* 76 (March 1984): 494.

Selik, R. M., J. W. Ward, and J. W. Buehler. "Trends in Transfusion-Associated Acquired Immune Deficiency Syndrome in the United States, 1982 through 1991." *Transfusion* 33, 11 (1993): 890–893.

Sentinel. "HIV News: Public Health Releases New AIDS Figures." February 23, 1994.

————. "Baltimore: AIDS Doctor Lured with $12 Million." March 25, 1995.

Serraino, D., et al. "The Classification of AIDS Cases: Concordance between Two AIDS Surveillance Systems in Italy." *American Journal of Public Health* 85, 8 (August 1995): 1112–1114.

"Sex, Drugs and Consequences: An Evening Special." ABC-TV. Broadcast June 6, 1996.

Shannon, G. W., G. F. Pyle, and R. L. Bashur. *The Geography of AIDS: Origins and Course of an Epidemic.* New York: Guilford Press, 1991.

Shapin, S. "History of Science and Its Sociological Reconstructions." *History of Science* 20 (1982): 157–203.

Shapin, S., and S. Schaffer. *Leviathan and the Air-Pump: Hobbes, Boyle, and the Experimental Life.* Princeton, N.J.: Princeton University Press, 1985.

Shilts, R. "How AIDS Is Changing Gay Lifestyles." *San Francisco Chronicle,* May 2, 1983: 1, 5, 7.

————. *And the Band Played On: Politics, People and the AIDS Epidemic.* New York: St. Martin's Press, 1987.

Simon, P. A., et al. "Income and AIDS Rates in Los Angeles County." *AIDS* 9, 3 (1995): 281–284.

Smallman-Raynor, M. R., and A. D. Cliff. "Acquired Immune Deficiency Syndrome (AIDS): Literature, Geographical Origins and Global Patterns." *Progress in Human Geography* 14, 2 (1990): 157–213.

Sonnabend, J. A. "The Etiology of AIDS." *AIDS Research* 1, 1 (1983).
———. "Review of AZT Multicenter Trial data obtained under the Freedom of Information Act by Project Inform and ACT-UP." *AIDS Forum* 1, 1 (January 1989): 9–15.
———. "Fact and Speculation about the Cause of AIDS." *AIDS Forum* 2, 1 (May 1989).
———. *Why AIDS Research Has Left So Many Promising Leads Unexplored.* Unpublished document from the files of J. A. Sonnabend, M.D., 1991–1992.
———. "The Debate of HIV in Africa." Letter. *Lancet* 355 (June 2000): 2163.
———. "Epidemiologic Differences in the HIV Epidemic in Africa Compared to the U.S. and Europe." Paper presented at the Twelfth International Conference on AIDS, July 2000, in Durban, South Africa.
Sonnabend, J. A., and S. Saadoun. "The Acquired Immunodeficiency Syndrome: A Discussion of Etiologic Hypotheses." *AIDS Research* 1, 2 (1984): 107–120.
Sonnabend, J. A., S. S. Witkin, and D. T. Purtillo. "Acquired Immune Deficiency Syndrome (AIDS)—An Explanation for Its Occurrence among Homosexual Men." In *The Acquired Immune Deficiency Syndrome and Infections in Homosexual Men,* ed. P. Ma and D. Armstrong. New York: Yorke Medical Books, 1984: 409–425.
———. "A Multifactorial Model for the Development of AIDS in Homosexual Men." *Annals of the New York Academy of Science* 437 (1984): 177–183.
Stevens, C. E., et al. "HTLV-III Infection in a Cohort of Homosexual Men in NYC." *Journal of the American Medical Association* 255, 16 (April 25, 1986): 2167–2172.
Stine, G. J. *AIDS Update 1994–1995.* Englewood Cliffs, N.J.: Prentice Hall, 1995.
Stites, D. P., A. I. Terr, and T. G. Parslow. *Basic and Clinical Immunology.* 8th ed. East Norwalk, Conn.: Appleton & Lang.
Stoler, A. L. "Making Empire Respectable: The Politics of Race and Sexual Morality in 20th-Century Colonial Cultures." *American Ethnologist* 16, 4 (November 1989): 634–660.
Strobel, G., and S. Dickman. "Does HIV Pick on Naive Immune Cells." *New Scientist,* May 6, 1995: 16.
Strohman, R. C. "An Open Letter on the HIV-AIDS Hypothesis: Scientific Community Has Shut Out Dissenting AIDS Theories." *Daily Californian,* April 1, 1993: 4.
Swirsky, D., and S. N. Weber. "HIV and AIDS." *Nature* 347 (September 27, 1991): 324.
Tesh, S. N. *Hidden Arguments: Political Ideology and Disease Prevention Policy.* New Brunswick, N.J.: Rutgers University Press, 1988.
Thacker, S. B., et al. "The Surveillance of Infectious Diseases." *Journal of the American Medical Association* 249, 9 (March 4, 1983): 1181.
Thomas, P. A., et al. "Trends in the First Ten Years of AIDS in New York City." *American Journal of Epidemiology* 137, 2 (January 15, 1993): 121–133.
Thompson, J. B. *Ideology and Modern Culture.* Stanford, Calif.: Stanford University Press, 1990.
Treichler, P. A. "AIDS, Homophobia, and Biomedical Discourse: An Epidemic of Signification." In *AIDS: Cultural Analysis, Cultural Activism,* ed. D. Crimp. Cambridge: MIT Press, 1988: 31–70.
———. "AIDS and HIV Infection in the Third World: A First World Chronicle." *Remaking History.* Seattle: Bay Press, 1989: 31–86.
———. "AIDS, Africa, and Cultural Theory." *Transition* 51 (1991): 86–103.
———. "AIDS, HIV, and the Cultural Construction of Reality." In *The Time of AIDS: Social Analysis, Theory, and Method,* ed. G. Herdt and S. Lindenbaum. London: Sage Publications, 1992: 65–100.
———. "Seduced and Terrorized: AIDS and Network Television." In *A Leap in The Dark: AIDS, Art, and Contemporary Cultures,* ed. A. Klusacek and K. Morrison. Montreal, Quebec: Véhicule Press, 1992: 136–151.
———. *How to Have Theory in an Epidemic: Cultural Chronicles of AIDS.* Durham, N.C.: Duke University Press, 1999.
Turner, B. *The Body and Society, Explorations in Social Theory.* Oxford: Basil Blackwell, 1984.
———. *Medical Power and Social Knowledge.* London: Sage Publications, 1987.
Turshen, M. *The Politics of Public Health.* New Brunswick, N.J.: Rutgers University Press, 1989.
———. "Women and AIDS in Africa: A Health Policy View." *Association of Concerned Africa Scholars Bulletin,* Fall 1992.
Vaughn, M. "Syphilis and Sexuality: The Limits of Colonial Medical Power." *Curing Their Ills: Colonial Power and African Illness.* Stanford, Calif.: Stanford University Press, 1991: 129–154.

————. "Syphilis in Colonial East and Central Africa: The Social Construction of an Epidemic." In *Epidemics and Ideas: Essays on the Historical Perception of Pestilence,* ed. T. Ranger and P. Slack. Cambridge: Cambridge University Press, 1992.

Village Voice. "Michael Callen, 1955–1993." January 11, 1994: 1, 22.

Volberding, P. A. "Review of Clinical Guidelines." San Francisco General Hospital Medical Center. *AIDSFILE* 7, 3 (September 1993).

Von Glasersfeld, E. "An Introduction to Radical Constructivism." *The Invented Reality: How Do We Know What We Believe We Know? Contributions to Constructivism.* New York: W.W. Norton, 1984: 13–40.

Waitzkin, H. "A Critical Theory of Medical Discourse: Ideology, Social Control, and the Processing of Social Context in Medical Encounters." *Journal of Health and Social Behavior* 30 (June 1989): 220–239.

Waldby, C. *AIDS and the Body Politic: Biomedicine and Sexual Difference.* London: Routledge, 1996.

Walker, M. *Dirty Medicine: Science, Big Business, and the Assault on Natural Health Care.* London: Slingshot Publications, 1993.

Wallace, J. I., et al. "T-cell Ratios in Homosexuals." *Lancet,* April 17, 1982: 908.

Wallis, R. *On the Margins of Science: The Social Construction of Rejected Knowledge.* Keele: University of Keele, England, UK 1979.

Washington Post. "'Map of AIDS' Deadly March Evolves from Hepatitis Study: Blood Samples of Gay Men Prove Invaluable." February 1, 1987.

————. "AIDS: Apples, Oranges . . ." March 12, 1994: A20.

Watney, S. *Policing Desire: Pornography, AIDS, and the Media.* Minneapolis: University of Minnesota Press, 1987.

Waugh, M. "Historical Developments in Gay Health and Medicine." *International Journal of STD & AIDS* 7 (1996): 71–76.

Weeks, J. "AIDS: The Intellectual Agenda. Moral Panic (1982–5)." *Against Nature: Essays on History, Sexuality and Identity.* London: Rivers Oram Press, 1991: 118–120.

Weiss, R. A., and H. W. Jaffe. "Commentary: Duesberg, HIV, and AIDS." *Nature* 345 (June 21, 1990): 659–660.

Wiley, J. A., and S. J. Herschkorn. "Homosexual Role Separation and AIDS Epidemics: Insights from Elementary Models." *Journal of Sex Research* 26, 4 (November 1989): 434–449.

Winkelstein, W., Jr. "The Natural History of Acquired Immune Deficiency Syndrome (AIDS) in Homosexual Men." Principal Investigator, RFP-NIH-NIAID-MIDP-83–11. Original proposal from the files of Dr. W. Winkelstein, 1983.

————. "Dissenting Scientists: Earth Is Not Flat." *Daily Californian,* April 13, 1993: 4.

Winkelstein, W., Jr., D. M. Lyman, et al. "Sexual Practices and Risk of Infection by the Human Immunodeficiency Virus: The San Francisco Men's Health Study." *Journal of the American Medical Association* 257, 3 (January 16, 1987): 321–325.

Winkelstein, W., Jr., N. S. Padian, et al. "Homosexual Men." In *The Epidemiology of AIDS,* ed. R. A. Kaslow and D. P. Francis. New York: Oxford University Press, 1989, pp. 117–135.

Winkelstein, W., Jr., M. Samuel, et al. "The San Francisco's Men's Health Study: III. Reduction in HIV Transmission among Homosexual/Bisexual Men, 1982–1986." *American Journal of Public Health* 76, 9 (June 1987): 685–689.

Wood, R. W. Letter to the editor, *New England Journal of Medicine,* April 15, 1982: 932–933.

Wood, W. B. "AIDS North and South: Diffusion Patterns of a Global Epidemic and a Research Agenda for Geographers." *Professional Geographer* 40 (1988): 266–279.

Wright, P., and A. Treacher. *The Problem of Medical Knowledge: Examining the Social Construction of Medicine.* Edinburgh: Edinburgh University Press, 1982.

Young, I. *The AIDS Dissidents: An Annotated Bibliography. Volume One.* Metuchen, N.J.: Scarecrow Press, 1993.

Zaiwang, J., et al. "Immunodeficiency in Patients with Hemophilia: An Underlying Deficiency and Lack of Correlation with Factor Replacement Therapy or Exposure to HIV." *Journal of Allergy and Clinical Immunology* 83, 1 (January 1989): 165–170.

Zero Patience. Zero Patience Productions, 560 West Forty-Third Street. New York City, 1993.

Index